CW01670307

Fraser's The Behaviour and Welfare c
3rd Edition

FSC
www.fsc.org
MIX
Paper from responsible sources
FSC® C022174

Fraser's The Behaviour and Welfare of the Horse, 3rd Edition

Christopher B. Riley BVSc(Hons), PhD, Diplomate ACVS
Professor of Equine Clinical Studies and Registered Specialist in Equine Surgery
School of Veterinary Science, Massey University
New Zealand

Sharon E. Cregier PhD (Walden), FIASH (Hon, Edinburgh)
University of Prince Edward Island
Canada
and
North American Editor Emerita, Equine Behaviour.

Andrew F. Fraser MRCVS, MVSc†
Formerly Professor of Surgery (Veterinary)
Memorial University of Newfoundland Canada
and
Formerly Editor-in-Chief, Applied Animal Behaviour Science

CABI

CABI is a trading name of CAB International

CABI
Nosworthy Way
Wallingford
Oxfordshire OX10 8DE
UK

Tel: +44 (0)1491 832111
E-mail: info@cabi.org
Website: www.cabi.org

CABI
WeWork
One Lincoln St
24th Floor
Boston, MA 02111
USA

Tel: +1 (617)682-9015
E-mail: cabi-nao@cabi.org

A catalogue record for this book is available from the British Library, London, UK.

Library of Congress Cataloging-in-Publication Data

Names: Riley, Christopher B., author. | Cregier, Sharon E., author. | Fraser, Andrew F., author.
Title: Fraser's the behaviour and welfare of the horse / Christopher B. Riley, BSc, BVSc(Hons), MSc, PhD(Saskatchewan), Diplomate ACVS, MANZCVS, Professor of Equine Clinical Studies and Registered Specialist in Equine Surgery, School of Veterinary Science, Massey University, New Zealand, Sharon E. Cregier, PhD (Walden), FIASH (Hon, Edinburgh), University of Prince Edward Island, Canada and North American Editor Emerita, Equine Behaviour, Andrew F. Fraser, MRCVS, MVSc, Formerly Professor of Surgery (Veterinary), Memorial University of Newfoundland, Canada and Formerly Editor-in-Chief, Applied Animal Behaviour Science.
Other titles: Behaviour and welfare of the horse
Description: 3rd edition. | Wallingford, Oxfordshire ; Boston, MA : CAB International, [2022] | Revised edition of: The behaviour and welfare of the horse / Andrew F. Fraser. end ed. c2010. | Includes bibliographical references and index. | Summary: "This classic book provides a comprehensive overview of equine behaviour, an outline of current advances in our understanding, as well as offering insights into contemporary and future challenges for improving horse welfare and safety"-- Provided by publisher.
Identifiers: LCCN 2021052218 (print) | LCCN 2021052219 (ebook) | ISBN 9781789242102 (hardback) | ISBN 9781789242119 (paperback) | ISBN 9781789242126 (ebook) | ISBN 9781789242133 (epub)
Subjects: LCSH: Horses--Behavior. | Animal welfare.
Classification: LCC SF281 .F73 2022 (print) | LCC SF281 (ebook) | DDC 636.1--dc23/eng/20211025
LC record available at https://lccn.loc.gov/2021052218
LC ebook record available at https://lccn.loc.gov/2021052219

References to Internet websites (URLs) were accurate at the time of writing.

ISBN-13: 978 1 78924 210 2 (hardback)
978 1 78924 211 9 (paperback)
978 1 78924 212 6 (ePDF)
978 1 78924 213 3 (ePub)

DOI: 10.1079/9781789242133.0000

Commissioning Editor: Caroline Makepeace
Editorial Assistant: Emma McCann
Production Editor: Marta Patiño

Typeset by SPi, Pondicherry, India
Printed and bound in the UK by Severn, Gloucester

Contributors

Dr Sharon E. Cregier PhD (Walden) FIASH (Hon, Edinburgh)
Cheiron's Court
P.O. Box 1100
Montague
PE Canada C0A 1R0,
Email: cregierboth@gmail.com

Associate Professor Erica K. Gee BVSc, PhD, Diplomate ACT
School of Veterinary Science
Massey University
Private Bag 11222
Palmerston North, New Zealand 4442
Email: e.k.gee@massey.ac.nz

Dr Rebecca Husted BS PhD
Technical Large Animal Emergency Rescue®, Inc.
1787 Georgia 18
Macon, GA 31217, USA
Email: delphiacres@hotmail.com

Associate Professor Barbara Padalino DVM, PhD, Celta
Dipartimento di Scienze e Tecnologie Agro-Alimentari
University of Bologna
Viale Fanin, 50 - 40127
Bologna, Italy
Email: barbara.padalino@unibo.it

Ms Gemma Pearson BVMS, MScR, MRCVS
Equine Hospital,
Royal (Dick) School of Veterinary Studies
University of Edinburgh
Edinburgh, Scotland, UK
Email: gemma.pearson@ed.ac.uk

Professor Christopher B. Riley BVSc(Hons), PhD, Diplomate ACVS
School of Veterinary Science,
Massey University
Private Bag 11222,
Palmerston North, New Zealand 4442
Email: c.b.riley@massey.ac.nz

Professor Chris W. Rogers MAgrSc, PhD
School of Veterinary Science,
Massey University,
Private Bag 11222,
Palmerston North, New Zealand 4442
Email: c.w.rogers@massey.ac.nz

Professor Natalie K. Waran PhD
Faculty of Education, Humanities and Health Science
Eastern Institute of Technology,
Hawke's Bay, 501 Gloucester Street,
Taradale, Napier, New Zealand 4112
Email: nwaran@eit.ac.nz

Preface

Since the publication of the second edition there has been a rapid expansion of research into domesticated equine behaviour, and a paradigm shift in the world view of their welfare, from simply meeting basic needs, to promoting a life worth living. For decades the implementation of animal welfare principles has been underpinned by the Five Freedoms. Freedom from hunger and thirst, discomfort, pain, injury or disease, to express normal behaviour, and from fear and distress remain important. However, since the publication of the second edition, the application of the Five Domains framework has gained significant momentum. Encompassing behaviour, nutrition, health and environment (each are addressed in this third edition), a fifth dimension seeks to explore the mental state and well-being of the horse. As described in the chapters in this book, we must acknowledge that the mental state of the horse affects every aspect of its physical welfare, and that horses experience emotional and subjective responses to stimuli that affect the quality of their life experiences. As we acknowledge in this book, research into the emotional needs of horses is difficult and in its early stages of development. However, in the future, meeting the emotional needs of the horse may very well be regarded as important as meeting its physical needs.

The pursuit of endeavours that improve our understanding of the why of equine behaviour has led to best practices that promote the mental and emotional well-being of the horse. Increasingly practices encompassing principles of equine learning theory, such as those promoted by the International Society for Equitation Science, are actively encouraged for horse training. Several of the internationally recognized authors of chapters in this edition continue to play key roles in the translation of research into all aspects of our interactions with the domesticated horse, including veterinary practice.

With the passing of the editorial torch in this third edition, it should be recognized that the ground-breaking first and second editions have inspired generations of equine scientists and veterinarians with a genuine interest in the behaviour and the improvement of the welfare of our equine companions. Translated, this has in some way stimulated at least some of the recent work reviewed in this book. Naturally, this has led to a much greater task assembling and summarizing this explosion of knowledge into one volume. To that end, the third edition brings together a truly international cadre of authors from both hemispheres, three continents and five countries. The authors have sought to generate evidence-based summaries and recommendations, drawing on both their considerable professional experience, and the published works of researchers and practitioners from all continents, many countries, and many professional disciplines. Whereas in the past much of equine training and husbandry has been underpinned by traditional knowledge and practices, the way forward for improving the welfare of the horse, and the realization of the Five Domains, must be through the translation of evidence-based research onto practice for all.

C. B. Riley
New Zealand
February 2022

Table of Contents

In Tribute xi

1 Development and Assessment of Equine Behaviour 1
Natalie K. Waran, Gemma Pearson and Andrew F. Fraser

2 Sensory and Neurologic Faculties 24
Christopher B. Riley

3 The Neurological Underpinnings of Behaviour 36
Christopher B. Riley

4 Behavioural Homeostasis, Daily Rhythms and Advances in Monitoring 50
Barbara Padalino

5 Ingestion, Elimination and Comfort 61
Christopher B. Riley

6 Kinetic Behaviour and Athletic Performance 81
Chris W. Rogers

7 Spatial Factors 96
Chris W. Rogers

8 Equine Transport 103
Barbara Padalino and Christopher B. Riley

9 Reproduction and Breeding 124
Erica K. Gee

10 Mare and Foal Dynamics 138
Erica K. Gee

11 Foal Function and Welfare 147
Christopher B. Riley

12 Development and Social Behaviour 166
Natalie K. Waran, Gemma Pearson and Andrew F. Fraser

13 Undesirable Behaviour and Stress 179
Gemma Pearson, Natalie K. Waran and Andrew F. Fraser

14 Humane Control, Training and Husbandry 195
Christopher B. Riley

15 Evacuation and Rescue Welfare 210
Rebecca Husted

Index 229

In Tribute

Andrew F. Fraser
1927 – 2021

In the mid-1960s, Andrew Fraser, a lifetime horseman, was full of questions about how and why animals determine what they do and how they interact with humans. Searching for information at a leading veterinary library, he was told: 'None of our old gentlemen would approve the purchase of such non-veterinary literature'.

It was a dismissiveness that launched a sea-change. He resolved to do the work himself. Inspired by Ruth Harrison's 1964 *Animal Machines*, and the 1965 *Brambell Report*, Andrew Fraser gathered cohorts. Their scheme began with the founding of the Society for Veterinary Ethology (now the International Society for Applied Ethology) and its galloping horse icon. The publishing of its proceedings in the *British Veterinary Journal* followed. Elsevier's *Applied Animal Ethology* (now *Applied Animal Behavior Science*) was established in 1974 under Andrew Fraser's editorship. Speaking tours, larded with Andrew Fraser's tact, humour, and professional acumen followed, resulting in South Africa and New Zealand's veterinary schools incorporating animal ethology into their curricula. The Society for Veterinary Ethology was invited to the Council of Europe's Expert Committee on the Protection of Animals, advised Britain's Ministry of Agriculture, and influenced Codes of Practice worldwide. Novices, too, benefitted, as Andrew Fraser fostered *Equine Behaviour*, a volunteer quarterly accepting observations from scientists and horsemen of all levels. The world had been introduced to the myriad qualities and attributions of animals.

In his remaining years, well seasoned to the challenge of bureaucratic obstacles, he won protected status for the Newfoundland Pony. Five hundred, and their Celtic heritage, unlike the thousands before them, were saved from slaughter.

Tenacious in his resolve, Andrew Fraser and his distinguished colleagues built the case that man had a moral duty toward animals. All this activity dislodged the traditional pathogenic approach to animal care. With a broadened understanding of the why and how of animal behaviour, and recognition of the animal's cognitive abilities and sentience, the scatter-shot approach to animal health faded. The rigid structure of reductionist behaviourism was being dismantled. Professionals were accepting ethology as a necessary tool for the veterinarian. More refined and timely diagnoses resulted, benefitting veterinarians' credibility. The social license to have animals in care and training was invigorated and endorsed.

The horse held a special place in Andrew Fraser's life. He once referred to its nobility. He dedicated his life to increasing our understanding of its nature and needs. Today, the study and application of animal ethology has improved diagnostics, training, relationship building, and more humane treatment. Veterinarians, trainers, and handlers of all levels are forever in debt to one man's tenacious curiosity. Now generations of practitioners can provide better care for the animals in their keeping, the very thing Andrew Fraser was hoping for when he began his life quest.

His breadth of knowledge was such that it took seven contributors to this third edition of *The Behaviour and Welfare of the Horse* to cover the scope he prepared single-handedly. Today, his works take pride of place in veterinary libraries worldwide ... even in the one that first refused 'such non-veterinary literature'.

Sharon E. Cregier, PhD FIASH (Hon., Edin.)
Christopher B. Riley, PhD Diplomate ACVS

1 Development and Assessment of Equine Behaviour

Natalie K. Waran PhD[1]*, Gemma Pearson BVMS, MScR, MRCVS[2] and Andrew F. Fraser MVSc, MRCVS[3]

[1]*Eastern Institute of Technology, Hawke's Bay, New Zealand;* [2]*The University of Edinburgh, Midlothian, Scotland, UK;* [3]*Carbonear, Newfoundland, Canada*

The Process of Evolution	2
Innate Behavioural Patterns and Environment	2
Changes in Form or Type	2
Initial Learning	3
Domestication	4
Inherent Capability in Learning	6
Homeostasis and Survival	6
Appraisal of Behaviour in Horses	7
Methods for Appraising Behaviour	8
Open-field tests	8
Specific behavioural tests used in veterinary studies	9
Critical Appraisal of Behaviour	10
Behaviours Associated with Clinical Conditions	10
Locomotory Behaviour	11
Ontogeny of Behaviour: Instinct	11
Instinctive behaviour	12
Release of innate responses	12
Sensitive periods and imprinting	13
Early Experience	13
Ontogeny of Behaviour: Learning	14
Classical conditioning	14
Operant conditioning	15
Non-associative learning: habituation and desensitisation	15
Motivation, Reinforcement and Punishment	16
Emotionality and Intelligence	18
Cognitive Bias	18
Behaviour and Equine Welfare	19
One welfare	19
References	21

*Corresponding author: nwaran@eit.ac.nz

 Fraser's the Behaviour and Welfare of the Horse (eds C.B. Riley, S.E. Cregier and A.F. Fraser)
DOI: 10.1079/9781789242133.0001

The Process of Evolution

When the behaviour of the domestic horse is studied, both objectively and realistically, ethology is being applied to a subject that is not entirely a product of natural selection. Variations have been used in the creation of breeds by generations of horse breeders. Nevertheless, this animal's great inheritance is its natural past, which deserves appreciation because that is the source of much of its behaviour today (Clutton-Brock, 1999).

Darwin concluded that the evolution of a species occurred through selective processes (Jones, 2001). These determine which individuals are most able to survive and reproduce, and consequently to participate in the continuation of the species. The norms of horse behaviour today are the natural heritage of a long history of evolution before human control. Horses were subjected to nature's control for some 8 million years before their domestication. During those times there was natural selection, in which some individuals were ultimately more successful at living and breeding than others, depending on their genes. This is the process of differential reproduction, whereby evolution occurs as a result. Ethology has an interest in natural selection. Behavioural and physical (i.e. visible) characteristics of a living thing (phenotype) must be distinguished from its genetic make-up (genotype). The evolutionary process produces changes if phenotype and genotype are both involved and adaptations, or differences in traits, increase the fitness of its carrier.

What is selected is the whole make-up of the living organism, including its variations and genes, and its behavioural fit into its ecological niche. The state of overall fitness is achieved through behaviour, structure and niche, and their constant interaction with each other. Applied ethology is interested in the animal's dynamic wholeness. The applied ethological perspective of evolution is both holistic and traditional. It recognises that behaviour and structure have their own environmental needs and motivational components for survival (Lorenz, 1965).

Innate Behavioural Patterns and Environment

Horses are born equipped with 'ingrained' or, more accurately, instinctive responses that provide them with survival advantages. These are fixed action patterns of behaviour carried through generations in the species' genetic code. These inherited behavioural attributes are common to all individuals in a species, although there may be differences in how these are expressed within individuals. Fixed behaviour patterns are not variations but are 'fixed' in the given species – possibly as endpoints of evolution, serving as cornerstones in the long-term support of the species. They are not learned and consist of certain complex responses usually triggered by a simple sensory signal. An example of this is the foal's responses immediately after being born, such as standing, teat-seeking and sucking from the teat, and then when on its feet, following the dam. All are triggered by simple sign stimuli such as the feel of the mare licking it, the attraction the foal has to the smell of the inguinal wax (hence the term 'waxing up') between the teats and a heightened sensitivity to the temperature gradient that will attract them to the right place for milk. Once near the teat, the foal is instinctively attracted to objects of the 'right' shape. Once on the teat, the 'suck reflex' ensures that the foal gets colostrum quickly to aid his survival. The foal is also born with an instinctive attraction for large moving objects (usually the mare) and will follow her once able to move independently. This means that under natural circumstances, the mare and foal can very quickly re-join the herd.

Changes in Form or Type

Novel features in a species can arise from genetic changes, such as mutations, occurring during cell division in the reproductive process. Such a variety might or might not be suited to the parental niche. If forced to move to a new niche, where it becomes geographically isolated, the mutant character would be perpetuated in homozygous form. This would allow a new form of the species to continue to reproduce unchanged. This phenomenon occurs in many species, including Equidae (see Table 1.1).

Table 1.1. Classification of equine species.

Classification	Species	Common names
Order Perissodactyla (odd-toed ungulates)	*Equus caballus*	Horse (domestic)
Suborder Hippomorpha	*Equus asinus*	African wild ass (and domestic donkey)
Superfamily Equoidea Family Equidae	*Equus burchelli*	Common zebra

The present array of horse types suggests that this has occurred periodically, resulting in phenotypic differences, including for example, ponies, heavy horses and the so-called 'hot-blooded' horse breeds (see Fig. 1.1 for varietal extremes). Through mutation, the latter type of horse, notably the Arabian, became more reactive and more athletic compared with the 'cold-blooded' type. Archetypal characters (both physical and behavioural) are retained and persist in a mutant. This genetic inheritance contributes to the success of the mutant form as a derivative with archetypal attributes. The origin of archetypal behavioural attributes lies in the phenomenon of epigenesis, whereby fixed designs are accurately and actively able to continue their developmental functions through successive generations. For example, a newborn foal, transferred suddenly from an intrauterine environment to a completely new environment to which it must quickly adapt, is equipped with 'fixed' action patterns, such as standing and finding the teat, both being essential instinctive behaviours for foal survival (Robinson, 2007).

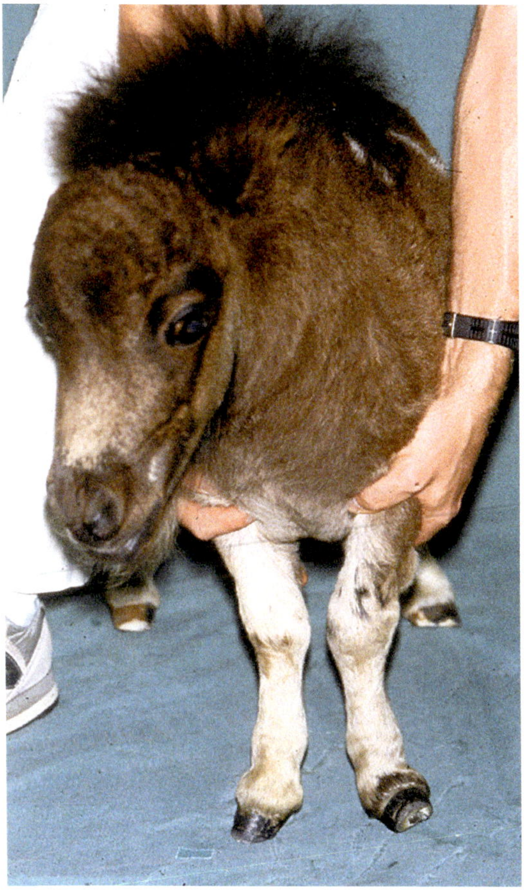

Fig. 1.1. Varietal extremes. Young American miniature horse. Photo: C.B. Riley.

Initial Learning

During the early development phase, the mare and her newborn react to one another instinctively and reciprocally. The birthing process triggers the onset of maternal behaviour, and the smell and taste of the uterine membranes and fluids attract the parturient mare to lick the foal clear of membranes and clean of fluids. While doing so, the sensorium of the foal is being 'imprinted' with the mare's details. Thereafter, it efficiently recognizes and remembers significant details about her. Similarly, the mare quickly identifies her progeny and accepts it as something to be protected. The evolved and innate abilities to learn quickly are thereby well illustrated in both neonate and adult.

Evolutionary processes dictate that parents care only for their own offspring, and reproduction occurs only between members of the same species. Such attachments in horses depend on the critical timing of first impressions in the neonatal foal (Bateson and Horn, 1994). The timing of the sensitive period during which the mother–offspring bond is formed is closely matched to the period when the possibility of error is very small, such as before the newborn has a chance to meet members of any species other than that of the mother.

The neonate foal relates to its mother not as a complex organism but as a unitary stimulus. Parturient mares usually isolate themselves from the herd before giving birth. This means that the first large moving object seen by the newborn will be its own dam. Although the foal can be quite easily confused by other large moving objects, it also receives, through touch, 'thigmotaxic' stimuli that enable it to recognize its dam. Through the contact of its muzzle with the ventral surfaces of the dam's body, it learns the identity and location of this vitally important region and eventually finds the dam's udder and food (see Fig. 1.2). The mare's behaviour becomes gradually modified through experience to increase the efficiency of her task of watching over the foal, thus granting her reproductive success (see Fig. 1.3).

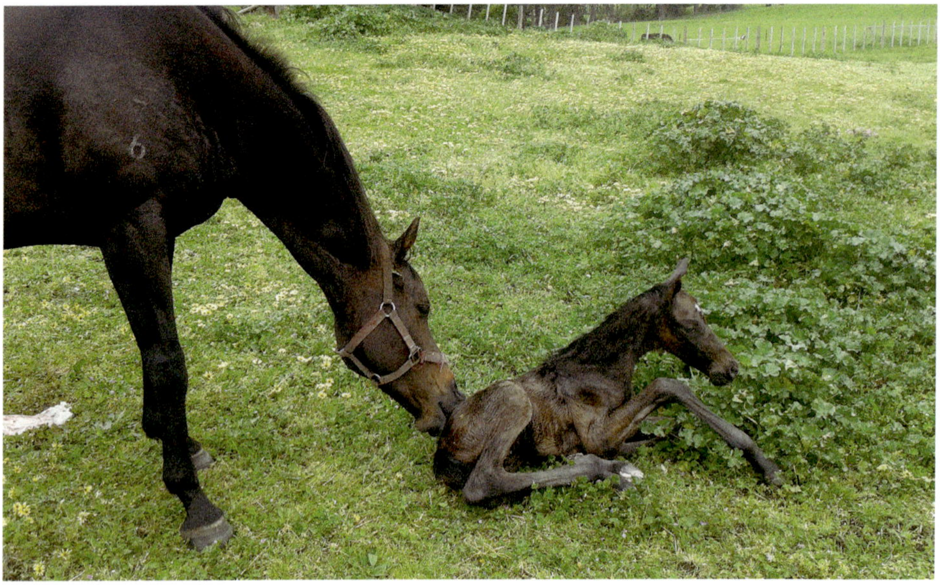

Fig. 1.2. Tactile exploration of the newborn foal by the mare. Reciprocity by the foal will follow once she is standing. Photo: C.B. Riley.

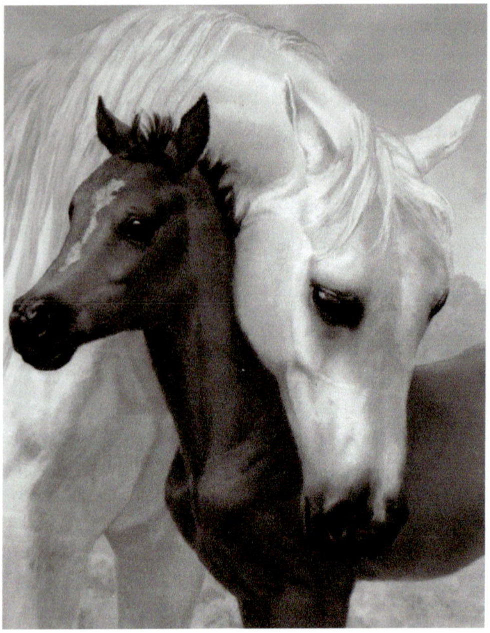

Fig. 1.3. Mare with reproductive success. Anonymous artist.

Domestication

Variation through selection as a result of domestication leads to the realization that many genetic mutations are non-adaptive in the evolutionary sense. Breeds with non-adaptive characters have appeared and have been kept true by continuous human selection for specific useful attributes, with the possessors of such mutations being complemented by human agency so that they can survive and reproduce. There are many non-adaptive phenotypic variations, such as coat colour, that play no essential part in the survival of the domesticated species. The true unit is the species as a whole, including variations, as well as the environmental niche and incidental factors within that niche.

For the complete success of the species, behavioural development in relation to environmental pressures play a central role in ensuring that the animal is able to adapt during its own lifetime. Environmental features provided by the husbandry system exert influences that determine whether the horse can adapt behaviourally to the system. Various environmental circumstances have been studied. Changes in behaviour, and ultimately in physical conditions, result directly or indirectly from environmental adaptation. The adaptive mechanisms of horses living under various environmental conditions have shown differences in response to housing, enclosure and the immediate environment. Some responses are maladaptive, and some vary between breeds and individuals. Adaptation is evident in respect of thermoregulation and ingestion (Herdt, 2007).

The temperature at which the so-called cold-blooded type of horse maintains a normal body surface temperature (the thermo-neutral zone) seems to be roughly from –10 to +20 °C, whereas warm-blooded horses can tolerate higher temperatures up to +30 °C. Ranges will be affected by other external factors such as wind and rain. Under extremes of temperature, horses use behavioural methods in attempting to control their temperatures. The most easily recognizable evidence of adaptive behaviour in horses is the movements directed towards thermoregulation and related aspects of body care. These include sheltering, shade-seeking, inactivity, etc. An early behavioural adaptive change during high temperatures is a reduction in food intake. This may arise not only from the shade-seeking activities of the animal but also from a reduced desire for food. Consequent results are an alteration in grazing behaviour and a general decline in all activity. Such an alteration in behaviour may indicate a welfare problem (Dawkins, 2004).

Taste and imitation play important parts in grazing behaviour, and this ensures that the requisite elements are consumed by a horse in appropriate quantities and suitable type to maintain health (McGreevy, 2004). Adaptive seasonal changes in eating indicate that grass palatability has been altered. Seasonal palatability varies markedly on 'unimproved' pasture. Horses generally prefer grass that is high in leafiness, greenness and nitrogen content. Sugar, organic acids and fats are preferred, whereas tannins and alkaloids are avoided. Variation in food choice by ponies is explained by the abundance of plant species at different stages of the growing season. As a rule, a drop in the percentage of time spent feeding on a species of grass can be attributed to a dearth of that grass or to the growth of a preferred one. The exceptions to this rule occur in summer and autumn, when certain leaves, such as beech (in the Northern Hemisphere), are increasingly consumed by horses. In the Camargue, in southern France, a long-term study of horses has shown a marked seasonality in use made of plants. Deep-water rushes, which are high in protein, form the main summer food, while perennials and legumes are dominant in the diet at other times.

Much contemporary controversy centres on the extent of behavioural adaptation that has taken place in farm animals because of the restrictions of husbandry. Opinions have been commonly expressed in support of a notion that adaptation is inevitable in the face of continuing husbandry pressure. Some believe that many generations of selection for productivity have resulted in animals being docile to a level that would be disastrous in the wild but essential under domestication. Docility is, however, adaptive behaviour and is chiefly the result of selection and individual management, where there is the capacity for such adaptation. The influence of domestication is not detrimental to animal well-being if the techniques of domestication allow the animal to adapt to a humane system (Riolo *et al.*, 2001).

Innate behaviour and expression are two different factors. While the phenotypic expression can be environmentally modified, the brain circuitry and chemistry of the genetic programme will persist in the animal despite it being domesticated. There has been an assumption that much adaptation in respect of domestication has taken place over recent centuries. This assumption of general behavioural adaptation in domestication leans on two contingent assumptions. First, a general potential for further (and possibly faster) adaptation must exist to cope with any change in husbandry. Secondly, adaptation to confinement has been largely achieved already through exposure to conventional husbandry. The main and two contingent assumptions have failed to take certain facts into account, including the following:

1. Species attributes are characteristic and fixed in the species and are liable to quick change only by a mutation in an individual.
2. Varietal (or breed) attributes are the features on which domestic selection has been concentrated.
3. Behaviour is phenotypic.
4. Adaptation is not inevitable.

In the adaptation controversy, there has been a failure to make a distinction between varietal (i.e. of the breed) behavioural attributes – some of these have flourished and others have disappeared as a result of selection – and specific (i.e. of the species) behavioural attributes – most of which have persisted. Specific behavioural attributes, and in particular those of maintenance, must persist of necessity since they are bound in with much critical physiology. It is important to recognize the fact that (genetic engineering apart) while domestic selection can eliminate some behavioural varietal traits and propagate others, it cannot create any totally new genetic attributes.

Many domesticated changes in horses have undoubtedly occurred by full use of fortuitous mutation, such as heaviness or smallness. By exclusion of variability, much refinement of characteristics has also been achieved in breed features. This has been done using genetic material already present. Deliberate elimination of innate behaviour has not been a major objective, and no claim of its significant removal can be made with scientific justification. No convincing proof has been advanced showing the elimination of any equine behaviour essential to survival. On the contrary, much evidence shows that such behavioural potential still exists in highly bred domestic horses not subject to survival pressure. Today's horse keepers and breeders are clearly left with products of evolution and are obliged to act as curators, not as creators. As Kilgour and Dalton (1984) famously concluded: 'Domestication has not greatly altered the species-specific behaviour patterns of farm animals'.

Inherent Capability in Learning

Learning is the modification of an animal's behaviour as a result of previous experience and is an example of an evolutionary system of great adaptive significance. There are a number of different forms of learning providing a means for animals to adapt to changing circumstances during their own lifetime. It has been observed that untrained adult horses, on the first attempt to halter them, react negatively and vigorously to this form of control. If the animals are released after a 15 min session and then subjected to a haltering session after an interval of several days, they will respond differently and individually. Some may show fewer negative reactions to being handled and be more likely to accept the control of the halter, whilst others may be more difficult to handle. Each horse will have a different subsequent reaction as a result of its own experience of the event, illustrating that the type of learning (sensitization or habituation) that has taken place relates to the animal's individual perception of the handling.

Interestingly the impact of such an event on an individual relates to internal and external factors. The different genetic make-up of the horses interacting with the animals' previous experiences will ensure that the handling experience described above has a different emotional impact on each horse, resulting in a different behavioural response. Two schools of thought can be identified with regard to the issue of genetic effects versus environmental influences on behaviour. This conflict has been variously described as instinct versus learning, nature versus nurture, or endogenous versus exogenous determination of behaviour. A compromise synthesis is now generally recognized, in which all phenotypes are seen to be derived from the interaction of an organism's genes with its environment. Behaviour, of course, is as much a phenotype as any physical characteristic.

Although the relative contributions of genotype and environment vary considerably, neither is ever without input. Even when behavioural phenotypes, such as temperament, differ with regard to the interaction between experience and genotype, some contribution from each factor always takes place.

A useful way of recognizing the interaction of genetics and environment in the production of behaviour is to realize that behaviour is not contained in a complete form within genes. Genetic codes for behaviour do not have the capability of independent manifestation as behaviour without an environmental context. The genetic nature of behaviour, even that which is 'fixed' in the animal, is like a template. Through this, a clear pattern can only be produced if the appropriate stimulus is applied within a specific environmental situation. The genetic basis of behaviour varies in degree of specificity. Some behavioural templates are precise and detailed, while others are vague in outline and more general in form. An example of the precise genetic basis of behaviour is seen in the fixed behavioural patterns performed by newborn foals during the postnatal period.

Homeostasis and Survival

In addition to reproductive success, the establishment of homeostasis through feeding and related behaviour is vital to survival (Robinson, 2007). At the level of the individual animal, it is of the highest importance and takes the form of behaviours directed towards maintenance. It is now better appreciated that maintenance behaviour is very extensive and comprehensive. Formerly, this was considered to be limited to the basic needs for life. The needs of the living animal are continuous; however, they include more than those most basic items such as food, water and shelter. The integration of activities is represented in the unitary behaviour that gives the individual and its species much of its ethos. It is suggested that maintenance is the essence of homeostasis (Table 1.2).

In the domestic situation, homeostasis is often dictated by husbandry systems. This is achieved by manipulating methods of management in such

Table 1.2. Example of an ethogram of maintenance behaviour in the horse.

Category	Varied features	Function
Reaction	Reflexes, responses in general, fight or flight	Defence
Ingestion	Grazing, drinking, chewing, browsing	Nutrition
Body care	Rubbing, rolling, scratching, nibbling	Hygiene
Motion	Natural gaits, play, comfort shifts	Exercise
Rest	Drowsing, idling, lying, sleeping	Restoration
Association	Affiliation, bonding, herd unity	Companionship
Exploration	Attention, curiosity, wandering	Learning
Territorialism	Affinity for home base and home range	Security

ways that animal self-maintenance is facilitated. This is the objective of traditional animal husbandry and good animal care. Given its freedom in an appropriate environment, the domestic horse is still able to care for itself. The survival successes of feral and liberated horses speak volumes for the innate behavioural resources of these animals, which have been retained through hundreds of generations of domesticated breeding and selection. Perhaps now, more than ever before, the evolutionary heritage of domesticated horses can be appreciated (Bateson, 2003). The recognition of inherent behaviour, either precise as a pattern or variable as a process, should form the basis of a modern ethical approach to horse husbandry (Christiansen and Forkman, 2007).

Appraisal of Behaviour in Horses

When looking at a particular behaviour pattern or response, behavioural scientists ask four questions: how did the behaviour evolve; what is the biological function of the behaviour; what causes it to occur; and how did it develop in that animal? These 'Four Whys' were developed by Nobel Prize winner and one of the fathers of ethology (the scientific study of animals *in their natural environments*), Professor Niko Tinbergen. They are the framework upon which all aspects of horse behaviour can be explored and explained. Research related to the social, sexual, perinatal, parturient, maternal, developmental, maintenance and abnormal behaviour in horses, has provided valuable information that can be applied to ensure the well-being of the horse. Although the application of research findings to the management of horses in captive conditions is challenging for practitioners and students, advances are being made that benefit horses. It is recognized that veterinarians, equine practitioners, and owners need to understand the nature of horses, including the development of behaviour if they are to manage them effectively and humanely (Budiansky, 1997).

The objective measurement of equine behaviour is essential to ensure that assessments are reliable. However, these are often most suited for research conditions. For more practical use, veterinary clinicians tend to develop their own procedures for making behavioural assessments of animals, including a general appraisal of horse reactivity or general demeanour and taking a thorough behavioural history in relation to the specific individual case or a group (Gore *et al.*, 2008).

For safety and to ensure the welfare of the horse, its attitude, disposition and temperament should be assessed before any handling of the animal is attempted. The animal's perception and awareness of its general environment should also be noted. In particular, the subject's appreciation of sense-directed stimuli must be determined. Sensations such as vision, sound and position must be appraised. Ear and eye movement can be good indicators of emotional state. Recent studies have suggested that the animals' facial expression, including nostril tightening, eye wrinkles, exposure of the eye orbit and blink rate are all useful for determining level of arousal and emotional state (Waran and Randle, 2017). Spontaneous behaviour such as the horse's willingness to move, as well as the nature of its posture and gait, are also important considerations, as is the inclination to initiate contact with the handler. An evaluation must also be made of various reflex responses, both general (such as the response to sound) and specific (such as the response to a local stimulus, e.g., pressure, on a given site on the body). Reflex responses to localized stimuli, such as tapping below the jaw, may also be noted if there is a need to determine significant reactivity. Within an adequately extended examination period, acts of normal behaviour should become noticeable. These might include behavioural items of self-maintenance, such as feeding (or response to an offering of food) and body care. Illness, in general, can inhibit grooming and stretching reflexes. Acts of normal body care, such as 'comfort shifts', evacuation and self-grooming, in long behavioural examinations are especially significant because such normal behaviours often reduce or cease as a first or early sign of illness.

Methods for Appraising Behaviour

Behavioural appraisals are of value in judging the physical and mental health of the animal. General reflexes should not be studied only as isolated phenomena but as actions of the whole animal. Pandiculation (holistic stretching after arousal or rising) is an action pattern of common occurrence seen in healthy foals and, to a lesser extent, in adult horses. Differences in responses occur between breeds (Ligout *et al.*, 2008; Lloyd *et al.,* 2008).

In a study of posture in behavioural appraisal, it must be remembered that many postural abnormalities are not shown unless the horse is at rest or minimally disturbed in its usual stable. For this reason, patient and quiet observation of the animal may be necessary before any abnormality of posture can be detected. As a rule, the behavioural examination is best performed in a quiet space or enclosure, with limited light, where distractions will be minimal. Tranquillization should be avoided and parts of the examination, such as forced running, which could stimulate the animal, should be postponed until the end.

In determining the suitability of a horse for a given role, its characteristic behavioural repertoire is of paramount importance (Seaman *et al.*, 2002). For this to be determined reliably, a broad range of behavioural responses and performances should be appraised. Again, in the course of convalescence from an illness, the behaviour of self-maintenance returns to the animal's behavioural repertoire. An extended period of behavioural examination of the animal in its bedded premises is usually necessary for convalescence to be appraised by the behavioural method. Some outdoor methods allow the behaviour of horses to be studied in test situations without demanding 'artificial' conditions imposed upon them. These tests can allow a critical appraisal to be made on a horse, or horse group, with minimal manipulation, allowing behaviour to occur in a fairly spontaneous manner. Such methods include the use of data recorders on the horse, passing through a chute or a simple maze. Even fearfulness can become evident in this method (Lansade *et al.*, 2008).

There are a variety of objective methods used for assessing equine behaviour that are more applicable to a research setting. These range across observational field studies of horse social behaviour, time budgets, frequency and type of interactions to more specific measures made of horse choices, strength of preferences and cognitive biases in controlled tests under laboratory conditions. In all cases, behavioural assessments are conducted using the scientific method, ensuring that measurements are made and their interpretation is robust.

Open-field tests

The 'open-field test' is a basic ethological method (Lehner, 1996) used to determine the responses of animals to a novel environment including various stimuli. In the open-field test, which in some instances could be more aptly termed the 'closed-field test', the animal is liberated into an enclosure that permits extensive movement. In the horse's case this is often an arena, a small paddock, or a large pen. The total ground area or floor space is subdivided by actual regions or imaginary dividing lines, allowing for measurements related to movement within the pen, or around a specific object in the pen to be recorded. During a pre-determined time period after the animal is released into the open field, a record of the time spent within specific areas of the pen, the amount of the enclosure covered and explored, and the animal's general behavioural responses, including changes in reactivity, are made. Various measures can be combined to provide scores for each animal's 'open-field' response, and these can be related to other measures made of the animal's social behaviour, position in the social hierarchy or other such measures to provide an overall assessment of the animal's temperament (see Visser *et al.,* 2001). While the open-field test is principally applied in experimental situations to one animal, equivalent methods of behavioural assessment can be applied under natural and practical situations to groups (Martin and Bateson, 2007).

From a practical point of view, horse behaviour in the paddock is useful for understanding how space is utilized, as well as the frequency and patterns of maintenance activities such as feeding, resting and evacuating. These studies reveal the level of organization of behaviour performed by horses, even under confined conditions within the paddock. Even when they are highly restricted in paddocks, horses will attempt to use specific areas and resources for body care, social behaviours and self-maintenance. Such studies can help with providing information to ensure that husbandry conditions are consistent with good welfare.

Specific behavioural tests used in veterinary studies

There are several simple behaviour tests that can provide practical information regarding horse responses. These include:

The stimulus response test. This is where a specific stimulus is presented to an animal, and the reaction is recorded and used to determine the significance of the stimulus at that time. This method has been profitably used in noting the effects of 'teasing' on oestrus display, or determination of libidinal sensitivity in the stallion, for example. Breeding soundness should be based to a considerable extent on evidence of normal reproductive behaviour. Such behaviour often hinges on the occurrence of overt oestrus. The primary character of oestrus is, of course, receptivity to mating. The intensity of oestrus may vary considerably in mares. The appraisal of oestrous behaviour is therefore essential in horse breeding, although the normal female mating state has both behavioural and physiological elements (Table 1.3).

Incident frequencies and bout lengths. Recording the number of performances and/or the length of a specific response within a given period of time can provide information about the importance of that behaviour to the animal within a specific context. Behaviour frequency and bout length measurements have been put to good use investigating frequencies of avoidance and aggression between individuals within social groups. In addition, this method can be used to identify the significance of behaviour that is apparently abnormal and warrants improved definition and diagnosis.

Table 1.3. Varieties of oestrus manifestations in mares.

Character of oestrus	Common duration	Nature of behavioural display	Urinary ejaculations
Normal heat	>3 days	Frequent and complete	Numerous and copious
Weak heat	<3 days	Occasional and incomplete	Absent
Silent heat	>3 days	Occasional and partial without stallion; aggressive with stallion	Absent

Free choice tests. An animal is provided with a variety of resources to choose between and is provided with the time and space to determine the relative importance of each to them. The method has been used to understand the preference of an animal for given features of husbandry, such as the way in which food is presented or the way the horse is managed. For example, Jørgensen *et al.*, (2016), used a free choice methodology to determine whether horses in a colder climate preferred staying outdoors, going into a heated shelter compartment or into a non-heated shelter compartment. By scoring the frequency of the horse's location and behaviour, they showed that horse breed, coat thickness and weather conditions all influence the horses' choice of housing environment.

Ethograms. Ethograms are structured lists of defined behaviours that can be used to provide information regarding the normal balance of behaviours shown by individuals or groups in a given situation. With these proportions established, excesses or reductions can be recognizable, and the information can be used to redress the balance. An excellent example of an established ethogram for normal behaviour in a free-living situation was developed by McDonnell (2003).

Observational studies. Sometimes an individual animal can be assessed behaviourally to the best advantage in its normal biological situation. For example, the vitality of the newborn foal can be determined by undisturbed observations of the behaviour of the animal at its birth site. The action patterns (such as time to stand and find the teat) that unfold in the young animal in such characteristic and predictable ways serve to show the vitality of the individual neonate. Both the order and the time of behavioural events give a general picture of the foal's viability and the progress of its postnatal maturation (Morresey, 2005). Under normal conditions and when undisturbed, head lifting and shaking will occur first, quickly followed by rotation of the body to sternal recumbency. Rising attempts soon follow, and a first, fully upright stance is normally attempted within 30 min and attained within 1 hour. The first successful suck of the active neonate foal is achieved when it is between 1 and

2 hours old. Delays in the behavioural schedule of development can be used as indicative of imminent clinical problems resulting from dysmaturity in the newborn (Russell and Wilkins, 2006). Another use of this method is in appraising the temperament of the horse. Certain reactive behavioural activities, including threat displays and challenges are common in adult horses (Jensen, 2001). These can be used to assess the horse's character.

Critical Appraisal of Behaviour

While the behaviour of a normal and healthy horse is clearly the concern of many people, it is often the veterinary surgeon or the animal scientist who is required to be able to identify and explain abnormal behaviour. Increasingly veterinarians are expected to understand the behaviours that reliably indicate conditions associated with distress, discomfort, pain and deprivation of behavioural needs. These conditions often lead to changes in behaviour that become problematic for the horse owner.

Stress is defined as the biological response elicited when an individual perceives a threat to its homeostasis. Stress can lead to a heterogeneous group of dysfunctions, the manifestations of which are many, but the main concern is that these behavioural responses can be subtle and may go under detected. Appreciation of this fact ensures that veterinary and equine scientists are equipped to guide horse users in recognizing the early signs of a problem and how to provide the optimum and acceptable conditions of maintenance and care to avoid the development of these negative emotional states. The changing roles of veterinarians and other equine industry professionals rely upon developing an understanding of applied ethology, learning theory and the appraisal of abnormal behaviour as an aid to diagnosis. At the present stage, it is impossible to deal with this topic comprehensively, but one can consider a number of clinical circumstances in which diagnosis can be established on the basis of changes in a horse's behaviour. Greater veterinary involvement in applied ethology is needed to support an improved understanding of the impact of disease within the discipline of welfare (Willeberg, 1997; Christiansen and Forkman, 2007; Fraser, 2008).

Behaviours Associated with Clinical Conditions

The postural characteristics of the horse are among the commonest behavioural features to change in diseased conditions. Therefore, it is essential to appreciate normal posture as a basis for recognizing postural abnormalities for clinical purposes (see Fig. 1.4). The following are the main circumstances under which horses adopt abnormal postures:

1. Mechanical conditions involving loss of support of stability by the animal.

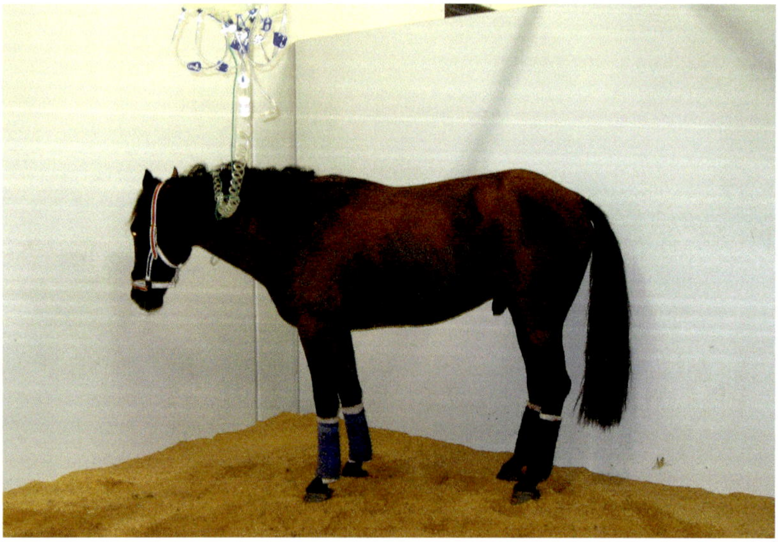

Fig. 1.4. Postural signs of compromised well-being of a horse with abdominal pain. Photo: C.B. Riley.

2. Neurological conditions with inadequate neural function to maintain muscular tone.
3. Painful conditions making it uncomfortable for the animal to maintain its natural posture. In addition, there can be permanent adaptive changes to pain, that the animal may have acquired as a result of prior experience of any disabling circumstances.

These three circumstances are further considered below.

Mechanical conditions. Mechanical conditions influencing postural behaviour are many, and the following few examples are given as illustrations. For example, fracture of the third metacarpus (cannon bone) in the horse makes it impossible for the animal to take any weight at all on the affected leg. Fracture of the humerus also leads to a lack of mechanical support and a grossly altered posture and abnormal limb position. Severance of both flexor tendons in the horse leads to a sinking of the fetlock and a turning up of the toe. Congenitally contracted tendons in foals also make normal posture impossible. Limb injuries, including an increasing number of fractures can respond in many cases to therapy and rehabilitation, allowing normal limb function to be restored (Stubbs *et al.*, 2013).
Neurological conditions. Neurological conditions that can create abnormal postures include radial paralysis following, for example, prolonged recumbency during anaesthesia. A lesion in the cervical vertebrae causes the condition of 'wobbler syndrome' in the horse, the main characteristics of which are ataxia and stiff neck (Gore *et al.*, 2008).
Painful conditions. The behaviour of a horse in pain has certain specific features that are recognisable. Painful conditions causing abnormal posture in horses include laminitis and osteoarthritis, where the animal will assume positions to help ease discomfort in the affected limbs. Permanent adaptive changes to pain, as a result of neuropathic changes, may also arise in a condition such as laminitis. On rare occasions, animals that have experienced laminitis learn to ease the pressure and pain through adopting a characteristic 'pointing' foreleg position. This is accompanied by the hind legs of the animal being brought further forward.

The facial expression in pain is often quite characteristic and has been documented in the equine grimace scale (Dalla Costa *et al.*, 2014). The 'pain face' is associated with the ears being held stiffly backwards, orbital tightening, tension above the eye areas and prominent strained chewing muscles. In addition, attention may be given to one area of the body, such as looking at the flank where there is a specific site of pain as is the case for horses experiencing colic. With persistent pain horses may also show unusual recumbent behaviour, while at other times, they adopt an unusual stance. Horses may back into a corner of a stall/loose box, or are observed standing, pushing their heads against a wall when an uncomfortable or painful condition is present. Horses suffering from abdominal pain can appear restless, lying down frequently and repeatedly rising after short intervals of recumbency. In between these periods of recumbency, a horse with colic may scrape at its bedding with a forefoot while slowly pivoting around on its hind legs. Thoroughbred horses suffering azoturia sometimes scrape up mounds of wood shavings provided as bedding and then stand with their back legs on these mounds (Mills, 1991).

Locomotory Behaviour

When the locomotor behaviour of a horse is to be examined, it should be singled out and observed in good light, moving about on a clean, dry and level surface. The horse should be led by hand at different gaits when a special examination of locomotor behaviour is carried out. If appropriate it can then be allowed to move freely to observe free action (Fig. 1.5). Abnormalities of posture and gait may indicate a neurological condition (Oliver and Lorenz, 1993). Some alterations of mental state, such as depression, disorientation or hyper-excitability, can accompany some locomotor signs. Assessment of gait should take account of every aspect of gait, such as length of stride, whether too long or too short. A painful skeletal lesion gives a short stride with a reduced support phase and is often unilateral; the commonest form of this is a 'limp'. In the wide range of clinical veterinary textbooks (see Back and Clayton, 2013), there is extensive detail on all clinical dysfunctions affecting equine mobility.

Ontogeny of Behaviour: Instinct

Horse behaviour develops through a combination of instinctive and learned responses. Instinctive behaviours appear to be pre-programmed, or genetically encoded, but are subject to modification through experience. Choices emerge with environmental challenge and experience. Maintenance and reproductive motivations, e.g., hunger, thirst, comfort,

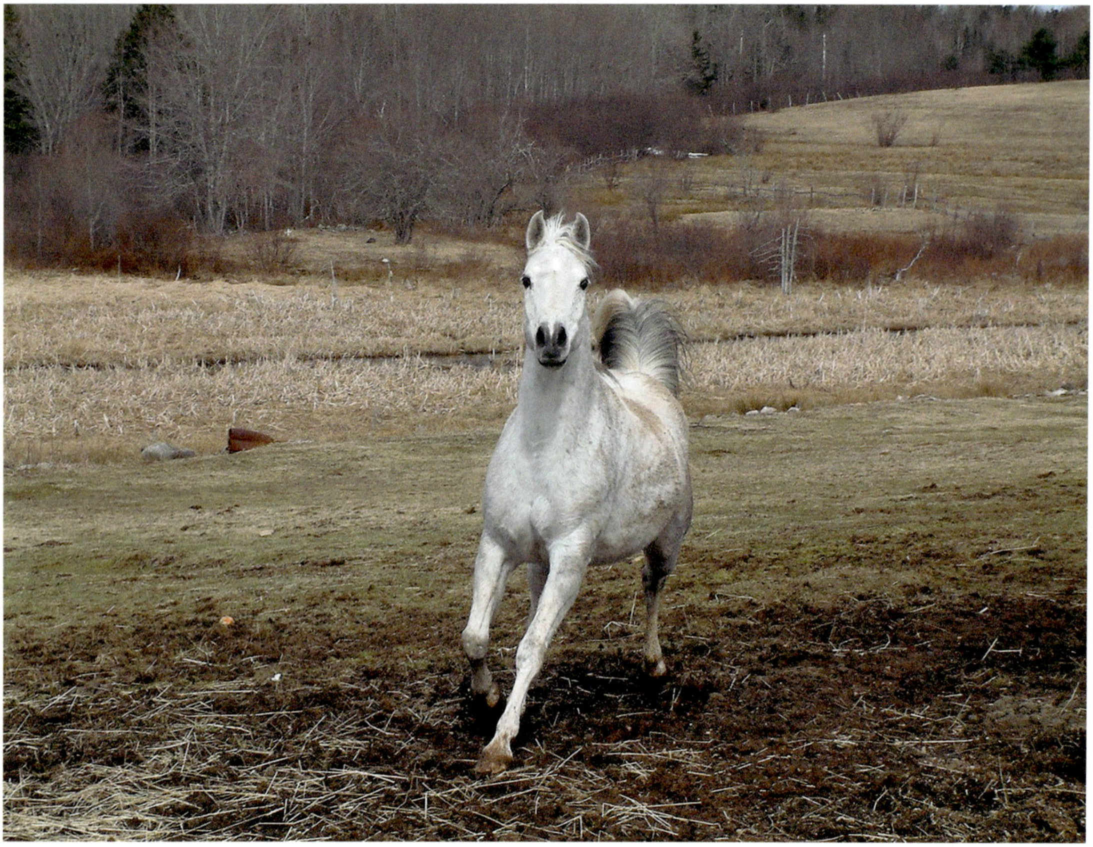

Fig. 1.5. Spontaneously running Arab horse turned out into the pasture. Photo: C.B. Riley.

motion, association and sexual motives, switch and change priorities. Feeding and reactive and reproductive behavioural motives, in particular, are modified by the experience and environmental circumstances of a horse.

Instinctive behaviour

Lorenz (1965) and other early ethologists described instincts or innate forms of behaviour in various vertebrates. Innate behaviour is that element of behaviour that has been inherited. This inherited basis of behaviour may be modified during the life of the animal, according to its experiences with its environment. The evolved genetic basis ensures that the animal is equipped with a repertoire of adaptive responses that can be utilized without essential prior experience. The precise nature of innate behaviour allows us to recognize readily that such behaviour can be elicited in the proper circumstances without prior experience. For example, many of the neonate's functions are predetermined. Some innate behaviours may not be revealed until the animal is an adult and mature, as, for example, in most kinds of maternal behaviour. The adult horse's characteristic sexual behaviour is largely determined by genetic factors. However, it is important to recognize that, even with this fixed foundation, innate behaviour can be changed as the animal acquires information regarding the success or otherwise of a given response.

Release of innate responses

Much of the 'priming' of innate behaviour occurs in the endocrine system, and the coordination of action patterns is dependent on activation of nerve centres, e.g., the hypothalamus. In classical ethology, the releasing of innate actions requires specific stimuli, essentially sign stimuli or releasers.

Certain theories exist in connection with releasers. A releaser is defined as any specific feature in an animal's environment that prompts an innate response. Behavioural characters that are peculiar to the equine species can thus be set in motion by certain stimuli. The theory of the innate releasing mechanism (IRM) has grown from this hypothesis. The IRM is physiological, built into the animal and inactive until it becomes appropriately stimulated. The appropriate stimulus in the environment is considered to be the key that unlocks the appropriate action pattern.

In this theory, releasers act upon the IRM by issuing a simple sign stimulus. The IRM should allow an animal to automatically respond to a behaviourally relevant stimulus that the animal will not have previously encountered. One particular type of releaser that plays an important part in determining behaviour is the social or sexual releaser. Such a releaser may be an animal's odour, shape, sequence of movements, variety of sounds or general display; it serves the specific function of eliciting a particular response in another member of the same species. The role of such releasers is considerable in the mating and nursing behaviour of horses, where instinctive movements are necessary to ensure individual and the species' fitness and survival (Kiley-Worthington, 1999).

Sensitive periods and imprinting

Imprinting is a unique form of behavioural development, where a critical feature of the environment becomes highly significant to an animal within a specific early period of its life, referred to as the critical or sensitive period. A modified concept of this phenomenon has been suggested to be applicable to equine early development (Miller, 2003), although this is somewhat controversial. Some trainers have made use of this period when the foal is particularly aware of environmental stimuli to carry out what they call 'imprint training'. Proponents claim that early handling of the foal (in the first days after birth), getting them used to sounds and equipment such as clippers, and acquainting them with the application of ropes and mild pressure in areas where leg and rein aids will be used, leads to young horses that have learned to tolerate rather than struggle against humans and to cope with the sorts of stimuli that are frequently part of the horse's working life. Of course, with the foal's welfare in mind, such early training needs to be done extremely carefully to not negatively impact the relationship between foal and dam. Some obscure influences of imprinting can persist for extended periods in areas of behaviour such as mating orientation. Male animals, for example, may attempt to mount individuals of a different species with which some degree of imprinting may have occurred in a critical period of development. It's not only the offspring who have an inbuilt preference at certain times during development. There is also thought to be a sensitive period following parturition when the dam quickly learns the identity of her newborn and develops a rapid attachment. In contrast, other young, even if similar, are rejected and hostile behaviour exhibited towards the alien. Such behaviour in mares may amount to extreme aggression in many cases. When the maternally sensitive period has passed, adoption of fostered young by learning is more protracted and less certain. Such maternal behaviour is strongly and quickly motivated to establish parental care (Clutton-Brock, 1992).

There are other examples of sensitive periods in development, such as the socialization period, during which young animals are highly sensitized to enable them to acquire knowledge of the normal social behaviour of their own species. For horses, the socialization period occurs as soon as the foal starts to interact with other foals and dams in the herd. During puberty, this is important for the development of sexual preferences and behaviours. Often young stallions that do not gain appropriate orientation at this critical time have some delay in learning the motor skills of mounting and mating.

Early Experience

The effects of early experience on the development of adult behaviour are significant. When horses are raised as orphaned animals, their later behaviour differs from the reactive characteristics of most normally reared horses; they are often difficult to restrain and to train, for example. At the same time, foals reared exclusively in their mother's company usually adopt the reactive tendencies of the mother and acquire the mother's temperamental characteristics. Foals raised without human contact before weaning, such as may occur in free-living animals, may have difficulty in accepting handling by humans in their later life. They appear to be fearful and insecure under human control. Acquisition of undesirable behavioural states can be avoided by positive and structured early handling, although this must always be carried out by experienced personnel so as not to inadvertently elicit undesirable responses in the young animal. Ideally, this should begin early in the foal's life, with some advocating for the first day after birth. Through gradually habituating the foal to gentle handling, it will learn that there is no danger in being contained by human force and that short separation from its dam is not traumatic. During this time, the foal can be carefully touched all over to learn acceptance of human contact. Sessions of touching, bodily restraint and brief separation from the mother allow the foal to habituate to human presence and accept control over its behaviour. After it is weaned, such early experience aids in its handling (Zentall, 1996).

During the paediatric period, the total effects of experience are compounded. The development of emotions, the opportunity to pursue exploratory behaviour, the social experiences of the young animal and the development of its physical and physiological apparatus all combine to influence the animal's reservoir of acquired behaviour. Post-weaning environmental experiences, including the method of weaning used (Waran *et al.*, 2008), also play their part in developing the behaviour of the subject in subsequent adult life. Experimental processes continue into this period, and senses continue to develop (Houpt, 1991). A study of the many factors capable of affecting a horse's behaviour must include the various early experiences that can permanently affect the behaviour of that individual, even into its adult life. Environmental factors and social forces have a much more powerful and durable influence when applied in early life than similar ones experienced in adult life (Forkman, 2002). Investigatory activities, from which much learning is derived, continue throughout life, though they tend to be more obvious in the young animal. Good habits are dependent on familiarity with a wide range of husbandry features that provide optimal conditions for the animal. Exposing foals to essential husbandry procedures, such as haltering, can prove to be helpful in their adaptations. Many routines become established as the basic pattern of management, and it is highly desirable to allow the animal to acquire experience of these routines before they become enforced procedures. Much learning in young foals is by observation, and they learn more readily by watching their mothers than by watching others. Their mothers, of course, permit close investigation by their own young. Grazing horses, again particularly young ones, learn from others such things as food selection and location, paths and routes, watering places and shelters. Such learning is of critical importance in the ability of the young horse to integrate successfully with its environment and home range. Visser *et al.* (2003) found that learning ability in young horses was variable between horses but consistent in individuals.

Ontogeny of Behaviour: Learning

The biggest changes in a horse's behaviour occur as a consequence of the experiences it has. Scientists define learning as a relatively permanent modification in behaviour as the result of personal experience, and for the most part, learning occurs gradually with repetition. Learning enables an animal to shape its responses in line with its own environmental challenges. While the horse can acquire certain behavioural methods of adapting to its circumstances and environment, it can readily acquire maladjusted forms of behaviour. Husbandry factors can give rise to behavioural anomalies, and many items of abnormal behaviour are of diagnostic value in the identification of defective husbandry.

Learning is, therefore, a part of each domestic horses' development. The animal depends on learning and memory to cope with the circumstances of the environment that it experiences, not only at the moment of the experience but also in later circumstances of a similar nature. Learning theory outlines the various forms of learning and how they occur, but the most relevant to horse training and management are habituation and associative learning.

There are two main types of associative learning: classical and operant or instrumental, and together these form the basis of the main way in which horses learn about their environment and their handlers, and are trained under saddle.

Classical conditioning

A response is termed conditioned when a stimulus, other than the natural or originally effective one, can bring about the response. The normal, or originally effective, reflex eliciting stimulus is termed the unconditional stimulus. The unconditioned stimulus (such as food) elicits a natural (unconditioned) reflexive behavioural response (such as salivating) because it has become closely associated in time and space and serves as a good predictor. The outcome (i.e. feeding) associated with the stimulus reinforces the animal's behavioural response. Some stimuli result in positive outcomes; some are negative from the animal's point of view. Either way, the behavioural responses are reinforced due to the consequences to the animals. Reinforcement relates to the increase in the likelihood of a behaviour occurring again in relation to a stimulus being given/applied (positive) or removed (negative). Positive reinforcers are stimuli that the subject will work to attain, and negative reinforcers are stimuli that the subject will work to reduce or end. Positive and negative reinforcers are also described as primary or secondary. In mating, for instance, it could be said that the unconditioned stimulus is the general form of the stationary mare, but it is observed that many other stimuli, in time, elicit a full behavioural response in the stallion. In the case of stallions under restrained husbandry, leading the animal out towards the customary service area will, in time, act as if it were the sexual stimulus, eliciting a conditioned response. When conditioned stimuli have been established, they can be very effective in stimulating the animal's responses.

The classical procedures in conditioning are those that involve the repetition of the same sequence of stimuli. Routines of husbandry are suited to the establishment of classical conditioning, although this may not always be desirable. In conditioning, a state of generalization is common where actions occur in response to a variety of unrelated stimuli or have only a loose connection with the primary stimulus. The numerous daily routines of animal husbandry create many generalized states of conditioning, such as the sound of food preparation.

Examples of classical conditioning in horse husbandry and training are numerous. Stud horses become sexually activated when haltered to be led out by their grooms for breeding purposes; horses at grazing will run to a trough/neigh when someone appears with a bucket; and when stabled often develop a door-banging problem.

Operant conditioning

A major type of learning utilized in equine handling and training is instrumental or operant conditioning. It is, in effect, trial and error learning and is the learning that occurs from the numerous empirical activities generated by exploratory and investigative behaviour. Operant conditioning is also called instrumental learning or conditioning since the behaviour is the instrument by which the reward, or reinforcement, is obtained. Training animals is an operant task: the trainer may wait until the animal produces the desired activity or manipulate the environments such that the performance of the behaviour is required. Once performed, the behaviour can be positively or negatively reinforced on a specific reinforcement schedule (i.e. constantly or intermittently, depending upon the stage of training). Shaping behavioural responses in this way ensures that the animal gradually learns the associations between its behavioural responses to reliable stimuli or signals and the desirable consequences. In their training, horses rely upon operant conditioning for learning behaviours that are not natural, innate actions. Through systematically applying a stimulus such as bit pressure through the rider's application of the reins, the horse will learn the reinforcing consequences through its own actions or responses. When pressure is released as soon as the horse responds to bit pressure in the desired way (e.g., slowing down), we term that negative (removal) reinforcement. When a horse increases its responses to something that has been added or provided such as a carrot or a soothing stroke, we call that positive reinforcement. Learning theory is the term used to describe what we know about how animals absorb, process and retain information through the association between stimulus–response–reinforcement, together with the emotional and environmental factors that influence this. The relatively new field of equitation science (Goodwin *et al.*, 2009) argues that successful and humane training relies on the trainer developing an understanding of the correct application of learning theory, horse ethology, physiology and biomechanics.

Non-associative learning: habituation and desensitization

Habituation is the elimination of responses that are not imperative or biologically meaningful, and as such, it serves to ensure that the horse conserves its energy. It may be a simple form of learning, but it is important in allowing a horse to filter out non-vital information, enabling it to conserve energy and to focus on more significant things in the environment. Habituation in the natural environment may include reducing reactivity to other harmless species that graze alongside the herd, or the sound and sight of the wind moving the trees. Use of this natural phenomenon can be made during training by ensuring that horses become accustomed to the variety of unnatural or potentially frightening stimuli they need to deal with throughout their working lives. Examples include the sight or feel of the saddle and girth, the rug being thrown over and onto the horse, and the sound of traffic on the road. All of these and many more are stimuli that horses need to habituate to, and so it is important that they are presented in a non-threatening and consistent manner. Habituation of horses to the many circumstances of their use is clearly an important factor in their training, for rider safety and horse welfare (Appleby and Hughes, 1997; Waran and Randle, 2017).

Desensitization is where, through gradual and positive exposure, the horse becomes more familiar and more relaxed and accepting of naturally fear- or stress-eliciting stimuli or circumstances such as loud noises and flapping objects. The objective is not to flood the horse by forcing it to accept the presence of something feared but rather to reduce fear through systematic exposure over time, taking into account the horse's responses in deciding when to move to the next phase of training. Desensitization is often used for dealing with horses where there is an established fear response in relation to a management procedure such as injection or worming. Desensitization of needle-shy horses requires a planned approach, ensuring that the horse is given the time and space to change its response to something that it has become increasingly fearful of.

Motivation, Reinforcement and Punishment

For any learning to occur, the horse must be motivated and his response must be reinforced in some way. Motivation occurs due to internal and external conditions known as causal factors. For example, if the horse is hungry, it is internally more motivated to find food, and if food items are present, it will be externally motivated to try to get to that food. Whether or not an animal performs a behaviour is not only influenced by how motivated it is to perform that particular response but also by the strength of any conflicting motivation to perform other competing responses. This is extremely relevant to the horse training and handling situation because fearful or stressed horses will be more highly motivated to protect themselves, often involving an escape response, than to learn any new behavioural responses that the rider may be trying to develop. In addition, the horse must be sufficiently motivated to learn a new association. For example, if food is used as a reward, the animals must be hungry or the food item must be recognized as of high value by the horse.

Another important element is how learning is rewarded, or more correctly, reinforced. Reinforcement maintains the association and ensures that the behavioural response becomes strongly associated with a particular signal and persists. Reinforcers are termed positive and negative – but, in both cases, they serve to increase the chance that the behaviour will be performed again. For example, a positive reinforcer is one that is 'added in' to increase the chance that the animal will perform the behaviour again. This is normally something the horse is naturally attracted to, such as a tasty food item or providing some social contact. Negative reinforcement (not to be confused with punishment) involves applying an unpleasant or mildly aversive stimulus (such as leg pressure) and removing it when the horse performs the desired behaviour (moving forward). In working with horses under saddle, this pressure-and-release system is practical, where positive reinforcement often is not.

It is important not to leap to conclusions about the terms used in learning theory. These are borrowed from psychology and are not intended to describe good or bad types of signals from the horse's point of view. Negative refers to the removal or 'taking away' a stimulus that has been used as a signal and positive means 'adding in' a stimulus. In positive reinforcement training, we often provide the horse with a food treat once he has performed the response to the signal, so adding something to help the horse remember the association. This is often harder to apply when training horses under saddle, which is why negative reinforcement is usually used. An example of the correct use of negative reinforcement in horse training is when rein or rope pressure (the stimulus, signal or aid) is applied to slow the horse's forward movement (pull back on reins) or increase the horse's forward movement (a pull forward on the lead rope) (see Fig. 1.6). When being trained, the horse has to learn the association between a tightened rein, causing pressure through the various parts that the bridle has contact with, and the desired slowing response.

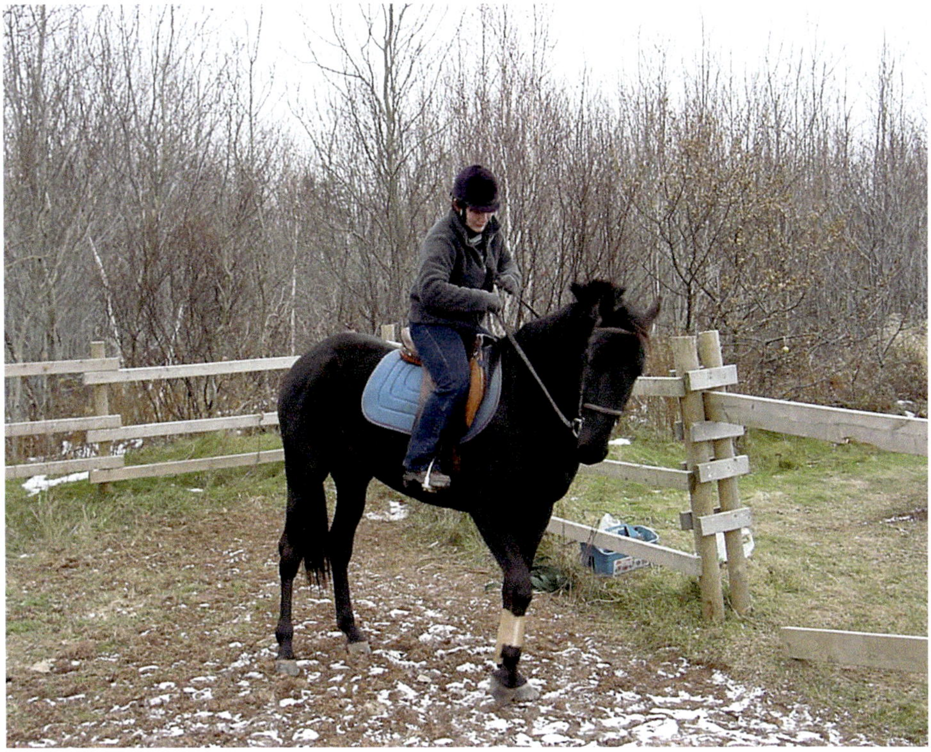

Fig. 1.6. Negative reinforcement – the pressure applied through the reins is released as soon as the horse slows. Photo: Natalie Waran.

To get to this point, the horse's slower movement (the desired response or action to that signal) must be reinforced so that as soon as the horse starts to slow its legs, the rein pressure is released (taken away). The reward or the reinforcement is the release of the rein pressure. The same formula can be applied to the establishment of the rider's leg signals. The reason the horse makes a good association is that as soon as he moves 'off the leg aid', the rider removes the leg pressure immediately.

In horse training we use both positive and negative reinforcement to incentivize the horse to perform and to maintain the performance of a specific response to a given signal. However, there are some interesting results that suggest that positive training techniques may increase the speed of learning. Positive interactions shown towards the handler during training improve retention of the association in the longer term (Sankey *et al.*, 2010). It may be that a combination of positive and negative reinforcement serves best for ensuring a positive learning experience and long-lived associations. Heleski *et al.*, (2008) found that the situation was safer and less stressful for the handler when positive reinforcement is used along with rope pressure for training horses to perform a fear-provoking task such as crossing a tarpaulin on the ground.

Regardless of whether one or the other type of reinforcer is used, it is crucial that the reinforcement is applied (or removed) immediately the desired behaviour is performed (within a couple of seconds) in response to a specific signal. In horse training, the goal is to get the association so well entrenched through repetition, good timing of release of, or provision of, the reinforcer, so ensuring that the horse needs only the lightest signal (for example a light pressure on the rope if wanting them to lead) to elicit the required response.

Finally, it is worth noting that in learning theory terminology and practice, negative reinforcement and punishment are not the same things. Negative reinforcement involves increasing the tendency to perform required responses through removing an applied pressure on the horse as soon as it performs the desired response, and this can be delivered effectively and humanely, enabling the horse to learn a specific relationship between an aid and required behaviour. On the other hand, punishment is pressure applied to a horse during an on-going behaviour and is used to 'stop' the behaviour after it has already begun or occurred. The problem with using a punisher is that the horse is being expected to make an association between behaviour that has already happened or is happening, using a fear-provoking and sometimes painful action by the handler/trainer. Since horses are not good at making retrospective associations, training using punishment is at least ineffective and at worst unethical and inhumane. If a punisher is to be used to deal with an ongoing behaviour, it needs to be applied immediately or within two seconds of the start of the behaviour for it to be effective. This is often hard when on board a horse and with the rider trying to maintain balance. However, it can be effectively applied in problem situations when on the ground. For example, if a horse attempts to bite the handler, where the handler emits a loud 'no' to distract the horse momentarily and then provides the horse with a more appropriate response that can be rewarded, such as asking the horse to reverse a step negatively reinforced by a release of the head-collar rope as the horse steps back.

Emotionality and Intelligence

Animal intelligence is a controversial and much-debated topic. How to define it and whether it exists as it does in humans is of increasing interest. Studied attempts have been made to make appraisals of animal intelligence on the implicit assumption that animals and their behaviour could be better understood through proper comprehension of their intelligence. The assumption was faulty. Although intelligence in mankind is well understood and, in many cases, affects human behaviour, it cannot be assumed that intelligence in animals is of an identical nature. It can now be recognized that intelligence in horses is more general than specific and that its role in behaviour is apparently a supportive one based on essential sensory perception. Nevertheless, animal intelligence does exist, although it is difficult to define and often referred to as cognitive ability.

While various methods are often used to measure cognitive ability in animals, it would appear that the length of time that an animal can remember a specific training signal or command could be taken as some measure of intelligence. However, Hanggi (2003) argues that horses have more advanced learning capabilities than previously assumed. Some horses seem to learn with greater facility than others, and variation in intelligence could be argued to be shown in this way. Intelligence could also arguably be demonstrated when the horse learns to ignore irrelevant stimuli, just as it also becomes sensitized to significant stimuli. This permits the behavioural developments that make discrimination possible. The animal's integration with its domestic environment is facilitated by this ability to compare and contrast, based upon its previous learning and the skills acquired. Most horses can accurately discriminate between stimuli and evaluate them, e.g., they can differentiate sounds, visual features of special significance, identities of people and so on. This ability appears to improve with experience (Domjam, 1998).

Environmental conditions such as constant confinement and behavioural restriction can impact negatively on cognitive ability and so-called intelligence, affecting horses. While a horse's physical condition may be preserved in the stable, its emotional (nervous) condition is likely to be adversely affected by the chronic restriction. In many cases, if the restrictive husbandry is constant, the animal's natural activities become redirected, so to speak, into abnormal action patterns. More simply, restriction negatively affects their behaviour and their emotional state leading to changes in their ability to learn. In constant close confinement, horses can suffer affective dysfunctions. The typical dysfunctions usually occur in mouthing (Sambraus, 1985), marking time and reacting, but affective states can also appear in adverse features of temperament or disposition.

A traditional form of restriction used on horses is 'breaking-in' for human use. The term says much about the animal's affected spirit. Such evoked submissive responsiveness in the horse is achieved forcibly. Today there is increasing awareness of the alternative method of inducing compliance in the horse by humane manipulation of the animal's nature. Willing compliance is preferable to imposed submission since it is more likely that leads horses to develop in their conventional tasks by using intelligent responses (see Figs 1.7–1.9).

Cognitive Bias

An interesting emerging area of research involves measuring the judgment bias of animals to objectively

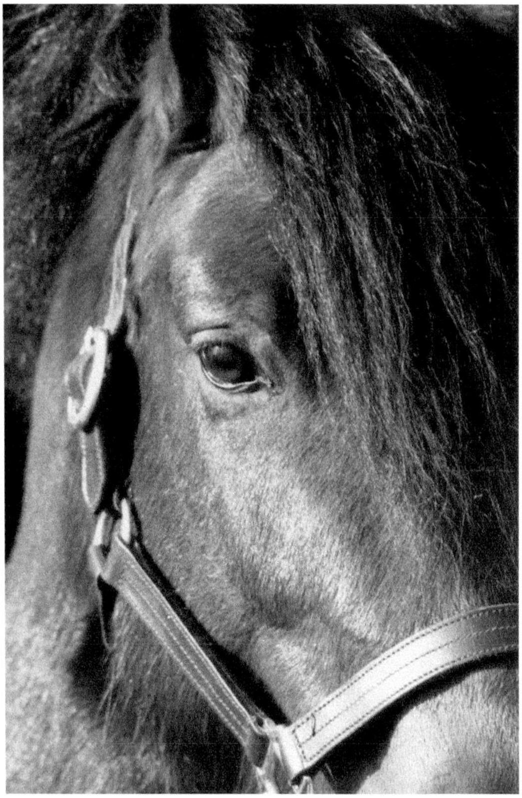

Fig. 1.7. Normal eye expression in watchfulness. Photo: Melanie MacDonald.

assess their emotional states. Emotions are intense, short-lived affective responses to situations and events that have some important significance in the life of an animal. They can be both positive and negative. One way to determine the mental state of an animal is suggested to be through cognitive bias testing, that is, assessing the impact on cognitive processes such as learning speed and choices of its mood or emotional state. One of the cognitive measures is to assess how animals interpret ambiguous stimuli or 'opportunities' that lie somewhere in between those sure to give a reward and those sure not to. The decisions in ambiguous situations can be biased by the underlying mood state. Animals in a more positive mood will expect something positive to happen when confronted with ambiguous stimuli (optimistic bias). In contrast, animals in a more negative mood will not expect something positive to happen (pessimistic bias). In humans, individuals in a positive mood state will be more attentive to positive events, be more optimistic, learn more easily and memorize more effectively. Studies of this phenomenon in horses have shown promising results regarding the impact of training and housing methods. Not surprisingly, horses exposed to more restricted environments showed more pessimistic responses in bias tests, suggesting that their welfare is likely to be impaired (Henry *et al.*, 2017). In a practical sense, this may prove useful for horse keepers, recognizing that the choices a horse makes reflect its emotional state, which in turn is affected by its previous experiences, good and bad.

Behaviour and Equine Welfare

Equine welfare is a complex area for study, but it is essential that horse owners and practitioners are familiar with behavioural indicators of poor and good welfare states. Welfare is not confined to measures of physical health but includes the assessment of mental well-being and behavioural opportunities. Good welfare is not simply the absence of negative experiences, but rather is primarily the opportunity for and expression of positive behaviours indicating underlying positive mental states such as pleasure. Although the assessment of equine welfare has traditionally relied on measures of negative states such as pain, distress, fear and discomfort, increasingly reliable indicators of positive emotions are being developed, such as play, mutual grooming and facial expressions. The equine nature is expansive from its massive inheritance and its cumulative experiences. Its immediate circumstances create an additional factor in the determination of its behaviour. As a result, no two horses are exactly alike in general conduct. Every horse is unique in its nature: in its character, temperament, personality and individual behaviour. It follows that horse welfare is axiomatic and that the management of each horse should be in accord with its particular individuality. Therefore, knowledge of equine behaviour, in general, is fundamentally required in modern horse care.

One welfare

For a prey species such as the horse, fear is a powerful motivator because it is an unpleasant emotional experience. Anything that removes the horse from experiencing that unpleasant feeling is strongly reinforced and will be repeated. This is why when a horse has had a bad experience and has responded

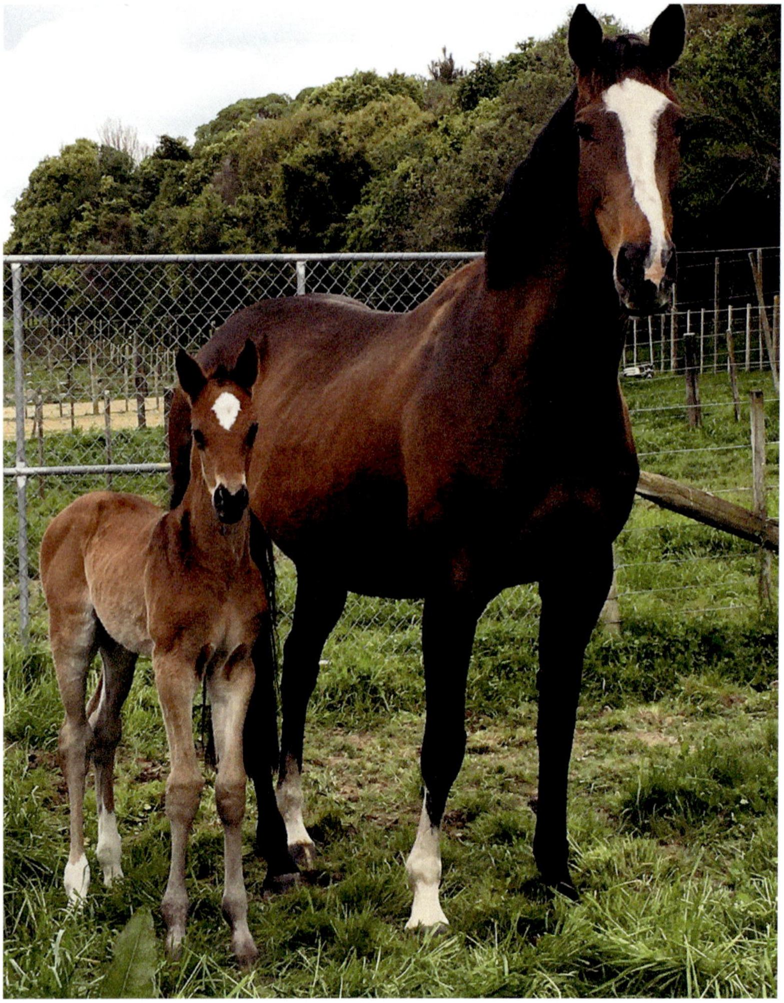

Fig. 1.8. Colt and mare showing full attention. Note the orientation of body, dilated nostrils, pricked-forward ears and watchful eyes. Photo: C.B. Riley.

almost instinctively to protect itself, he will refine and repeat his response so that he is able to anticipate and react to cues that enable him to anticipate and avoid the frightening situation in future. In horse handling and training, humans exert a considerable impact on their horse's behaviour and emotions. It stands to reason that methods of handling and training based on provoking fear that may lead to short-term success will also produce animals with behavioural responses and fear memories that are not desirable for horse and human safety in the long term. Unfortunately, many problem behaviours develop because horses are extremely good at rapidly learning from successfully dealing with something that causes a negative feeling. Common fear-provoking events leading to a learned behaviour often result in horses acquiring undesirable responses such as unwillingness to enter a trailer, especially when coming home from a show, rushing when showjumping and refusing to be caught in the field. Increasingly those involved with horses are being asked to recognize that coercive riding and handling techniques not only compromise the horse's welfare, but also put horse and rider at a greater risk of injury resulting from the horse's fear reactions. It is of increasing concern that professionals such as equine veterinarians carry a high risk of sustaining an occupational

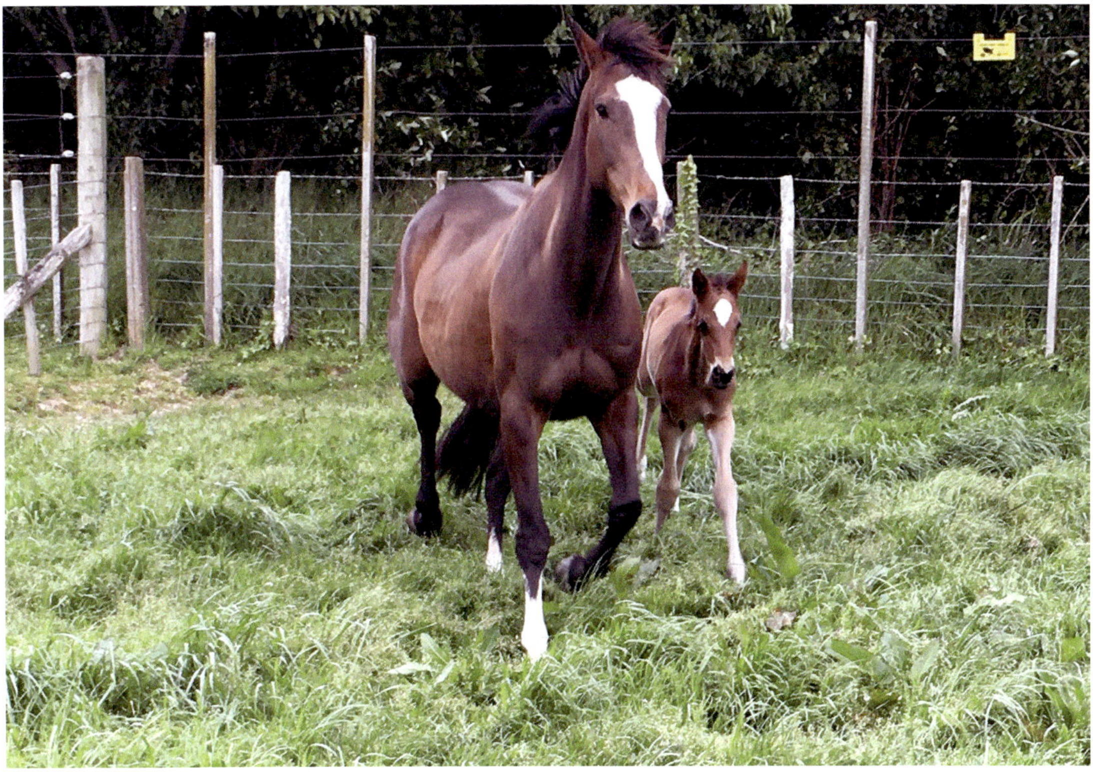

Fig. 1.9. Foal watching and learning while moving in step with his dam. Photo: C.B. Riley.

injury as a result of the fear/pain response of the horse they are attempting to treat (Pearson, 2016). Improving understanding of equine behaviour and effective use of learning theory amongst horse owners, veterinarians, and other equine professionals is essential for ensuring good welfare for all.

References

Appleby, M.C. and Hughes, B.O. (eds) (1997) *Animal Welfare*. CAB International, Wallingford, UK.

Back, W. and Clayton, H.M. (2013) *Equine Locomotion-E-Book*. Elsevier Health Sciences.

Bateson, P. (2003) The promise of behavioural biology. *Animal Behaviour* 65, 11–17.

Bateson, P. and Horn, G. (1994) Imprinting and recognition memory: a neural net model. *Animal Behaviour* 48, 695–715.

Budiansky, S. (1997) *The Nature of Horses*. The Free Press, New York, pp. 211–234.

Christiansen, S.B. and Forkman, B. (2007) Assessment of animal welfare in a veterinary context – a call for ethologists. *Applied Animal Behaviour Science* 106, 203–220.

Clutton-Brock, J. (1992) *Horse Power: A History of the Horse and the Donkey in Human Societies*. Harvard University Press, Cambridge, MA, pp. 192.

Clutton-Brock, J. (1999) *A Natural History of Domesticated Mammals*. Cambridge University Press, Cambridge.

Dalla Costa, E., Minero, M., Lebelt, D., Stucke, D., Canali, E. and Leach, M.C. (2014) Development of the horse grimace scale (HGS) as a pain assessment tool in horses undergoing routine castration. *PLoS ONE* 9(3), e92281.

Dawkins, M.S. (2004) Using behaviour to assess welfare. *Animal Welfare* 13, 53–57.

Domjam, M. (1998) *The Principles of Learning and Behaviour*, 4th edn. Brooks/Cole, London.

Forkman, B.A. (2002) Learning and cognition. In: Jensen, P. (ed.) *The Ethology of Domestic Animals*. CAB International, Wallingford, UK, pp. 51–64.

Fraser, A.F. (2008) Veterinarians and animal welfare – a comment. *The Canadian Veterinary Journal* 49(1), 8.

Goodwin, D., McGreevy P., Waran N. and McLean A. (2009) How equitation science can elucidate and refine horsemanship techniques. *Veterinary Journal* 181, 5–11.

Gore, T., Gore, P. and Griffin, J.M.L. (2008) *Horse Owner's Veterinary Handbook*, 3rd edn. Wiley Publishing Inc., Hoboken, New Jersey.

Hanggi, E.B. (2003). Discrimination learning based on relative size concepts in horses (*Equus caballus*). *Applied Animal Behaviour Science* 83(3), 201– 213.

Heleski, C., Bauson, L. and Bello, N. (2008) Evaluating the addition of positive reinforcement for learning a frightening task: a pilot study with horses. *Journal of Applied Animal Welfare Science* 11(3), 213–222.

Henry, S., Fureix, C., Rowberry, R., Bateson, M. and Hausberger, M. (2017) Do horses with poor welfare show 'pessimistic' cognitive biases? *Naturwissensch aften* 104, 8.

Herdt, T.H. (2007) Gastrointestinal physiology and metabolism (Section IV). In: Cunningham, J.G. and Klein, B.G. (eds) *Veterinary Physiology*. Saunders Elsevier, Amsterdam.

Houpt, K.A. (1991) *Domestic Animal Behaviour for Veterinarians and Animal Scientists*, 2nd edn. Iowa State University Press, Ames, Iowa.

Jensen P. (2001) Parental behaviour. In: Keeling, L.J. and Gonyou, H.W. (eds) *Social Behaviour in Farm Animals*. CAB International, Wallingford, UK, pp. 59–82.

Jones, S. (2001) *Darwin's Ghost. The Origin of Species Updated*. Anchor Canada, Random House of Canada Ltd, Toronto.

Jørgensen, G.H., Aanensen, L., Mejdell, C.M. and Bøe, K.E. (2016) Preference for shelter and additional heat in horses exposed to Nordic winter conditions. *Equine Veterinary Journal* 48, 720–726.

Kiley-Worthington, M. (1999) *The Behaviour of Horses*. J.A. Allen & Co. Ltd, London.

Kilgour, R. and Dalton, C. (1984) *Livestock Behaviour: A Practical Guide,* 1st edn. CRC Press, New York, pp. 334.

Lansade, L., Bouissue, M.F. and Erhard, H.W. (2008) Fearfulness in horses: a temperamental trait, stable across time and situations. *Applied Animal Behaviour Science* 115, 182–200.

Lehner, P.N. (1996) *Handbook of Ethological Methods*, 2nd edn. Cambridge University Press, Cambridge.

Ligout, S., Bouissou, M.F. and Boiviu, X. (2008) Comparison of the effects of two different handling methods on the subsequent behaviour of Anglo-Arabian foals towards humans and handling. *Applied Animal Behaviour Science* 113, 175–188.

Lloyd, A.S., Martin, J.E., Bornett-Gauci, H.L.I. and Wilkinson, R.G. (2008) Horse personality: variation between breeds. *Applied Animal Behaviour Science* 112, 369–383.

Lorenz, K. (1965) *Evolution and Modification of Behaviour*. University of Chicago Press, Chicago, Illinois.

Martin, P. and Bateson, P. (2007) *Measuring Behaviour*, 2nd edn. Cambridge University Press, Cambridge.

McDonnell, S. (2003) *A Practical Field Guide to Horse Behavior: The Equid Ethogram*. The Blood Horse Inc., Lexington, KY.

McGreevy, P. (2004) *Equine Behaviour*. Saunders, Edinburgh, UK.

Miller R. (2003) *Imprint Training of the Newborn Foal.* Western Horseman Publishing.

Mills, N.J. (1991) Mound making in azoturia cases. *Veterinary Record* 128, 215.

Morresey, P.R. (2005) Prenatal and perinatal indicators of neonatal viability. *Clinical Techniques in Equine Practice* 4, 238–249.

Oliver, J.E. and Lorenz, M.D. (1993) *Handbook of Veterinary Neurology*, 2nd edn. W.B. Saunders, Philadelphia, Pennsylvania.

Pearson, G. (2016) Equine learning theory and the horse-veterinarian interaction. MScR thesis. University of Edinburgh, UK.

Riolo, R.L., Cohen, M.D. and Axeford, R. (2001) Evolution of cooperation without reciprocity. *Nature* 414, 441–443.

Robinson, N.E. (2007) Respiratory function (Section VIII) and homeostasis (Section IX). In: Cunningham, J.G. and Klein, B.G. (eds) *Veterinary Physiology*. Saunders Elsevier, Amsterdam.

Russell, C.M. and Wilkins, P.A. (2006) Evaluation of the recumbent neonate. *Clinical Techniques in Equine Practice* 5, 161–171.

Sambraus, H.H. (1985) Mouth-based anomalous syndromes. In: Fraser, A.F. (ed.) *Ethology of Farm Animals, World Animal Science*. Elsevier, Amsterdam, pp. 381–411.

Sankey, C., Richard-Yris, M.A., Henry, S., Fureix, C., Nassur, F. and Hausberger, M. (2010) Reinforcement as a mediator of the perception of humans by horses. *Animal Cognition* 13, 753–765.

Seaman, S.C., Davidson, H.P.B. and Waran, N.K. (2002) How reliable is temperament assessment in the domestic horse (*Equus caballus*)? *Applied Animal Behaviour Science* 78, 157–191.

Stubbs, N., Menke, E. Back, W. and Clayton, H.M. (2013) Rehabilitation of locomotor apparatus. In: Back, W. and Clayton, H.M. (eds) *Equine Locomotion*, 2nd edn. Saunders Elsevier, Edinburgh, UK, pp. 381–418.

Visser, E.K., van Reenen, C.G., Hopster, H., Schilder, M.B.H., Knaap, J.H. *et al.* (2001) Quantifying aspects of young horses' temperament. Consistency of behavioural variables. *Applied Animal Behaviour Science* 74, 241–258.

Visser, E.K., Van Reenen, C.G., Schilder, M.B.H., Barneveld, A. and Blokhuis, H.J. (2003) Learning performances in young horses using two different learning tests. *Applied Animal Behaviour Science* 80, 311–326.

Waran, N. and Randle, H. (2017) What we can measure, we can manage: The importance of using robust welfare indicators in Equitation Science. *Applied Animal Behaviour Science* 190, 74–81.

Waran, N.K., Clarke, N. and Farnworth, M. (2008) The effects of weaning on the domestic horse (*Equus caballus*) *Applied Animal Behaviour Science* 110(1–2), 42–57.

Willeberg, P. (1997) Epidemiology and animal welfare. *Epidemiologie. Santé Animale* 31, 3–7.

Zentall, T.R. (1996) The analysis of initiative learning in animals. In: Hayes, C.M. and Galef, B.G. (eds) *Social Learning of Animals: The Roots of Culture*. Academic Press, San Diego, California, pp. 221–243.

2 Sensory and Neurologic Faculties

CHRISTOPHER B. RILEY BVSc(HONS), PHD, DIPLOMATE ACVS*

Massey University, Palmerston North, New Zealand

Introduction 24
Senses 24
  Vision 24
  Hearing and balance 27
  Olfaction and taste 29
  Touch, somatic sensation and pain 31
Neurologic 32
  Memory 32
  Intelligence 33
  Emotionality 33
Welfare Summary 34
References 34

Introduction

The endpoints of the modern evolution in horses are evident in the sensory faculties that stimulate reflex actions, responsiveness to underfoot conditions, effective flight, shyness, specific gregariousness, emotionality, food preferences, kinetic learning ability and memory. These faculties rest on vision, hearing, smell, taste and touch, resulting in responses underpinned by the horse's instinctive, behavioural and emotional make-up (Schrimpf *et al.*, 2020). Their senses are reviewed here in summary form to show certain links with behaviour and welfare, both equine and human.

Senses

Vision

In contrast to its Eocene forest-dwelling forebears, the modern horse has its eyes located on the lateral aspects of its forehead (MacFadden, 2005). Some breeds have a slightly more lateral orbital location than others. The visual system of the foal is already well developed at birth, as expected for a precocious species (Ström *et al.*, 2018). However, a normal menace response (aversion to an object rapidly approaching the eye) may take up to 2 weeks to develop after birth, despite normal pupillary responses to light. The visual field of the horse is considered panoramic because of the anatomical location of the eyes, no doubt an evolutionary response to predator detection in an open plains environment, engaging its flight response when danger is perceived.

The quality of the visual field varies. For a horse standing straight and looking directly forward, there is a binocular field of vision for up to 65–75° and a larger approximately 140° field of monocular vision for each eye (Fig. 2.1). One trade-off with the monocular field of vision is limited depth perception. However, if a potential threat is identified, the horse quickly tilts its head or turns its neck to assess the potential threat with its binocular vision. They have a blind spot immediately behind the croup (rear) with a small range of marginal vision on either side, but this is rapidly overcome by a

*Corresponding author: c.b.riley@massey.ac.nz

 Fraser's the Behaviour and Welfare of the Horse (eds C.B. Riley, S.E. Cregier and A.F. Fraser)
DOI: 10.1079/9781789242133.0002

simple turning of the head and neck and refocusing (Timney and Keil, 1999).

The horse has some limitations associated with its field of vision. It has difficulty in focusing its eyes on objects less than 0.6 m (2 ft) in front of its face and greater problems with visual accommodation (i.e. focusing on objects directly in front of it). When focused on objects immediately within this vicinity, it may momentarily lose the ability to consciously observe the rear and to the sides. Its monocular vision means that it may simultaneously see different objects on either side of its face. So, when the horse is trying to focus on a nearby stationary object using its monocular vision on one side and turns its head, the object has the appearance of moving from the initial side of the face and then suddenly reappearing in the visual field of the other eye. That is, moving objects sail into view while stationary ones appear to jump into it in response to the horse's own motion. Therefore, the horse may unexpectedly check its head up or away, despite being stationary. Alteration of the head position may be required to bring a stationary item into clear view (Fig. 2.2). The smaller the item, the more likely the horse perceives this object as coming unexpectedly into its visual field, causing it to shy away. There are also simple anatomical limitations that prevent the horse from seeing above its eyebrows or at its mouth. In the latter case, the horse may use odour and touch (including vibrissae) to evaluate feedstuffs.

The wider field of vision combined with high sensitivity to movement and dynamic flight response has conveyed evolutionary advantages to the horse in detecting and escaping from predators. These peculiar advantages and disadvantages of the horse's vision explain a good deal of its behaviour in response to a perceived threat from the rear. For this reason, riders and handlers should take extra care when approaching the rear of the horse, as it may reflexively respond in surprise (flight, kick or buck), resulting in human injury through no fault of the horse. In many situations, the horse uses its head and neck movements to help focus the eyes and overcome some of the challenges described above.

If the horse raises its head, it sees better at a middle distance, but its long-range vision is relatively poor. If it lowers its head, close objects come into sharper view. By moving its head in a lateral direction to one side or the other, the horse focuses on

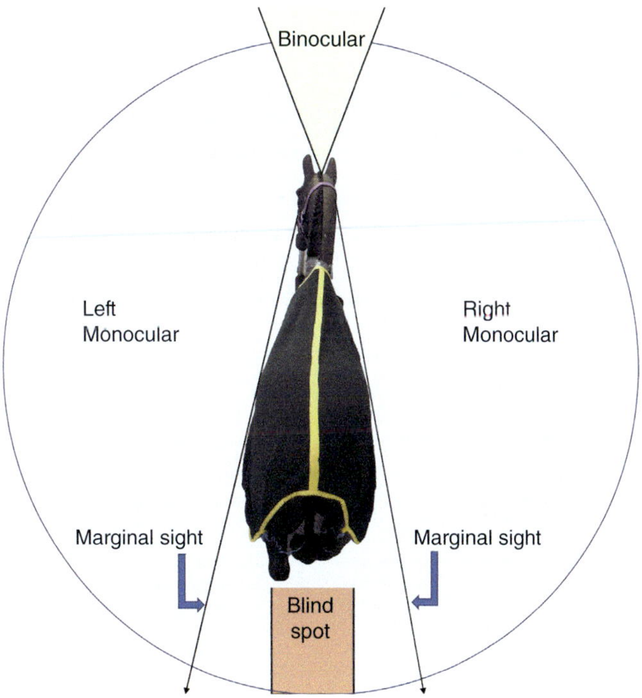

Fig. 2.1. The equine field of view. Illustration: author.

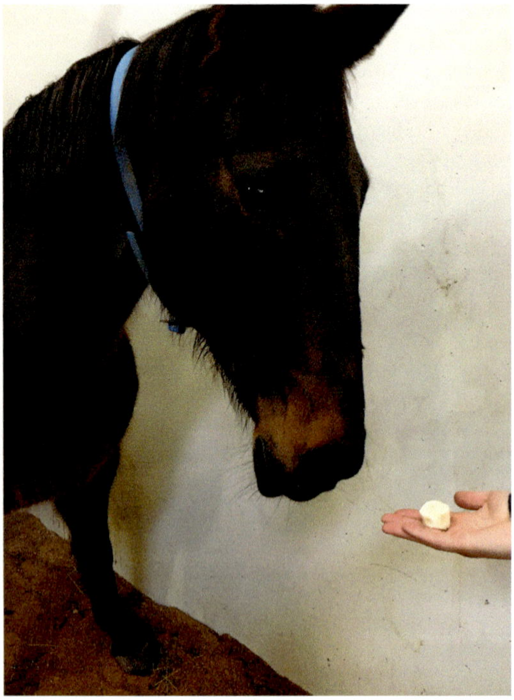

Fig. 2.2. Altering head position to see better a novel food item placed directly in front of the face. Photo: author.

specific items without altering the aperture of the pupil within the eye. When the horse puts its face perpendicular to the ground by flexing its poll, it obtains its best forward or frontal field of vision. Poll flexion is a common form of head carriage in horses with a high-stepping action. This gives the best possible vision of the ground immediately ahead. At slower travel rates, such as the slow to a medium trot, this is a suitable style of going. When the horse is cantering or galloping and is required to see objects at a greater distance, the horse raises its head at the cost of reducing side and ground vision. This is difficult for the horse when the ground is rough or unfamiliar.

An understanding of vision in the horse is linked to improving the rider or owner's understanding of equine perception. A consensus on the horse's capacity for colour vision has been slow to develop (Hanggi *et al.*, 2007), and only recently have improvements in the scientific understanding of equine vision been applied to benefit their welfare. Horses are dichromats, meaning that there are two types of photopigments within the retina (in contrast to the three in humans) that allow them to see colour but not to differentiate them to the same degree as human eyes. They perceive colour similarly to colour-blind people. Markers used for fences and hurdles on racecourses in the United Kingdom are orange. This provides poor visibility and contrast for horses, whereas yellow, blue, and white are more readily appreciated depending on the background type or vegetation (Paul and Stevens, 2020). Furthermore, for fences (jumps), colour influences the perceived angle of the jump and distances jumped. Therefore, to improve equine safety and welfare jumps and other obstacles should be designed to reflect the colour perceptions of horses rather than those of their riders. Nevertheless, the visual acuity of horses and their perception should not be underestimated. They not only recognize and remember their caregivers when shown photographs, but also observe and respond to human body language (Ladewig, 2019).

From a welfare perspective, it is pointless and inhumane to admonish or punish a horse for a slight mistake or vision problem (Fraser, 2010). When these problems are thought to be other than associated with normal behaviour, the horse should be evaluated for ocular disorders, including opacities of the cornea or lens or inflammatory or degenerative conditions affecting the retina. It is also important to consider the welfare implications of human interventions that intentionally interfere with the visual field of the horse. The three most common interventions include the application of a fly mask across the face, the use of blinkers or blinders to restrict lateral (monocular) vision and blindfolding. The fly mask, a mesh attached to the halter of the horse, is designed to prevent injury or infection of the injured, inflamed, or sensitive eyes from flies and midges. Whereas they may provide protection and relief to these horses, little is known of their effects on the vision of horses or their optimal design. Blinders or blinkers are commonly used in carriage horses (Fig. 2.3) or horses engaged in driving sports, and less frequently in Thoroughbred racing. They serve to restrict the side and rear visual fields of the horse, in most cases restricting them to the binocular field of view. Their use has developed from the belief that they prevent horses from being distracted by the crowd or other unfamiliar events or objects that might otherwise distract or frighten. It has been argued that they are a welfare benefit to the horse by decreasing the stress associated with the perception of being chased

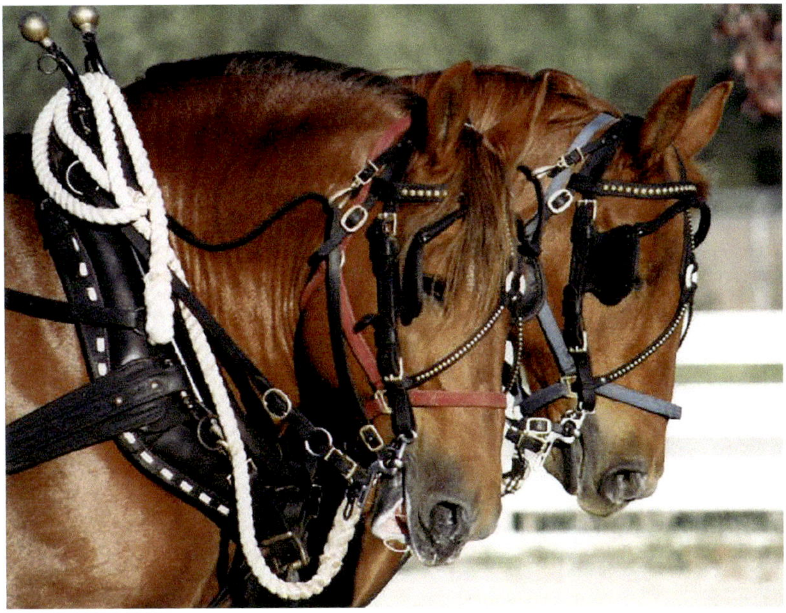

Fig. 2.3. A pair of draught horses in harness wearing blinkers. Photo: author.

(albeit by other horses) during a race, and, in the same breath, claimed that the whip is helpful in letting the horses know what is expected when they can't see what is behind. This is not supported by the evidence that shows that blinkers increase the stress of horses because they do nothing to eliminate strange or unusual noises that they cannot visually interpret (Dziezyc *et al.*, 2011). The welfare impacts of blinkers in carriage horses and racing requires critical review. Occasionally a blinker or eyecup is used for horses under veterinary care suffering from inflammation or other injury of the eye (Fig. 2.4). The tolerance of this device and the welfare of the horses is closely monitored. Blindfolding has been used to assist in the handling of difficult horses, the loading of horses for transport, and as part of the neurologic assessment of veterinary patients. Blindfolding has a negative effect on the postural stability of the horse, and in contrast to popular belief, it can make horses more nervous and difficult to handle (Parker *et al.*, 2004; Clayton and Nauwelaerts, 2014). Although there may be some situations where this practice assists with the welfare and handling of certain horses (e.g., in an emergency or urgent situation), it should not take the place of patient appropriate training for husbandry activities.

Hearing and balance

Hearing is critically important for the well-being of the horse as a flight animal. Horses have a good sense of hearing that, when paired with vocalization, facilitates appropriate behaviour when bonds are developing between breeding mares and stallions, broodmares and foals, and among herd mates (Briefer *et al.*, 2017). The pinnae are highly mobile, moving independently or in unison, facilitating the location of the source of sounds. They can swivel in a lateral arc of 180°, be directed forward-facing, or laid back and flat. They are laid back when interacting aggressively with other horses or species (including humans).

The anatomic composition of the external, middle, and inner ear structures is like other mammals, but there are some differences (Blanke *et al.*, 2014). The external ear consists of the auricle and external ear canal. The external ear canal has an outer cartilaginous section joined to a deeper osseous (bony) tube adjacent to the tympanic membrane (eardrum). This is lined by epithelium containing hair follicles, ceruminous and sebaceous glands, with the latter becoming fewer nearer to the tympanic membrane. The cerumen binds dust and dirt and contains antimicrobial substances. The ear canal is cleared of dust, dirt and insects by the horse quickly rotating or

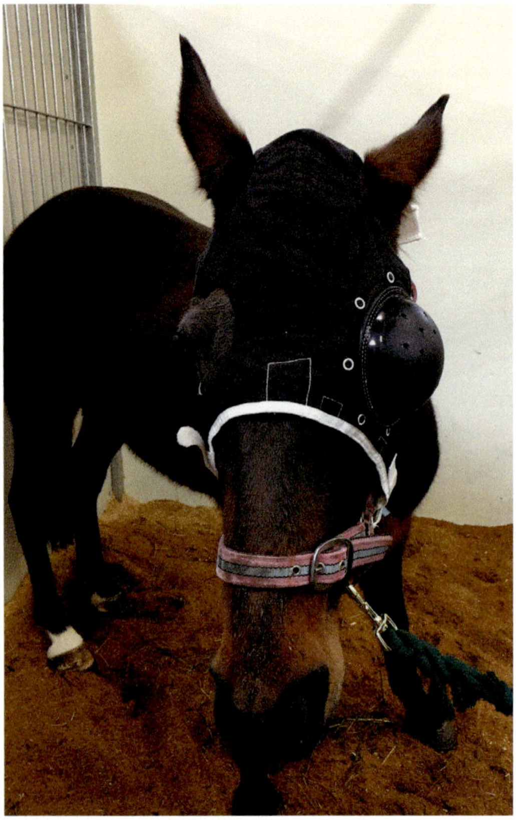

Fig. 2.4. An eye cup reduces the passage of light into a painful eye. Photo: author.

shaking its head. However, horses are unique in that they have inwardly directed rete pegs of epithelium in their ear canals not found in other mammals; these are assumed to play a role in self-cleaning the canal (Blanke *et al.*, 2014). The tympanic membrane and tympanic bulla are like that of other animals, except that the latter is comparatively small. The middle ear ossicles (malleus, incus and stapes) transfer mechanical energy from the tympanic membrane to the perilymph of the inner ear, and structures within the inner ear are comparable to other mammals. There are subtle differences in the musculature attached to the ossicles and fat that serves to dampen some electrical responses within the ear (Blanke *et al.*, 2014).

The inner ear contributes to the sense of position in equilibrium via impulses carried through the vestibular portion of the auditory nerve. Although not a hearing function, its role in equilibrium and posture is mentioned here because of its proximity to the other functional aspects of the ear. The inner ear is located within the petrous temporal bone, containing the bony labyrinth and its watery fluid called perilymph. The labyrinth has three parts: the centrally located vestibule adjacent to the middle ear, the cochlear and the three semicircular canals oriented in planes at 90° to each other. These canals align with the vertical, horizontal, and transverse planes with respect to the head. Fluid movements associated with the semicircular canals and vestibule are responsible for sensations of position and balance (i.e. equilibrium). Innervation is via the vestibular branch of the eighth cranial nerve. When the head moves, perilymph movement within the semicircular canals proportionately bends the hair cells of the canal system, signalling the brain to anticipate movement and sense position. It is a well-developed mechanism in the horse, allowing it to change direction quickly at speed. From a rider's perspective, this is particularly important in equestrian pursuits and road transport.

The high-frequency hearing range of horses (up to 33,000 Hz) extends far above that of humans (up to 20,000 Hz) but does not extend as low as our frequency range. Unlike humans that turn their head to see the source of a sound, horses first rely upon the motion of their ears to locate the source. That is, in responding to other animals or people, they raise the head and point the ears in the direction of the sound. A human with the horse may be less aware or not hear high-frequency sounds, causing the horse to display a freeze, fright or flight response. This means there is a disconnect between horse and rider in perception, with the rider frequently only becoming visually aware afterwards of what caused the disturbance. The rider or handler must determine the cause of the reaction rather than assuming that the horse is intentionally behaving poorly. In situations such as a parade or show, earplugs specifically designed for horses may be used when they are unduly agitated by these situations with complex background noise. These should be thicker than the wavelength being blocked, which is generally easier for high-frequency sounds while allowing for lower frequency sounds to be heard (Saslow, 2002). However, when applying any device that prevents the horse from receiving this input to advise it of possible danger, it is the responsibility of the rider, driver, or handler to be vigilant in protecting it in these situations. Although the research investigating the effectiveness of earplugs is limited, there is considerable variability in the function of commercially available equine earplugs (Figs 2.5a and b) (MacFarlane *et al.*, 2010).

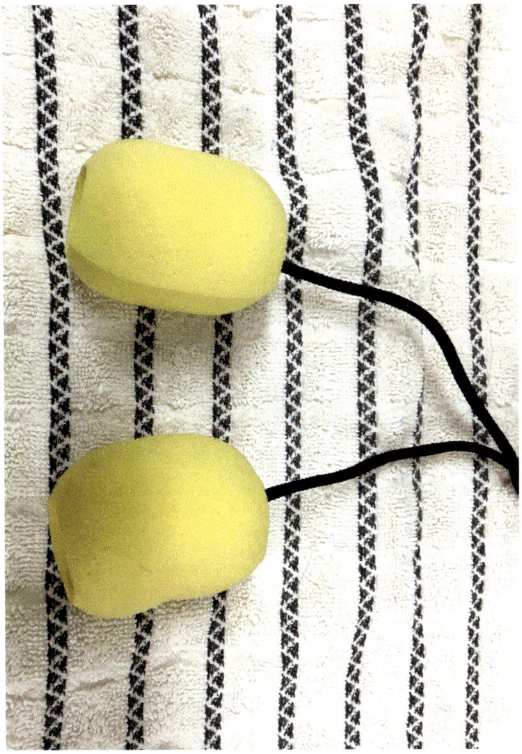

Fig. 2.5a. Compressible foam earplugs. Photo: author.

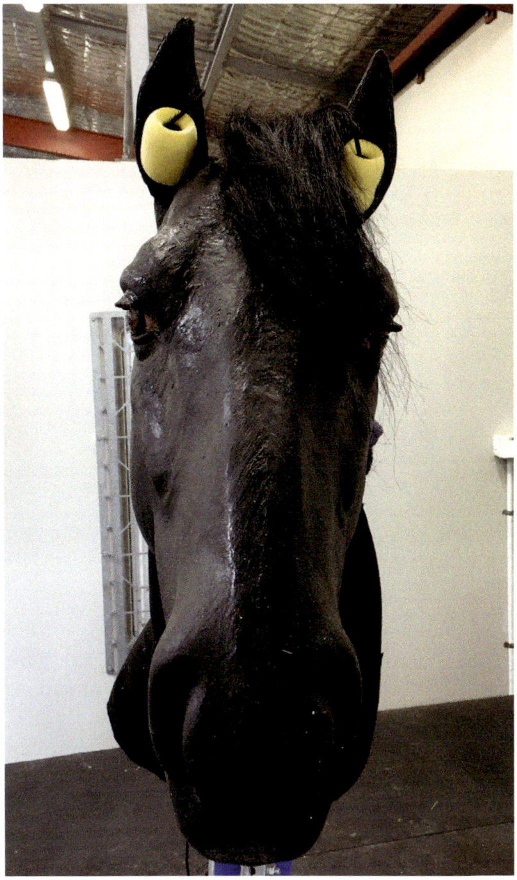

Fig. 2.5b. Placement of earplugs on an equine mannequin. Horses generally must be habituated or debilitated to accept them on first application. Photo: author.

Generally, horses and ponies communicate with both visual and auditory signals, apparently responding with equivalent efficacy to either cue (Prendergast *et al.*, 2016). We are only now comprehending the complexity of auditory signals that horses can interpret and the behavioural and emotional responses to these inputs. They can identify different familiar whinnies and accordingly react differently (e.g., respiration rate, head movements, the height of the head) to each horse and in each situation (e.g., separation or reunion) (Briefer *et al.*, 2017). They also respond differently to unfamiliar whinnies (e.g., increased locomotion), indicating a level of discernment not markedly different from our own. Not only do horses adequately hear human voices, but they also perceive changes in the pitch of the human voice associated with emotions such as excitement or fear (Saslow, 2002). They can differentiate between human laughter and growling, with the latter being more likely to cause horses to freeze for longer and adopt vigilance behaviours (Smith *et al.*, 2018) (Fig. 2.6). This means that emotional cues contained within the human voice can result in stress responses in the horse. Their response to human verbal cues may be moderated by associated visual ones, including facial expression. Horses associate positive verbal cues with positive facial expressions and negative cues with negative facial expressions (Nakamura *et al.*, 2018). Therefore, in stressful situations such as competition or horse rescue, attention and practice are required to maintain a calm human voice and facial expressions that are consistent with the tone of voice to the welfare benefit of the horse.

Olfaction and taste

Equine olfaction is important for social interactions, reproductive behaviour, detection and evaluation of feedstuffs, and with other cues, the detection of predators. These functions involve the olfactory mucosae and the vomeronasal organ.

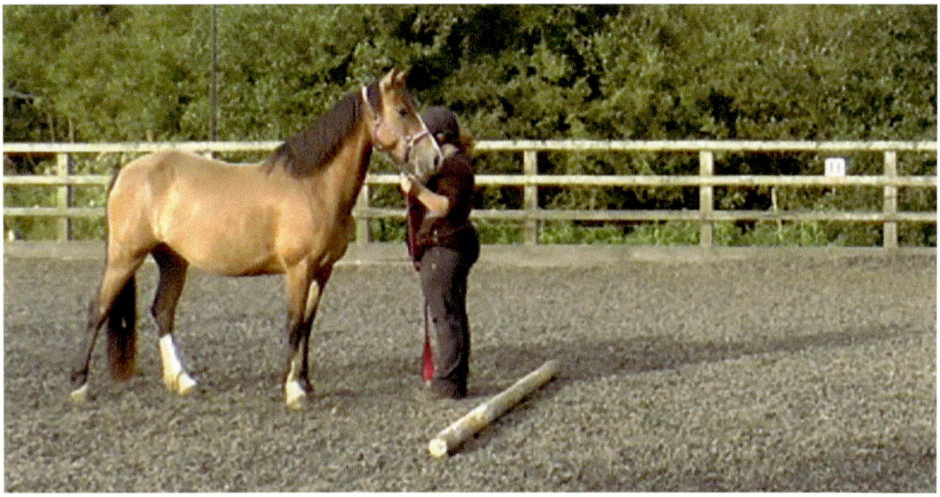

Fig. 2.6. This video still captures the horse frozen with its ears erect and forward in response to a sound broadcast from a loudspeaker in the background to the far right. Photo: Karen McComb.

The olfactory receptors and their associated neurons that generate the perception of smell are located in the mucous membrane of the upper caudal part of the nasal cavity. In smell, the airborne odorous substances enter the nose and then come in contact with carbohydrate-binding proteins (lectins) that protrude from glycolipids and glycoproteins on cell membranes in the microscopic hair-like structures on the receptor cells. The lectins vary widely in structure and concentrations, allowing for the interpretation of a broad range of olfactory stimuli (Lee *et al.*, 2016). The receptors in the olfactory mucosa bind with any odorous molecules entering in aerosol form, and the activation of the receptor cells is projected via the olfactory nerves to the main olfactory bulb within the brain. The olfactory bulb interacts with the telencephalon (cerebrum) that houses the intercalated structures required for the most complex and involved functions within the mammalian brain (Martinez-Marcos, 2009). Through sniffing, the horse intensifies the current of air in the nasal passage, moderating the contact between an odorous substance and the receptors in the mucosa.

The vomeronasal organ also detects odours but is particularly well developed (although not solely) to detect pheromones and other odours that underpin social relationships and reproductive status. It extends from 10 cm caudal to the nostrils to the middle of the second upper premolar teeth in the floor of the nasal cavity (König *et al.*, 2005). The organ is lined by sensory epithelium medially and non-sensory epithelium laterally. Glands within the organ secrete mucus and other substances onto its lumen, playing a role in detecting odour molecules by receptor cells within the sensory epithelium (Lee *et al.*, 2016). Its role in detecting pheromones is emphasized in the equine literature, but recent research has shown that both the olfactory epithelium and the vomeronasal organ process these sensory stimuli (Martinez-Marcos, 2009). Furthermore, they share some common pathway targets within the amygdala. Our understanding is incomplete, but it appears in some situations, such as the flehmen response, the nasal passages reflexively contract to direct airflow towards the opening of the vomeronasal organ during inspiration (König *et al.*, 2005). There is a misconception that this response only occurs in stallions. Females and foals of both sexes display this behaviour, with equivalent latency, duration and frequency (Weeks *et al.*, 2002).

Like most mammals, horses use smell and taste to identify and differentiate forages. These senses are utilized to preferentially discriminate between known and novel feedstuffs, usually towards those of higher nutritional value or palatability (Müller and Udén, 2007; Culda and Stermin, 2019). They may respond adversely to strange, unnatural odours or taste. Horses also choose feedstuffs based on remembering the odour of a preferred food even when it differs in composition or texture (van den Berg *et al.*, 2016a). This approach may be helpful when changing feedstuffs or when the caregiver is having difficulty introducing horses to less palatable feed. Preference testing can be used to identify the most appealing feedstuffs. Once horses are familiar with a specific high-quality feedstuff, they are less likely to smell it before intake (Tribucci *et al.*, 2013). Horses may utilize smell in concert with touch, particularly when hand-fed food is offered within their blind spot beneath the chin, and equally to use this to differentiate something that is not food (e.g. your hand) (Fig. 2.7).

Olfaction also plays a role in social interaction; this is not limited to the detection of oestrus in mares by stallions (Weeks *et al.*, 2002). Stallions use smell to differentiate between oestrus and dioestrus mares, directly or by sniffing their urine or faeces. In foals of wild equids, olfaction is associated with marking behaviour (Pluháček *et al.*, 2019). These foals are more likely to smell and eliminate over the faeces or urine of their own dam. Horses differentiate between their own faeces and that of others and spend more time sniffing the faeces of horses that have displayed aggressive behaviours towards themselves (Krueger and Flauger, 2011). Smell also plays a role in the establishment of the mare–foal bond following parturition, and within herds, horses are more likely to sniff the nose or bodies of their companions. Although other odours associated with biological fluids excreted by horses play a role, pheromones excreted within these fluids, the breath and skin, underpin much of this form of communication. As indicated above, they may communicate information related to sexual status, within-herd recognition, and recognition of other species. In terms of the latter, they detect and remember different people's scent and clothing (Próchniak *et al.*, 2017). In certain limited situations, specific odours can be used to decrease equine stress (Micera *et al.*, 2011).

In common with many other species, horses use taste as part of their food selection process. The taste buds are end organs in the mucous membranes of the mouth. Most of these are located on the anterior two-thirds of the tongue and contain molecular receptors that differentiate between sweet, bitter and salty flavours. These transfer information to the brain that is combined with sensory inputs from smell and touch (texture). This has benefits in ensuring that the appropriate nutrients are ingested but may also lead to over ingestion of preferred feedstuffs, particularly those rich in starch. Taste preferences in horses can be complex, and apart from the feedstuffs themselves, may be influenced by breed and sex. Arabian horses, for example, have a wider variety of feedstuffs than some other breeds, and mares prefer feeds containing molasses (Janczarek *et al.*, 2018). From a welfare perspective, the taste preferences of horses can be used to improve feed intake and to introduce novel feedstuffs in situations where familiar feeds are unavailable (van den Berg *et al.*, 2016b).

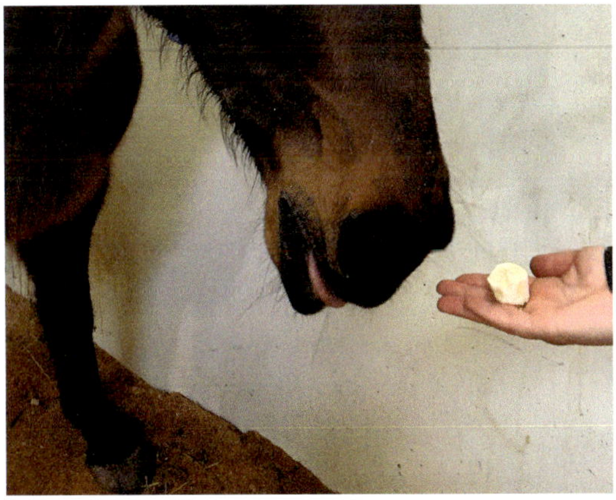

Fig. 2.7. The horse shown in Fig. 2.2 further explores the novel food item, dilating the nostrils to increase airflow for olfaction. Note the presence of the tongue between the lips in anticipation of tasting the banana. Photo: author.

Touch, somatic sensation and pain

Horses are very sensitive to touch and the stimulation of receptors that register in the brain as pain. These sensations are transmitted to the central nervous system by sensory nerve endings connected to numerous and varied nerve receptors within the somatic (e.g. skin, musculoskeletal tissues) and visceral structures. The receptors have specialized non-neural cells associated with nerve fibre endings. Specific receptors are related to the detection of temperature (heat and cold), pressure, some chemicals, blood pressure, movement (proprioception), touch and pain (nociception). Somatic sensation occurs mainly through touch and pressure from mechanical forces on hairs, the skin, deeper subcutaneous tissues, and changes in the loading and movement of joints (Hahn and Masty, 2015). In equine welfare, we are often concerned about pain, the central nervous system response that results from the stimulation receptors at the ends of certain small neurons.

The touch-pressure receptor organ is the pacinian corpuscle, located in the skin. The nerve terminal of the corpuscle is surrounded by layers of cells and extracellular fluid that, when disturbed by a mechanical force, generates an electrical stimulus that is transmitted to the brain. There is limited information about the equine response to touch. It appears that the systematic application of human touch can be therapeutic and decrease stress in horses (Birt *et al.* 2015; Haussler, 2018). Mechanoreceptors associated with joints and ligaments are activated by stretching, twisting or loading. The rate and degree to which these are stimulated provide information to the cerebrum and cerebellum about joint motion, limb and body position (proprioception). Conscious proprioception is interpreted in the contralateral cerebral cortex, whereas responses to subconscious proprioception are initiated within the ipsilateral cerebellum. Conscious responses include adjusting position, whereas unconscious responses are referred to as reflexive movement. When a temperature stimulus outside the homeostatic range occurs, changes in cell permeability and/or tissue damage (when temperature differences are severe) signal the brain, resulting in conscious and unconscious responses.

Pain is a subjective response to the noxious stimulation of nociceptors. These stimuli may result in tissue damage leading to the release of mediators (bradykinin, prostaglandins and others) that act upon specific receptors. These mediators facilitate pain sensation within the central nervous system and moderate the sensitivity of nerve endings in the affected region. Nociceptors respond to traumatic stimulation such as tissue-damaging pressure, intense heat, irritating chemical substances and skin abrasion. Electrical firing from the receptors increases as the severity of the stimulus intensifies unless these receptors are obliterated, as seen in full-thickness skin burns. Different nociceptors may stimulate specific and non-specific regions in the brain. Originally different nociceptors were thought to operate via separate specific pathways. It is now known these pathways substantially overlap in signal centres within the brain that initiate responses to pain (De Lahunta *et al.*, 2015). The cortex creates the perception of pain and makes the horse aware of the intensity and position of the pain stimulus. Non-specific pathways for nociception travel to the brainstem (and part of the thalamus) to initiate reactivity. These non-specific pathways connect with the limbic system, which plays a major role in integrating autonomic and endocrine responses plus the behavioural responses of aggression, defence, fear, and emotion. A painful sensory experience in conjunction with behavioural and emotional responses such as fear, anxiety, and unpleasantness persist in a horse's memory. Responses are complex and may emotionally prime horses in situations similar to one that led to their previous painful experience and creates challenges in training or utilising the horse for that activity. For example, a horse that sustains trauma during road transport may be difficult to load in future and requires a patient sensitive approach to retraining.

Neurologic

Memory

In common with other species, equine memory is related to experience and learning (see Chapter 1). Because of the focus on some of the negative consequences of memory, such as difficulty in handling or stereotypy, it is often falsely assumed that equine memory is selective for unpleasant events. However, a well-trained horse remembers its training for its lifetime. Persistent memories tend to fix habits, both positive and detrimental. Fixation of the latter may be associated with behavioural problems. Considerate handling and patient training when horses are young can provide the basis for memories that allow positive engagement with them later in life. Given the range of complex tasks required of the horse, particularly in equestrian activities such as dressage and eventing, they are clearly capable of remembering complicated sequences and tasks. As indicated above, memories are linked to significant behavioural and emotional responses, facilitated within the hippocampus and its links within the limbic system. Memories of pain and fear persist long after the unpleasant event. Horses require careful training and conditioning to overcome such experiences. The capacity for long-term memory is a key feature of a horse's learning and evolutionary fitness. Horses can remember their handlers and are capable of facial recognition over long periods of absence (Landsade *et al.* 2018), as well as human body language (Ladewig, 2019). They also remember different colours, symbols, and preferences for odours and flavours (Mejdell *et al.*, 2016).

Intelligence

When defining intelligence in non-human species, there is a tendency to anthropomorphize or compare with human intelligence. Definitions of intelligence vary but include the ability to learn or understand how to deal with new or trying situations, the skilled use of reason, or the ability to apply knowledge to manipulate one's environment or to think abstractly as measured by objective criteria. Some of these may be difficult to evaluate for the horse, but some of these concepts certainly apply (Hanggi, 2005; Ringhofer and Yamamato, 2017). Given the range of equestrian activities for which they have been trained, horses readily learn and understand new or trying situations. It has been suggested that measuring the amount of time the horse takes to learn tasks may indicate its intelligence (Mejdell *et al.*, 2016). However, in most situations, it is not possible to separate the effects of the trainer from the environment. Some horses can anticipate the commands of their riders or handlers; it is likely that they perceive body language changes that may precede a specific human action or behaviour (Ladewig, 2019). There are also natural behaviours underpinned by a combination of temperament and intelligence, contributing to its general behaviour (Table 2.1). Any attempt to assess equine intelligence must be made in context with both their evolutionary purpose and environment. It is likely that until we have meaningful and reproducible measures of non-human intelligence, people will attribute intelligence to a horse based on its temperament, ability to adapt to, learn, and anticipate our requirements, and its general behaviour. This will be influenced by factors that are intrinsic and external to the horse.

Emotionality

Most horse owners and caretakers believe that horses express emotions such as fear, joy, boredom, jealousy and pain. There is increasing scientific evidence supporting some of these beliefs (Hötzel *et al.*, 2019). Emotional responses in animals are associated with physiological arousal mediated via the hypothalamic–pituitary–adrenal axis and the autonomic nervous system. Equine emotional experiences are characterized in terms of their valence (e.g. pleasant or unpleasant sensation, rewarding or punishing, favourable or adverse) and the intensity or level of arousal they stimulate (Mendl *et al.*, 2010). From an evolutionary perspective, emotional responses confer survival advantages as an important part of behavioural motivation towards or away from a stimulus (Hall *et al.*, 2018). This supports group cohesion within the herds through activities such as mutual grooming. In free-ranging populations, these activities are important in reducing the threat from predators, maintaining social structures, and moving together to take advantage of optimal food sources. Within groups, positive emotionality reduces the risk of injury and reduces unnecessary energy expenditures. Herd composition and the behaviour of members within are linked to the emotional well-being of the individual. When individuals respond with emotions of either a positive or negative valence, there is a risk of short-term consequences and long-term impacts. Perhaps one of the more profound examples observed was recorded in an online video of donkeys responding emotionally to the death of a herd mate. Attempts by former donkey companions to rouse the dead donkey were accompanied by complex vocalizations and increased locomotor activities of an emotional nature (Anon., 2016).

Table 2.1. Behaviours reflective of equine intelligence that maintain well-being.

			Roles in well being	
Behaviour	Homeostatic features	Maintenance values	Short-range	Long-range
Fight	Aggression, agonistic acts and play	Self-assertion	Suppression of competitor	Control over resources of various kinds
Flight	Submissive withdrawal	Avoidance of threatful situations	Self-protection	Security of individual
Feed	Search, selection and ingestion of food	Self-maintenance in respect of visceral needs	Ingestion to repletion	Stabilization of hierarchies
	Consumption of water	Self-sufficiency in nutritional needs	Suppression of hunger	Building up body reserves and storage

Improving our understanding of emotionality in horses is gaining importance in a multidimensional consideration of welfare. The subjective interpretation for behaviours such as a mare nuzzling its foal, for playmates overlaying their heads upon each other, and in some cases, a horse putting its head on a person's shoulder have been interpreted as reflecting positive emotional states (Fraser, 2010). Whereas there may be some survival advantage for the first two examples, the survival advantage of the latter is less clear. Validated approaches to assessing equine emotions and the subjective experience of horses are limited, and an emerging field of equine welfare research. Assessment methods based on behavioural profiling and facial expressions have been used but rely upon subjective assessments that are difficult to validate and replicate (Wemelsfelder *et al.*, 2001; Lansade *et al.*, 2018). Superimposed on this difficulty is evidence that horses' emotions are influenced by the emotional state and facial expressions of the people working with them (Ladewig, 2019). Although scientifically evaluating the emotions of horses is difficult, based upon the available evidence, it must be assumed that interactions between humans and horses influence the emotional experience and behavioural responses of the latter. Therefore, care should be taken to minimize management inputs, handling, training and other experiences that stimulate negative emotional responses. Emotional responses such as fear and aggression increase the risk of human and equine injury.

Welfare Summary

There are significant differences between the senses and prioritization of their use between horses and people. Many horses may 'spook' at what we perceive as minor or innocuous factors suddenly coming into their vision. Adjustments to vision need quick changes of equine head position that may pose a risk to people nearby. A horse may be startled or distracted by high-frequency sounds and tend to respond with ear motion before orienting visually towards the source. Unlike humans, they may respond before or without seeing the source of the noise. It is therefore essential that the rider or handler understand these differences so that the horse is not punished for behaviours that are consequences of its natural design. In addition to physical and social aspects of welfare, it is increasingly apparent that attention is required to address their emotional welfare, as negative experiences result in short-term consequences and long-standing memories leading to future anxiety, fear or aggression.

References

Anon. (2016) An emotional goodbye to a dead donkey. Available at: https://youtu.be/LuxrhiicesU (accessed 31 August 2020).

Birt, M.A., Guay, K., Treiber, K., Ramirez, H.R. and Snyder, D. (2015) The influence of a soft touch therapy Flowtrition on heart rate, surface temperature, and behavior in horses. *Journal of Equine Veterinary Science* 35, 636–644.

Blanke, A., Aupperle, H., Seeger, J., Kubick, C. and Schusser, G.F. (2014) Histological study of the external, middle, and inner ear of horses. *Anatomia Histologica Embryologica* 44, 401–409.

Briefer, E.F., Mandel, R., Maigrot, A-L., Briefer Freymond, S., Bachmann, I. and Hillmann, E. (2017) Perception of emotional valence in horse whinnies. *Frontiers in Zoology* 14, 8.

Clayton, H.M. and Nauwelaerts, S. (2014) Effect of blindfolding on centre of pressure variables in healthy horses during quiet standing. *Veterinary Journal* 199, 365–369.

Culda, C.A. and Stermin, A.N. (2019) Horses' senses involvement in food location and selection. *Bulletin UASVM Animal Science and Biotechnologies* 76, 94–101.

De Lahunta, A., Glass, E. and Kent, M. (2015) General sensory systems: general proprioception and general somatic afferent. In: *Veterinary Neuroanatomy and Clinical Neurology*. Elsevier, St. Louis, Missouri, pp. 237–256.

Dziezyc, J., Taylor, L., Boggess, M.M. and Scott, M. (2011) The effect of ocular blinkers on the horses' reactions to four different visual and audible stimuli: results of a crossover trial. *Veterinary Ophthalmology* 14, 327–332.

Fraser, A.F. (2010) *The Behavior and Welfare of the Horse*, 2nd edn. CAB International, Wallingford, UK.

Hahn, C. and Masty, J. (2015) Overview of neuroanatomy. In: Furr, M. and Reed, S. (eds) *Equine Neurology*. Wiley Blackwell, Ames, Iowa. pp. 3–20.

Hall, C., Randle, H., Pearson, G., Preshaw, L. and Waran, N. (2018) Assessing equine emotional state. *Applied Animal Behaviour Science* 205, 183–193.

Hanggi, E.B. (2005) The thinking horse: cognition and perception reviewed. *AAEP Proceedings* 51, 246–255.

Hanggi, E.B., Ingersoll, J.F., and Waggoner, T.L. (2007) Color vision in horses (*Equus caballus*): Deficiencies identified using a pseudoisochromatic plate test. *Journal of Comparative Psychology* 121, 65–72.

Haussler, K.K. (2018) Equine manual therapies in sport horse practice. *Veterinary Clinics of North America Equine Practice* 23, 375–389.

Hötzel, M.J., Vieira, M.C. and Leme, D.P. (2019) Exploring horse owners' and caretakers' perceptions of emotions and associated behaviors in horses. *Journal of Veterinary Behavior* 29, 18–24.

Janczarek, I., Wilk, I., Piertrzak, S., Liss, M. and Tkaczyk, S. (2018) Taste preferences of horses in relation to their breed and sex. *Journal of Equine Veterinary Science* 64, 59–64.

König, H.E., Whissdorf, H., Probst, A., Macher, R., Voss, S. and Polsterer, E. (2005) Considerations about the function of the mimic muscles and the vomeronasal organ of horses during the Flehmen reaction. *Pferdeheilkunde* 21, 297–300.

Krueger, K. and Flauger, B. (2011) Olfactory recognition of individual competitors by means of faeces in horse (*Equus caballus*). *Animal Cognition* 14, 245–257.

Ladewig, J. (2019) Body language: Its importance for communication with horses. *Journal of Veterinary Behaviour* 29, 108–110.

Lansade, L., Nowak, R., Lainé, A-L., Leterrier, C., Bonneau, C. *et al.* (2018) Facial expression and oxytocin as possible markers of positive emotions in horses. *Scientific Reports* 8, 14680.

Lee, K-H., Park, C. Kim, J., Moon, C., Ahn, M. *et al.* (2016) Histochemical and lectin histochemical studies of the vomeronasal organ of horses. *Tissue and Cell* 48, 361–369.

MacFadden, B. (2005) Fossil horses: evidence for evolution. *Science* 307, 1728–1730.

MacFarlane, P.D., Mosing, M. and Burford, J. (2010) Preliminary investigation into the effects of earplugs on sound transmission in the equine ear. *Pferdeheilkunde* 26, 199–203.

Martinez-Marcos, A. (2009) On the organization of olfactory and vomeronasal cortices. *Progress in Neurobiology* 87, 21–30.

Mejdell, C.M., Buvik, T., Jørgensen, G.M.H. and Bøe, K.E. (2016) Horses can learn to use symbols to communicate their preferences. *Applied Animal Behaviour Science* 184, 66–73.

Mendl, M., Burman, O.H.P. and Paul, E.S. (2010). An integrative and functional framework for the study of animal emotion and mood. *Proceedings of the Royal Society B* 277, 2895–2904.

Micera, E., Moramarco, A.M. and Zarilli, A. (2011) Reduction of the olfactory cognitive ability in horses during preslaughter: stress-related hormones evaluation. *Meat Science* 90, 272–275.

Müller, C.E. and Udén, P. (2007) Preference for horses for grass conserved as hay, haylage or silage. *Animal Feed Science and Technology* 132, 66–78.

Nakamura, K., Takimoto-Inose, A. and Hasegawa, T. (2018) Cross-modal perception of human emotion in domestic horses (*Equus caballus*). *Scientific Reports* 8, 8660.

Parker, R., Watson, R., Wells, E., Brown, S.N., Nicol, C.J. *et al.* (2004) The effect of blindfolding horses on heart rate and behaviour during handling and loading onto transport vehicles. *Animal Welfare* 13, 433–437.

Paul, S.C. and Stevens, M. (2020) Horse vision and optical visibility in horse racing. *Applied Animal Behaviour Science* 222, 104882.

Pluháček, J., Tučková, V., King, S.R.B. and Šárová, R. (2019) Test of four hypotheses to explain the function of overmarking in foals of four equids species. *Animal Cognition* 22, 231–241.

Prendergast, A., Nansen, C. and Blache, D. (2016) Responses of domestic horses and ponies to single, combined and conflicting visual and auditory cues. *Journal of Equine Veterinary Science* 46, 40–46.

Próchniak, T., Rozempolska-Rucin′ska, I., Petrykowska, M., Zięba, G., S′laska, B. *et al.* (2017) Cognitive abilities of horses in terms of visual and olfactory perception. *Medycyna Weterynaryjna* 73, 48–52.

Ringhofer, M. and Yamamoto, S. (2017) Domestic horses send signals to humans when they face with an unsolvable task. *Animal Cognition*, 20, 397–405.

Saslow, C.A. (2002) Understanding the perceptual world of horses. *Applied Animal Behaviour* 78, 209–224.

Schrimpf, A., Single, M-S. and Nawroth, C. (2020) Social referencing in the domestic horse. *Animals* 10, 164.

Smith, A.V., Proops, L., Grounds, K., Wathan, J., Scott, S.K. *et al.* (2018) Domestic horses (*Equus caballus*) discriminate between negative and positive human non-verbal vocalisations. *Scientific Reports* 8, 13052.

Ström, L., Michanek, M. and Eksten, B. (2018) Age-associated changes in the equine flash visual evoked potential. *Veterinary Ophthalmology* 22, 388–397.

Timney, B. and Keil, K. (1999) Local and global stereopsis in the horse. *Vision Research* 39, 1861–1857.

Tribucci, A.M. de O., Brandi, A.R., Balieiro, J.C. de C., Titto, E.A.L. and Bueno, I.C. da S. (2013) Palatability of horse diets containing citrus pulp (*Citrus sinensis*) through the preference test. *Italian Journal of Animal Science* 12, e33.

van den Berg, M., Giagos, V., Lee, C., Brown, W.Y. and Hinch, G.N. (2016a) Acceptance of novel food by horses: The influence of food cues and nutrient composition. *Applied Animal Behaviour Science* 183, 59–67.

van den Berg, M., Giagos, V., Lee, C., Brown, W.Y, Caldwell-Smith, A.J. *et al.* (2016b) The influence of odour, taste and nutrients on feeding behaviour and food preferences in horses. *Applied Animal Behaviour Science* 184, 41–50.

Weeks, J.W., Crowell-Davis, S.L. and Heusner, G. (2002) Preliminary study of the development of the Flehmen response in *Equus caballus*. *Applied Animal Bevhaviour Science* 78, 329–335.

Wemelsfelder, F., Hunter, T.E.A., Mendl, M.T. and Lawrence, A.B. (2001) Assessing the 'whole animal': a free choice profiling approach. *Animal Behaviour* 62, 209–220.

3 The Neurological Underpinnings of Behaviour

Christopher B. Riley BVSc(Hons), PhD, Diplomate ACVS*

Massey University, Palmerston North, New Zealand

Introduction 36
Anatomy 37
Neurons 37
Neuroglia 39
Cerebral cortex 40
The Limbic System 42
Basal ganglia 43
Hypothalamus 43
Cerebellum 43
Brainstem 43
Spinal cord 43
Function 44
Autonomic system 44
Endocrine system – the chemical operators 45
Motivation 46
Summary 48
References 48

Introduction

The evolution of our understanding of equine behaviour and its effects on welfare is based on complex research often underpinned by an understanding of the anatomy and physiology of horses. This is no less true for the central nervous system (CNS) and its functional domains. The CNS deals with stimulation, sensory discrimination, motivation, learning, the inheritance of neural traits, and the release and control of action patterns (behaviour). The complex interactions associated with behaviour are made possible by the cells of the CNS and the electrical pulses that pass via the axons (nerve fibres) and dendrites to and from each neuron. All behaviour is rooted in the neurotransmission within, to and from the CNS interdependently with the endocrine system. The electrochemical transfers that occur across microscopic junctions between the connections of linked neurons are described straightforwardly. However, the complexity of the interrelationships between cell bodies is extensive, resulting in a vast signalling network throughout the horse. A study of the neural substrate and the mechanisms that control and interact with it assists us in comprehending how behaviour is regulated (Fig. 3.1) (McBride *et al.*, 2017). This chapter provides an overview of the complex nervous system and its endocrine partner, which is important in understanding normal behaviour patterns and anomalies.

*Corresponding author e-mail: c.b.riley@massey.ac.nz

  Fraser's the Behaviour and Welfare of the Horse (eds C.B. Riley, S.E. Cregier and A.F. Fraser)
DOI: 10.1079/9781789242133.0003

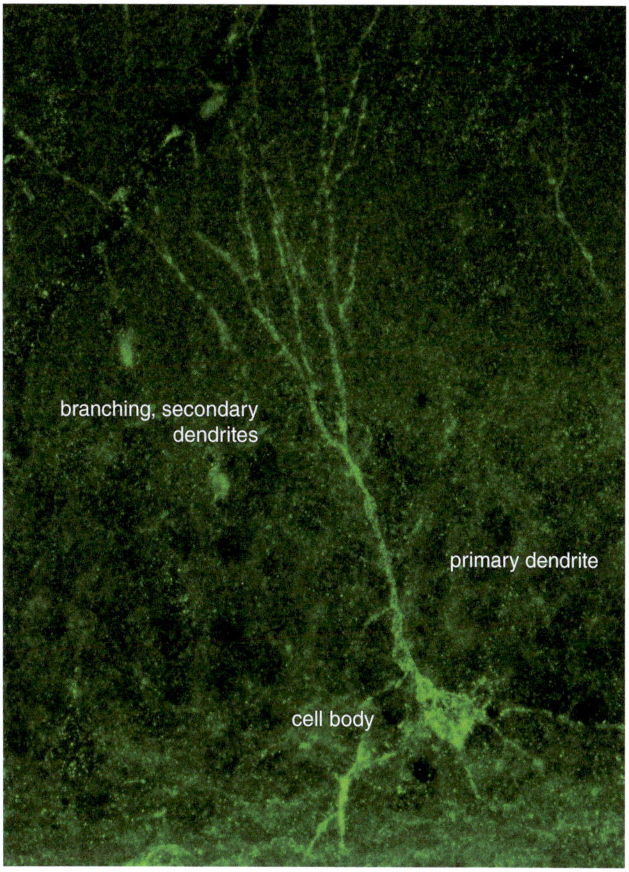

Fig. 3.1. Diagram of a complete neuron showing the cell body and dendrites. Photo: Jason N Snyder ("PSA-NCAM+ neuron" by Functional Neurogenesis is licensed with CC BY 2.0.)

Anatomy

Neurons

Neurons are the fundamental cellular components of the equine brain, spine and nerves. When sensory receptors are activated, depolarization within the nerve ending (axon) occurs, resulting in the transmission of electrochemical information to the neuron's cell body. This starts an integrated cascade of neural stimulation to neurons within the spine and the brain, initiating the subconscious and conscious responses on which behaviour is founded (Johnson, 2012).

Neurons typically consist of a cell body (soma) and a series of branching processes called dendrites that receive information from other excitable cells and receptors. In response to information, the output of the neuron is transmitted through a single process, the axon, which may later form collateral branches. The soma contains the Golgi apparatus and endoplasmic reticulum, but the mitochondria are contained within the soma and the axon. The neuron's endoplasmic reticulum has a cellular transport system originating in the lacunae within the Nissl bod ies. The granular Nissl substance is the site of protein and peptide synthesis, and its prominence within the neuron correlates with the high metabolic nature of the neuron. These substances are packaged within vesicles that migrate to the adjacent cell membrane and rupture into the synaptic space between associated neurons, facilitating communication through catecholamine, norepinephrine, and other substances (Fig. 3.2). Except for those located in the olfactory mucosa, most neurons cannot divide to multiply.

The branched projections of the neuron, the dendrites, receive input from many other neurons that

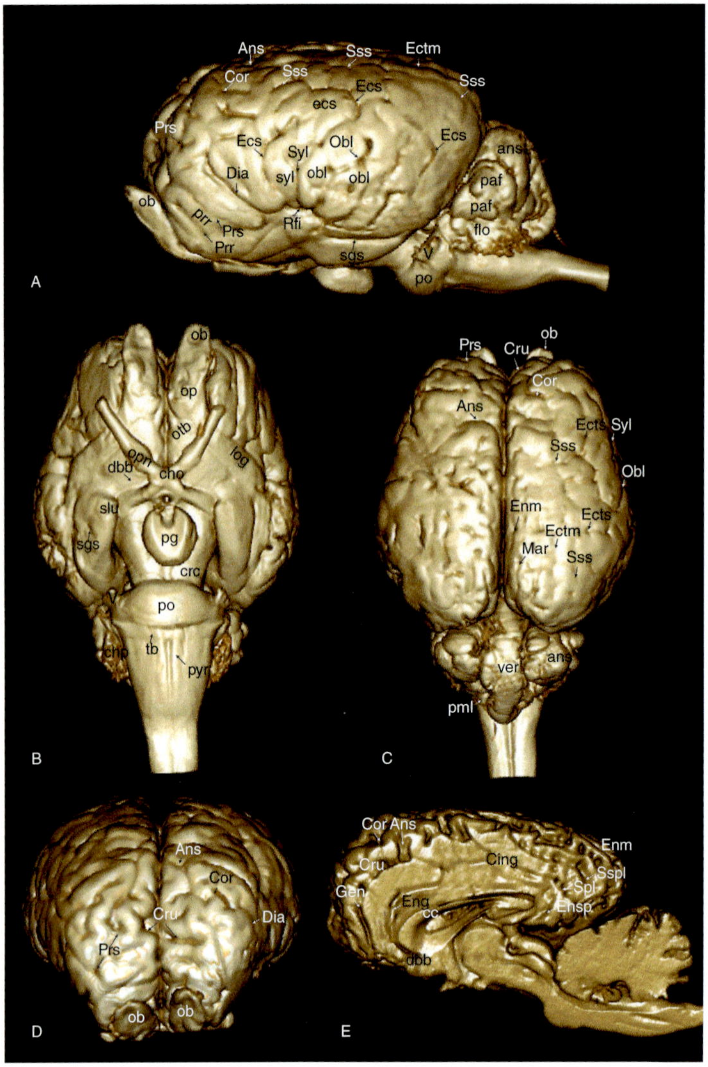

Fig. 3.2. 3D model of the equine brain based on magnetic resonance imaging. (A) Lateral view: Ans: ansate sulcus, ans: ansiform lobule, Cor: coronal sulcus, Dia: diagonal sulcus, Ecs: ectosylvian sulcus, ecs: ectosylvian gyrus, Ectm: ectomarginal sulcus, enrh: endorhinal sulcus, flo: flocculus, ob: olfactory bulb, Obl: oblique sulcus, obl: oblique gyrus, paf: paraflocculus, po: pons, Prr: prorean sulcus, prr: prorean gyrus, Prs: presylvian sulcus, Rfi: rhinal fissure, Sgs: sagittal sulcus, Sss: suprasylvian sulcus, Syl: sylvian fissure, syl: sylvian gyrus, V: trigeminal nerve. (B) Ventral view: cho: optic chiasma, chp: choroid plexus, crc: cerebral crus, dbb: diagonal band of broca, log: lateral olfactory gyrus, ob: olfactory bulb, op: olfactory peduncle, opn: optic nerve, otb: olfactory tubercle, pg: pituitary gland, po: pons, pyr: pyramidal tract, Sgs: sagittal sulcus, slu: semilunar gyrus, tb: trapezoid body. (C) Dorsal view: Ans: ansate sulcus, ans: ansiform lobule, Cor: coronal sulcus, Cru: cruciate sulcus, Ecs: ectosylvian sulcus, Ectm: ectomarginal sulcus, Enm: endomarginal sulcus, Mar: marginal sulcus, ob: olfactory bulb, Obl: oblique sulcus, pml: paramedian lobule, Prs: presylvian sulcus, Sss: suprasylvian sulcus, Syl: sylvian fissure, ver: vermis. (D) Frontal view: Ans: ansate sulcus, Cor: coronal sulcus, Cru: cruciate sulcus, Dia: diagonal sulcus, ob: olfactory bulb, Prs: presylvian sulcus. (E) Midsagittal view, Ans: ansate sulcus, cc: corpus callosum, Cing: cingulate sulcus, Cor: coronal sulcus, Cru: cruciate sulcus, dbb: diagonal band of broca, Eng: endogenual sulcus, Enm: endomarginal sulcus, Ensp: endosplenial sulcus, Gen: genual sulcus, Spl: splenial sulcus, Sspl: suprasplenial sulcus. (Schmidt *et al.*, 2019; CC BY.)

are transmitted to the soma. The average neuron receives excitatory or inhibitory input from hundreds of other neurons and thousands of synapses. A synapse is a point where the axon of one neuron functionally connects with another neuron, astrocyte or effector cell. The shared information is integrated, and the net result determines the response of the neuron. Some dendrites bristle with dendritic spines, membranous protrusions capable of interfacing with multiple axons. Therefore, one dendrite may communicate with hundreds of axons. The dendritic branching pattern of a neuron may increase or decrease. When young horses are learning within a stimulating or enriched environment, dendritic growth occurs.

The axon is a cytoplasmic process that propagates electrical impulses to or from the soma and range in length from a few millimetres between neurons (interneurons) to metres in length (e.g. in the equine limbs). Collectively, axons and dendrites are called neurites. Neurites are either afferent (carrying nerve impulses toward the CNS) or efferent (transmitting nerve impulses away from a soma). Efferent neurites usually have a constant cross-sectional area and are longer than afferent dendrites; afferent dendrites tend to taper. However, this may differ for sensory neurons. A sensory neuron of the lower equine limb has a long afferent neurite, a cell body located within the spinal ganglia, and an efferent neurite that synapses within the dorsal horn of the spinal cord. Because of their length and volume, most of the neuronal cytoplasm, neurotubules, mitochondria, vesicles, lysosomes and enzymes are contained within. Although the soma may be located a significant distance from the end of the axon, it still produces most of the peptides and proteins transported and used in the axon. The material moved to and from the soma along the length of the axon is transported via microtubules. This axon transport system relies upon the motor protein kinesin to move products from the soma down the axon and the motor protein dynein to move them along the length of the axon to the soma (Johnson, 2012).

Neuron types vary in the size of their soma, the length of the axons, and the complexity of dendrite branching. Although there are hundreds of different types of neurons, they fall within three main groups:

Sensory neurons. As part of the peripheral nervous system (PNS), they transmit information from the many different sensory nerve endings to the central nervous system.

Motor neurons. As part of the PNS, they transmit information from cell bodies within the CNS to somatic and visceral muscles.

Interneurons. Occurring most commonly within the CNS, they connect between neurons. Long interneurons may convey afferent or efferent information, and shorter ones may function to integrate information.

Neurons are connected and communicate with each other in two ways. The first involves chemical synapses where chemical neurotransmitters transit the 30–50 nm space between presynaptic and postsynaptic membranes. Chemical synapses are usually unidirectional and stimulate adjacent neurons to amplify the chemical signal in a cascading effect. Most synapses in the brain, and those at the neuromuscular junctions, are chemical synapses. When an action potential arises at a chemical synapse, it leads to the release of chemical neurotransmitters from the axonal terminus into the synaptic cleft. The neurotransmitter binds to the postsynaptic membrane stimulating chemically gated ion channels and inducing changes in the postsynaptic membrane potential and propagating information. The second mode of information transmission is via electrical synapses in which gap junctions form physical contact between adjacent cells. This system allows for faster conduction of membrane potential changes between neurons. Unlike chemical synapses, they do not amplify and are usually bidirectional.

Neuroglia

The neuroglia includes specialized non-neuronal cells in the CNS and PNS that maintain homeostasis, form myelin, and provide support and nutrition for the neurons. In the CNS, the neuroglia includes astrocytes, oligodendrocyte, ependymal cells and microglia. In the PNS, these are the satellite cells and Schwann cells (macroglia). Their morphology differs depending upon their location. Examples include the fibrous astrocytes of the white matter, the radial astrocytes of the cerebellum, and the protoplasmic astrocytes of the grey matter. Astrocytes contribute to maintaining the blood–brain barrier, blood flow regulation, neuronal nutrition, synapse insulation, intercellular communication and extracellular ion balance. They are also crucial in repairing the CNS and PNS following trauma, inflammation, or infection. The oligodendrocytes synthesize the myelin sheaths that insulate many axons in the CNS, either a single large axon or multiple small axons. Each Schwann cell only myelinates a single axon in the PNS. Myelin protects the axons and improves nerve impulse conduction. Adjacent myelin segments on the same axon are separated by 1 µm wide junctions called nodes of Ranvier, where iron channels propagate action potentials (electrical signals) along the axon. Approximately 20% of the glial cells are the microglia that form part of the immune defence of the CNS. These process damaged neurons, cellular debris and infectious organisms. They are crucial because the blood–brain barrier that separates the cerebrum and spinal cord from the rest of the body blocks antibodies from gaining access. Therefore, the microglia screen out foreign material and organisms and activate other immune cells within the CNS.

Cerebral cortex

During foetal development, the brain develops into the functional divisions of the brainstem, cerebrum (telencephalon) and cerebellum (dorsal metencephalon) (Fig. 3.2). The cerebrum has left and right hemispheres, each with inward folds called sulci, and external folds called gyri (Fig. 3.3) (de Lahunta *et al.*, 2015). Each gyrus corresponds with different functional parts of the brain and contains grey matter (neurons) superficially and white matter

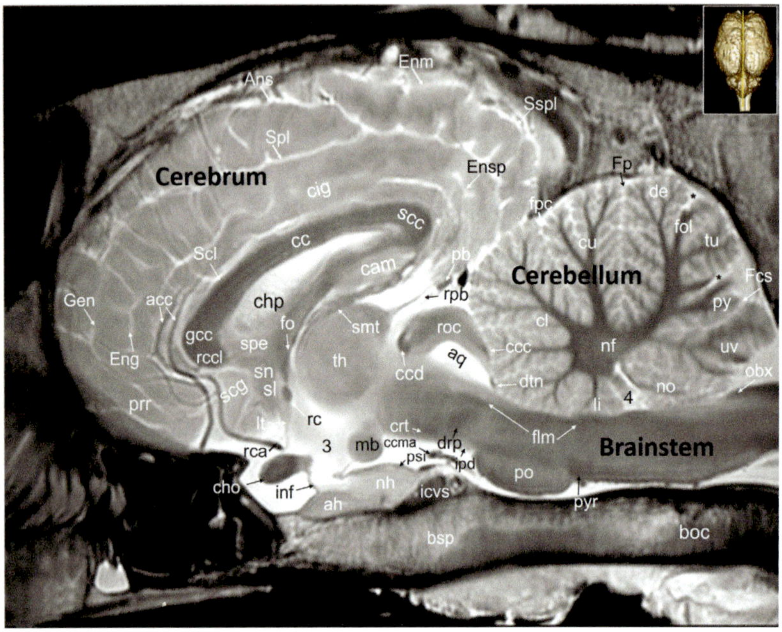

Fig. 3.3. Magnetic resonance image of the equine brain sectioned through the midline. acc: corpus callosum artery, ah: adenohypophysis, Ans: ansate sulcus, aq: mesencephalic aqueduct, boc: basioccipital bone, bsp: basisphenoidal bone, cam: ammon's horn, cc: corpus callosum, ccc: commissure of the caudal colliculus, ccd: caudal commissure, ccma: caudal communicating artery, cho: optic chiasm, chp: choroid plexus, cig: cingulate gyrus, cin: cingulum, cl: central lobule, crt: rubro-cerebello-thalamic tract, cu: culmen, de: declive of the vermis, drp: decussation of the rostral cerebellar peduncles, dtn: decussation of trochlear nerve, Eng: endogenual sulcus, Enm: endomarginal sulcus, Espl: ectosplenial sulcus, flm: medial longitudinal fasciculus, fo: fornix, fol: folium of the vermis, Fp: primary fissure, Fpc: praeculminate fissure, gcc: genu of the corpus callosum, Gen: genual sulcus, icvs: intercavernous sinus, inf: infundibular stalk, ipd: interpeduncular nucleus, li: lingula of the vermis, lt: terminal lamina, mb: mamillary body, nf: fastigial nucleus, nh: neurohypophysis, no: nodulus of the vermis, obx: obex, pb: pineal body, po: pons, prr: prorean gyrus, psi: pars intermedia of the pituitary gland, py: pyramis of the vermis, pyr: pyramidal tract, rc: rostral commissure, rca: rostral cerebral artery, rcc: radiation of corpus callosum, rccl: rostrum of the corpus callosum, roc: rostral colliculus, rpb: recess of the pineal body, scc: splenium of corpus callosum, Scf: secondary fissure, scg: subcallosal gyrus, Scl: sulcus of corpus callosum, sl: lateral septal nuclei, smt: stria medullaris thalami, sn: septal nuclei, Spl: splenial sulcus, Sspl: suprasplenial sulcus, th: thalamus, tu: tuber vermis, uv: uvula of the vermis, 3: third ventricle, 4: fourth ventricle. asterisk: blind-ending medullary branches, uncovered with cortex. (Schmidt *et al.*, 2019; CC BY.)

(axons) centrally. The cerebral cortex of the neopallium (grey matter) has six layers of neuronal cell bodies. The corona radiata (white matter) contains the myelinated axons of neurons connecting to and from the overlying cortex. Within the cortex are localized regions where sensory inputs are received, integrated and retransmitted. Accumulations of neurons within clusters generally perform the same function and, in the CNS, are called nuclei. Specialized areas of the cortex are primary sites for sensory reception, but signals are redirected to many areas of the brain, initiating the multitude of responses recognized as behaviour. These regions (cortices) reside within specific lobes of the brain (Table 3.1) and are fed sensory information from specific cranial nerves (Table 3.2). The cerebral cortex possesses four main primary sensory processing areas: the somaesthetic, visual, auditory and olfactory cortices.

The primary somatosensory cortex is located in the postcentral gyrus of the parietal lobe and is part of the somatosensory system. It contains neurons that respond to tactile sensation and is proportional in size to the density of cutaneous tactile receptors within the body surfaces. The horse has an extensive visual area in the occipital lobe of the cerebrum. Nerve fibres from the retina of the eye form the optic nerve, and information is initially

Table 3.1. Regions of the brain, their general functions and cranial nerve (CN) inputs. Source: Thomson and Hahn, 2012.

Anatomical regions and their components	Functional region	Primary functions	CN
Telencephalon (part of prosencephalon) cerebral hemispheres including hippocampus and basal ganglia	Forebrain	Receives, processes, and integrates sensory input Motor control Behaviour	I
Diencephalon (part of prosencephalon) thalamus hypothalamus subthalamus epithalamus metathalamus	Forebrain (caudal)	Relays sensory information between brain regions including structures of the endocrine and nervous systems Interacts with the limbic system to manage emotions and memories Controls arousal, awareness, autonomic functions, homeostatic regulation, circadian, seasonal reproduction activity Part of upper motor neuron system	II
Mesencephalon tectum (dorsal) cerebral peduncle (ventral) tegmentum substantia nigra crus cerebri	Midbrain (rostral brainstem)	Upper motor neuron nuclei Cranially projecting sensory inputs from limbs, body and head transit through it Caudally projecting motor outputs from the forebrain transit through it Arousal Reflexes associated with hearing and vision	III IV
Metencephalon	Pons (in brainstem) and cerebellum)	Pons: upper motor neuron nuclei Cranially projecting sensory inputs from limbs, body and head transit through it Caudally projecting motor outputs from the forebrain transit through it Arousal and awareness Cerebellum: coordination of motor functions	V
Myelencephalon	Medulla oblongata (caudal brainstem)	Upper motor neuron nuclei Cranially projecting sensory inputs from limbs, body and head transit through it Caudally projecting motor outputs from the forebrain transit through it Arousal Cardiovascular & respiratory control centres	VI VII VIII IX X XI XII

Table 3.2. The cranial nerves and their functions

Type of function	Cranial nerve name	Function	Number
Sensory	Olfactory	Olfaction	CN I
	Optic	Vision	CN II
	Vestibulocochlear	Balance and hearing	CN VIII
Motor	Oculomotor	Extraocular eye muscles Parasympathetic to the eye	CN III
	Trochlear	Extraocular eye muscles	CN IV
	Abducens	Extraocular eye muscles	CN VI
	Accessory	Pharyngeal and laryngeal muscles	CN XI
	Hypoglossal	Lingual (tongue) muscles	CN XII
Mixed	Trigeminal	Facial sensation Motor to muscles of mastication (chewing)	CN V
	Facial	Taste Motor to facial muscles (expression) Parasympathetic for salivation Parasympathetic for lacrimation (tearing)	CN VII
	Glossopharyngeal	Taste Pharyngeal sensation Swallowing muscles Parasympathetic for salivation	CN IX
	Vagus	Sensation pharynx and larynx Swallowing Parasympathetic for thoracic and abdominal organs	CN X

received at the visual cortex for processing and then on to other centres. The auditory cortex is part of the temporal lobe, processes auditory information, and has functions associated with hearing and vocalization. Auditory nerve impulses reach the thalamus and pons and pass to the cortex. The olfactory cortex in the forebrain receives input from the nasal cavity. It is further processed in the amygdala, orbitofrontal cortex and hippocampus that play roles in emotion, memory and learning (Hahn and Masty, 2015).

The Limbic System

The limbic system encompasses structures located on either side of the thalamus in the forebrain that interact heavily with the cortex. It is critical to the emotional experience of the horse as it functions to support emotion, behaviour, motivation, long-term memory and olfaction. There are interrelated portions of the frontal lobe cortex, temporal lobe, thalamus and hypothalamus, bringing the cortex together with certain regions within the midbrain. It operates to influence the endocrine system and autonomic nervous system. Interactions occur with the basal ganglia, subcortical structures located near the thalamus and hypothalamus that direct intentional movements. The system is also tightly connected to the prefrontal cortex, where motivation and pleasure are linked.

The limbic system enables horses to cope with and respond to the environment. Parts of the limbic system are concerned with primal activities related to food and sex. Others are related to emotions and feelings or are associated with spatial memory, learning and social processing. The hippocampus and the amygdala are the two main components of the limbic system. The hippocampus is important in spatial memory and provides for the emotional context of a sensory input via a feedback system. Other regions within the hippocampus are involved in the recall of spatial memories with particular effects on learning. There is an upsurge of neuron recruitment and the development of neural circuits and the hippocampus in response to training.

The amygdala is involved with many cognitive processes and encodes episodic memories, particularly those associated with an emotional event. It provides the horse with the ability to focus on some stimuli while ignoring others (attention). In humans, the cognitive functions relating to the evaluation of facial expression in social processing are important. Recent work demonstrating facial recognition by horses suggests that this is also true for horses (Lansade *et al.*, 2018; Lansade *et al.*, 2020).

Basal ganglia

The basal ganglia are subcortical nuclei in the forebrain and the top of the midbrain. These are interconnected with the cortex, thalamus, brainstem and other areas. Their primary function is to regulate the activities of the motor and premotor cortical areas so that voluntary movements are coordinated. For example, neurons whose activities relate to movements of the forelimbs are adjacent to those with activity related to hind leg movements, permitting coordinated movement through a variety of gaits (e.g. trot). These ganglia are associated with various functions, including habit learning, eye movements, cognition, emotion and the control of voluntary motor movements.

Hypothalamus

The hypothalamus is located at the base of the brain near the pituitary gland. It contains many small nuclei that play crucial roles in regulating body temperature and the synthesis and secretion of neurohormones (releasing hormones). Its functions are associated with the control of hunger and thirst, some aspects of parenting attachment behaviour, sleep, and circadian rhythms. It links the nervous system to the endocrine system via the principal endocrine gland of the body, the pituitary. This means that the hypothalamus, directly and indirectly, plays roles in the maintenance of most activities, including behaviour. Feedback mechanisms mean that the hypothalamus also responds to some of the endocrine activity that it initiates. The receipt of afferent stimulation provides the hypothalamus with input to maintain and regulate the activity of the pituitary gland. The hypothalamus is continuous, in the forward direction, with the limbic system.

Cerebellum

The cerebellum derives from the dorsal portion of the metencephalon and is located caudal to the cerebrum and dorsal to the fourth ventricle. The cerebellum is connected to the pons and medulla of the brainstem by three peduncles on each side of the fourth ventricle and by portions of the top of the fourth ventricle. Afferent axons pass through the middle and caudal cerebellar peduncles from the brainstem and spinal cord. The rostral cerebellar peduncle connects the cerebellum with the mesencephalon, with mainly efferent processes passing out of the cerebellum. The centre of the cerebellum contains an extensive network of white matter that penetrates the cerebellar cortex, where it connects with neurons (Hahn and Masty, 2015).

The cerebellum contains more neurons than the remaining areas of the brain combined. It has connections to many brain regions, including those involved in sensory systems, cognition, vocal communication and emotions. The cerebellum plays a major role in regulating motor activity, functioning to coordinate and control movements induced by the upper motor neuron system. This includes maintaining equilibrium and the management of muscle tone to maintain posture and body position during exercise and at rest.

Brainstem

The brainstem includes the diencephalon, mesencephalon, ventral metencephalon (the pons), and the myelencephalon (medulla) (Table 3.1). Neuronal axons project from the cerebral cortex to the brainstem, and neuronal axons project from the thalamus to the cerebral cortex. Although small relative to the size of the cerebrum, it is critical to the regulation of the heart and respiratory functions, controlling the rate of both. As listed in Table 3.1, it has extensive motor and sensory connections with the face and neck via the cranial nerves. The brainstem is critically important as the nexus for motor and sensory pathways from the cerebrum and cerebellum to the spinal cord and body, and from the body to the brain. Linked pathways include the corticospinal tract associated with motor function; dorsal column-medial meniscus pathway associated with fine touch, vibration sensation and proprioception; and the spinothalamic tract associated with pain sensation, temperature and coarse touch. It has a critical integrative function for motor and sensory inputs transmitted by the cranial nerves (Table 3.2).

Spinal cord

The spinal cord and brain are extensions of each other. The spinal cord is composed of white matter (axons and dendrites) that surrounds the grey matter (neurons and neuroglia). The left and right halves are divided by the dorsal median sulcus and ventral longitudinal fissure. The white matter consists of large bundles called funiculi, and these are formed from smaller bundles of white matter. These are the ascending and descending pathways that transmit sensory and motor information throughout the nervous system. The ascending pathways that commence in the spinal cord pass information to higher levels in the brain. The descending pathways that regulate motor activity originate in the higher levels of the brain, descending to the spinal cord segments. On either side, the divided segments of the spinal nerve roots enter and leave the spinal cord. The dorsal roots connect with the spinal cord at the dorsolateral sulcus, and the bundles of white matter between them are called the right and left dorsal funiculus. Nerve fibres located within these funiculi are primarily responsible for conscious proprioception, feeding inputs to the thalamus and forebrain. The dorsal funiculi are further divided into the fasciculus gracilis medially and fasciculus cuneatis laterally, carrying information related to conscious perception of the pelvic and thoracic limbs, respectively. The white matter between dorsal and ventral roots on either side, the lateral funiclus, contains the spinocerebellar tracts running from the spinal cord to the cerebellum; these support subconscious (autonomous) proprioception. The ventral funiculus between the ventral nerve roots is formed by a mixture of ascending and descending tracts, with the latter carrying upper motor neuron axons caudally located with the lower motor neurons in the spinal cord (Hahn and Masty, 2015).

The role of the spinal cord is complex in that it permits higher-order conscious function while maintaining autonomous reflex mechanisms. Spinal reflexes are quite numerous in equine behaviour. Reflex spinal arcs confer evolutionary advantages that are maintained but may be modified and controlled by superior reflex arcs involving the cerebrum. The scratch reflex is an example of coordinated cord reflex action. Specific motor reflexes involve the excitation of specific muscle groups and the inhibition of antagonistic muscles. For example, the stretch reflex involves excitation of the extensor muscles and inhibition of ipsilateral flexor muscles. Withdrawal reflexes are associated with the extension of the limb of the opposite or contralateral side of the body. Many neurons are common to these reflexes (i.e. ventral horn cells).

Function

Autonomic system

The autonomic nervous system is an involuntary mechanism that preserves a constant internal environment by innervating the heart and the smooth muscle of blood vessels and visceral structures. It has afferent, central and efferent components, and is subdivided into the craniosacral parasympathetic (rest and digest) and the thoracolumbar sympathetic (fight, flight) elements. The hypothalamus contains the autonomic upper motor neuron cell bodies.

Sympathetic innervation is provided through a network of paired neurons that synapse with each other in a ganglion before reaching the target of their innervation. The first neuron in the link is the presynaptic neuron of the sympathetic system, with its soma located in the lateral horn of the thoracic or lumbar segments of the spinal cord. The axon of the presynaptic neuron exits the spinal cord to synapse with a second neuron, the postsynaptic soma. Most sympathetic nerve endings release the neurotransmitter substance norepinephrine (noradrenaline), which is chemically similar to epinephrine (adrenaline) produced by the adrenal gland. Sympathetic nerve fibres are therefore referred to as adrenergic. Thus, the adrenal medulla resembles a ganglion of the sympathetic system in its roles. The release of norepinephrine at the adrenergic nerve fibre terminations prepares the horse for action or reaction.

Parasympathetic innervation arises from a similar network of paired neurons, but the presynaptic and postsynaptic somas are located in different parts of the system. The presynaptic parasympathetic somas occur in nuclei associated with specific cranial nerves and in the central portions of the spinal cord. The postsynaptic somas are located in the named ganglia associated with each of the specific cranial nerves and in terminal ganglia distributed in the body (Hahn and Masty, 2015). Most parasympathetic nerve endings release acetylcholine at synapses and nerve endings, and therefore are called cholinergic. After its synaptic release, acetylcholine amplifies the parasympathetic effects. Parasympathetic stimulation produces the vegetating effects of slower heart rate, lowered blood pressure, constriction of bronchi and increased gut activity for digestion.

The effects of the two aspects of the autonomic system oppose each other and are termed antagonistic. The autonomic system acts as a behavioural integrator. Its full role is in modulating the intensities of behavioural responses, including the emotional component of behaviour. Autonomic conditioning may last for years and requires little reinforcement. Any reinforcement to this system is powerful and may even occur in anticipation of circumstances (Olczak *et al.*, 2016). Sympathetic reactions are swift and precede somatic components of defence, alert, fight or flight. Autonomic innervation improves the acuity of olfaction, taste, hearing, touch and proprioception. In equine lives, the autonomic system is involved in agonistic reactions, self-determination, survival efforts, comfort-seeking and preparation for future circumstances.

Endocrine system – the chemical operators

The nervous and endocrine systems are cooperative and interdependent. Neural secretions and the priming effects of hormones on the brain process and regulate responses to external stimuli, translating elaborately organized phenomena into an outward behavioural response (Hahn and Masty, 2015). Either one or all of behaviour, environment and internal state can alter to cause a change in motivation and behaviour. These create complex situations of chemical activity in neuropeptides, hormones and pheromones, underpinning chemical communication within the body and between horses. Many equine bodily activities are governed by hormone production, mainly from endocrine glands. A brief outline of this system of chemical messengers is helpful for an appreciation of behavioural motivation.

Motivation is neuro-hormonally dependent. Hormones act on the CNS and PNS to prime the response of those neural systems programmed to function in the presence of the specific hormone. Many of these activated neural systems are not involved in routine behaviour. Hormone release requires stimulation, and the hypothalamus controls the secretions of both anterior and posterior pituitary lobes. It also governs releasing and inhibiting factors for feedback mechanisms, controlling cyclic phenomena and, ultimately, sexual behaviour.

Pituitary secretion is activated by the hypothalamus. Gonadotropin-releasing hormone acts on the anterior pituitary gland, causing it to produce and release luteinizing hormone (LH) and follicle-stimulating hormone (FSH). Both LH and FSH act upon the reproductive tract of either gender as their target, inducing the gonads to produce gametes and locally active hormones. Prolactin is produced in the anterior pituitary and also influences reproductive function. For example, it contributes to initial maternal behaviour in the dam. It also motivates grooming behaviours.

The posterior pituitary synthesizes oxytocin and vasopressin. Oxytocin contributes to milk release in the lactating mare and involution of the uterus following parturition. This hormone is also involved in male ejaculation and is used therapeutically for stallions to induce ejaculation (Cavalero *et al.*, 2019). Vasopressin (antidiuretic hormone) regulates the osmolality (the concentration of dissolved molecules including salts and glucose) of the blood and, therefore, the fluid volume within the blood vessels and tissues. It does this by regulating water retention in the kidneys. Within the carotid sinus and the left atrium of the heart are baroreceptors, centres that detect blood pressure. When these are activated by increasing blood pressure, nerve impulses from the baroreceptors to the CNS inhibit the secretion of vasopressin, increasing the renal excretion of water.

The two gonadotropic hormones from the anterior pituitary are essential to reproductive function and are produced in concert with one another in both sexes. In their behavioural roles, the sex hormones of the gonads are androgenic and oestrogenic in males and females, respectively. The levels vary in the female, creating cyclic ovarian activity and related behaviours in breeding mares. The production of gonadotropins in the male is steadier and more continuous. High levels of either androgens or oestrogens can inhibit the secretion of FSH and LH by feedback effected through the hypothalamus.

Corticotropin-releasing hormone (CRH) regulates the output of adrenocorticotropic hormone (ACTH). ACTH secretion is involved in sugar metabolism (glycogenolysis) and stress responses. ACTH causes the adrenal cortex to enlarge and produce a variety of corticosteroids, typified by cortisol. Blood cortisol concentrations rise in states of stress due to increased ACTH activity. ACTH is essentially the adaptive hormone for unusual circumstances. Its secretion increases during attempts at adaptation to environmental or husbandry problems (Nelson and Kriegsfeld, 2020). Steroids produced in the adrenal cortex generate glycogenesis by glucocorticoids. Of the adrenal cortical hormones (corticoids), cortisol is the most active and regulates carbohydrate metabolism to increase blood glucose to meet the energy expenditures associated with stressful events. The adrenal medulla is under close control by the limbic system and the hypothalamus in particular. The adrenal medulla synthesizes epinephrine. Epinephrine prepares the horse for gross physical activity in fight or flight situations, including temporarily increasing blood pressure in response to stress. In other words, increased epinephrine output is associated with agonistic events and alarm responses (Schulkin, 1999).

The small pineal gland, located in the groove between the two halves of the thalamus, produces melatonin. The output of this hormone is influenced by the light-dark photoperiod and is basic to seasonal phenomena in horses. Melatonin influences their diurnal and cyclic behaviour. It also influences the secretion of FSH and LH by the pituitary through a mechanism that is not well understood. The disconnect between the imposed breeding season for racing Thoroughbreds and Standardbreds and the natural breeding season as dictated by melatonin output contributes to welfare problems in these industries. However, melatonin secretion can be manipulated by housing animals with artificial light to induce earlier cycling. A blue light facemask has been developed that induces melatonin increases earlier with positive welfare effects on Thoroughbred foals and mares (Fig. 3.4) (Nolan *et al.*, 2017).

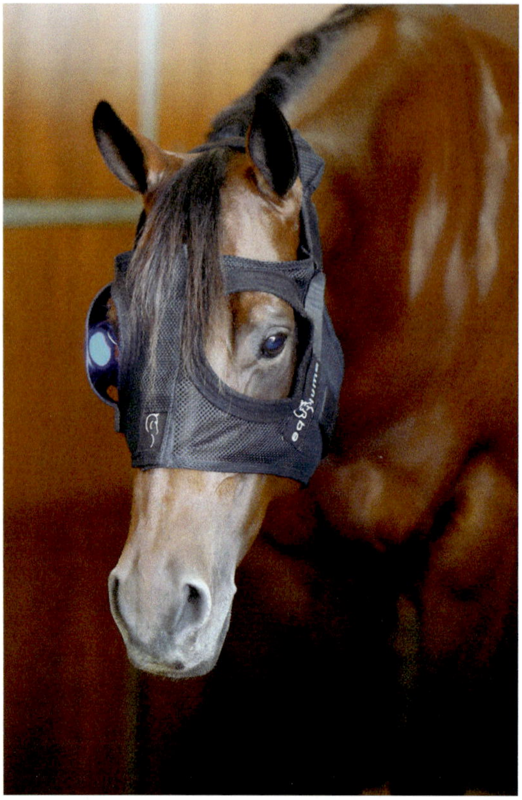

Fig. 3.4. A proprietary artificial light device used to manipulate melatonin secretion to induce earlier seasonal oestrus in the breeding mare. Photo: Amandine Lefevre, Equilume, NZ.

Thyroxine secreted by the thyroid gland influences energetic behaviour by affecting the metabolic pool of nitrogen and available energy. This hormone influences the activity of the gonads as well. Hypothyroid and hyperthyroid females sometimes have lengthened, irregular or arrested oestrous cycles.

The hormones associated with oestrous, dioestrus, pregnancy and parturition in the mare are discussed later in this book. Her reproductive cycle and behaviour, and the development of the periparturient mare–foal relationship, is greatly influenced by the hormonal–neurological axis.

Motivation

Motivation is a state of willingness through physiological and cognitive processes to undertake certain activities and plays a crucial role in learning (Olczak *et al.*, 2018). The motivational affective states encompass subjective states (feelings or emotions) that involve a positive (pleasant) or negative (unpleasant) effect, that are involved in motivating specific behaviours, and are plausible adaptations acquired through natural selection that are adaptive (Fraser and Duncan, 1998). Motivation can result from external or internal stimuli, triggering specific behaviours oriented towards achieving the desired result or reward. The motivation–reward system is highly dependent upon the limbic system. When dopamine levels increase, this leads to positive sensations in the brain and stimulates memory (learning) (Olczak *et al.*, 2016). Unfortunately, there are occasions when this system is ‘hijacked’, resulting in behaviours that are psychologically rewarding but adverse to the horse’s welfare (e.g., stereotypy). The emotional aspects of motivation and response are regulated by the limbic system. As described above, this highly interconnected group of brain structures are linked by neural pathways and other parts of the CNS. After afferent information is received from different afferent (sensory) routes, integration and processing of these signals within the limbic system results in a wide variety of autonomic responses and body actions constituting behaviour of numerous forms. These responses are affected by age, breed, heredity, gender, brain damage, illness and injury.

Three neural systems mediate the various emotional behaviours controlled by the limbic system. Following experimental stimulation of one area, the animal may actively approach a situation in a positive, exploratory manner. Stimulation of a second area may cause the animal to stop any behaviour it is performing. Stimulation of a third physiological area of the limbic system causes the animal to show marked aggressive change, either agitated from a calm state to an aggressive one or from the latter to docility. Alterations in the stimulation of the different limbic system areas are the foundation of our understanding of emotionally motivated behaviours.

Physiological and endocrinological studies have shown that the hypothalamus is an integrating region (Fraser, 2010). However, some neurophysiological activities are diverse in the organized control of their motivation. In the ethogram of the horse, there are two main categories of behavioural production. Firstly, phasic motivation of maintenance behaviour supports the bulk of the behaviour of horses concerned with such activities as ingestion, locomotion and social activities. Some physiological needs, such as resting, body care and thermoregulation, are also featured in the motivation of equine maintenance. Secondly, occasional forms of motivation also occur. These motivations are needed for dealing with occasional, specific and often critical circumstances. Examples include the introduction of a new role to a maiden mare with its first foal and the new role of a stallion when it starts its first breeding season. In these examples, motivation is provided hormonally to activate neural systems that are not involved in routine maintenance behaviours. Novel and emergency roles of behaviour must be present in the neuromechanism of the individual horse for activation when circumstances require them. In some situations, their activation never occurs if the appropriate motivation is not presented (e.g., castrating a colt before reproductive expression).

Self-stimulation behaviour is characterized by automatic and repetitive compulsion seen as an example of maladaptation, with negative consequences. Experimentally, the administration of amphetamine, which liberates amines, induces repetitive behaviour in animals, even when the stimulation no longer has a directly rewarding effect. A feature of the significance of amine neural fibres is that they can increase. This disrupts the reward system, and alternative neural pathways create stereotyped activity leading to consolidation and fixation of the aberrant behaviour. These discoveries fit with ethological findings on anomalous behaviour and explain their obvious characteristics (Fraser, 2010).

Neurophysiological research has established that motivational mechanisms of the brain are mediated by peptides. Changes in the chemical state of the brain can bias neuronal processes (Kandel *et al.*, 2012). Catecholamines are involved in controlling hormonal states. Their actions modulate sequential, step-by-step procedures, such as fixed action patterns of the more extended type, seen notably in reproduction. Catecholamines help trigger hormonal events, and then other hormonal processes continue the motivation. The catecholamine transmitters are triggered by normal action patterns and can carry the reward message returning from them. The biogenic amine system is the basis of the behavioural changes that facilitate the animal's achievement of homeostasis. The system can redirect behaviour in seemingly incongruous activities, which are capable of being strengthened in the neuronal substrate. The way the terminals infiltrate the cerebral cortex, mainly in its upper layers, indicates a pervasive influence of involuntary behaviour.

Control over motivation occurs under certain changes of season and husbandry. In a free state, horses aggregate in equid groups. Through systems of social organizations, harmony prominently features in their collective behaviour. Phenomenal features of group behaviour are synchrony and conformity of motives in the group, leading to social facilitation. A level of synchronous conformity is imposed on maintenance behaviours so that a herd will feed, move, react, associate, utilize territory, shelter and rest together. Group behaviour demonstrates cohesion, often reflecting a higher motivation than normally observed in the isolated behaviour of the individual.

Neuroethology has shown that some hormones underpinning motivation are controlled by catecholamines (Schulkin, 1999). Fibres containing these molecules pervade the critical brain regions and course through the nuclei. Changeability in the outlets of centres throughout the limbic system may underpin some ethological phenomena in horses, such as redirected drives, displacement activities and some abnormal behaviours. The substantia nigra, where one dopamine bundle has its main origin, controls motivation-rewarded behaviour and voluntary preferences to avoid noxious stimulation. The dopamine pathway carries incentive messages. The norepinephrine pathway carries motivation-reducing messages of satiety. Reward is implicit; both start and stop actions depend on whether there are incentive rewards or terminal consummatory rewards. Incentive rewards, such as the odour of food, utilize the dopamine pathways. Final rewards, such as the ingestion of food, act through the norepinephrine pathways.

Relationships between physiological, neural, and hormonal factors in motivation are coordinated in the hypothalamus. Nuclei governing feeding and drinking behaviour, including foraging and appetite, are located there. Stimulation of some hypothalamic areas of the limbic system elicits behaviour with a powerful emotional component. The medial hypothalamus exerts inhibition on the circuits, producing the fight-or-flight response. Therefore, the main structures involved in the control of emotion are predominantly located throughout the limbic system. The main units for consummatory behaviour are also located within the hypothalamus, although they also come under other controls. Emotional behaviour is the result of limbic stimulation.

Motivations in the horse are modified or directed by exogenous environmental stimulation, such as temperature, light intensity, day length, social factors and social circumstances. Endogenous stimuli also influence motivations (e.g., hormonal changes). Initially, appetitive behaviour is initiated by a period of seeking out a specific goal, such as food or any other goal associated with homeostasis. This behaviour is specific and searching, directed towards an appropriate goal (Fraser, 2010). The next component period emerges when the animal is presented with the targeted goal and initiates behaviours designed to satisfy the motivation. The behavioural classes of self-maintenance are all examples of consummatory behavioural processes, which can be regarded as expressions of emotive states, hunger, thirst, pain (or discomfort), fear and aggression (Olczak *et al.*, 2016).

Summary

The anatomic and functional organization of the equine central nervous and endocrine systems are complex. Although there are some differences from humans in these systems, the complexity and similarity in function of these systems in horses support the assumption that horses are behaviourally complex creatures capable of emotional and learned responses.

References

Cavalero, T.M.S., Papa, F., Schmith, R.A., Scheeren, V.F.C., Canuto, L.E.F. *et al.* (2019) Protocols using detomidine and oxytocin induce ex copula ejaculation in stallions. *Theriogenology* 140, 93–98.

de Lahunta, A., Glass, E. and Kent, M. (2015) Neuroanatomy gross description and atlas of transverse sections and magnetic resonance images. In: *Veterinary Neuroanatomy and Clinical Neurology*. Elsevier, St. Louis, Missouri, pp. 6–26

Fraser, A.F. (2010) *The Behaviour and Welfare of the Horse*, 2nd edn. CAB International, Wallingford, UK.

Fraser, D. and Duncan, I.J.H. (1998) Pleasures, pains and animal welfare: Toward a natural history of affect. *Animal Welfare* 7, 383–396.

Hahn, C. and Masty, J. (2015) Overview of neuroanatomy. In: *Equine Neurology*. John Wiley and Sons, Hoboken, New Jersey, pp. 3–29.

Johnson, C. (2012) Neurohistology, physiology and sciences supporting structures. In: *Veterinary Neuroanatomy: A Clinical Approach*. Elsevier Australia, Chatswood, NSW, Australia, pp. 17–29.

Kandel, E.R., Schwartz, J.H. and Jewell, T.M. (eds) (2012) *Principles of Neural Science*. Elsevier, Amsterdam.

Lansade, L., Nowak, R., Lainé, A-L., Leterrier, C., Bonneau, C. *et al.* (2018) Facial expression and oxytocin as possible markers of positive emotions in horses. *Scientific Reports* 8, 14680. doi:10.1038/s41598-018-32993-z

Lansade, L., Colson, V., Parias, C., Trösch, M., Reigner, F. *et al.* (2020) Female horses spontaneously identify a photograph of their keeper, last seen six months previously. *Scientific Reports* 10, 6302. doi: 10.1038/s41598-020-62940-w

McBride, S.D., Parker, M.O., Roberts, K. and Hemmings, A. (2017) Applied neurophysiology of the horse; implications for training, husbandry, and welfare. *Applied Animal Behaviour Science* 190, 90–101.

Nelson, R. and Kriegsfeld, L.J. (2020) *An Introduction to Behavioural Endocrinology*, 5th edn. Sinauer Associates, Sunderland, Massachusetts.

Nolan, M.B., Walsh, C.M., Duff, N., McCrarren, C., Prendergast, R.L. *et al.* (2017) Artificially extended photoperiod administered to prepartum mares via blue light to a single eye: Observations on gestation length, foal birthweight and foal hair coat at birth. *Theriogenology* 100, 126–133.

Olczak, K., Nowicki, J. and Klocek, C. (2016) Motivation, stress and learning – Critical characteristics that influence the horses' value and training method – A review. *Annals of Animal Science* 16, 641–652.

Olczak, K., Christensen, J.W. and Klocek, C. (2018) Food motivation in horses appears stable across different test situations. *Applied Animal Behaviour Science* 204, 60–65.

Schmidt, M.J., Knemeyer, C. and Heinsen, H. (2019) Neuroanatomy of the equine brain as revealed by high-field (3Tesla) magnetic-resonance-imaging. *PLoS ONE* 14(4), e0213814.

Schulkin, J. (1999) *Neuroendocrine: Regulation of Behaviour*. Cambridge University Press, Cambridge.

Thomson, C. and Hahn, C. (2012) *Veterinary Neuroanatomy: A Clinical Approach*. Elsevier Australia, Chatswood, NSW, Australia.

4 Behavioural Homeostasis, Daily Rhythms and Advances in Monitoring

Barbara Padalino DVM, PhD, Celta*

University of Bologna, Bologna, Italy

General Concepts 50
Time Budget 51
Inactive Behaviour 53
Active Behaviour 54
Feeding behaviour 54
Explorative behaviour 54
Social behaviour 54
Grooming 55
Play 55
Locomotory behaviour and exercise 55
Technological Advances for Monitoring Behaviour and its Rhythms 56
Slow and automatic feeders 56
Wearable heart rate monitors 56
Wearable electroencephalography 57
Equiwatch system 58
Pedometers, accelerometers and wearable GPS 58
Welfare Implications 58
References 58

General Concepts

Equine welfare could be viewed as a small and restricted area of study unless one looks more closely at the daily life of the horse, inside and out. Appreciating the specific phenomena of a horse's day-to-day existence suddenly broadens the field of welfare exponentially. This chapter focuses on the importance of striving for homeostatic stability in a horse's daily behaviour and rhythms. Ensuring that this knowledge is available to horse people contributes to equine welfare.

The life-sustaining process for all living organisms is homeostasis, the maintenance of constant internal conditions or the physiological balancing of systems and functions, physiology being the study of how these parts function and relate to one another. Cellular homeostatic phenomena and homeostasis occur at the level of organs within whole and multiple systems (Heidemann, 2007). Motivated behavioural processes are used to attain general physiological stability, whole-body homeostasis and social balance. These processes are under the control of the cerebral defence system, essentially, the limbic system. The view taken here is that the animal's limbic system and the autonomic and endocrine systems vitally and collectively support comprehensive well-being.

*Corresponding author: barbara.padalino@unibo.it

DOI: 10.1079/9781789242133.0004

The ramification of the three systems – limbic, autonomic and endocrine – creates a vast network of influential forces (see Chapter 3). From the frontal and prefrontal cortex, through all its numerous parts, to the hypothalamus, the limbic system has roles of profound importance in sustaining life and controlling physiological activities. The autonomic nervous system ensures bodily operations without conscious input and has a self-balancing capability in its two opposing subdivisions, the parasympathetic and the sympathetic. The endocrine system secretes hormones into the blood, carrying chemical messages of instruction throughout the entire body. It ensures the balanced maintenance of the animal with appropriate activities. This balance among behaviours during the day creates a particular time allocation for each essential activity during the day and night-time budgets.

Homeostasis often occurs in fluid cycles that characterize biological rhythms (Palmer, 2002). One of the most robust and best-studied classes of biological rhythms is that associated with the alternation of day and night (Piccione *et al.*, 2008). A daily rhythm corresponds to a regular oscillation of behavioural and physiological variables over a 24-hour period (Refinetti *et al.*, 2007). In mammals, the daily clock, located in the suprachiasmatic nuclei, regulates the metabolism and coordinates physiological functions, ensuring the organism is synchronized with its environment (Vitaterna *et al.*, 2001; Froy, 2011). Daily rhythmicity is influenced by external factors, known as 'Zeitgeber' (i.e. timing-cues), such as ambient temperature and light–dark cycle (Piccione and Caola, 2002). The light–dark cycle is the dominant Zeitgeber entraining the daily rhythmicity of physiological and behavioural processes (Piccione and Caola, 2002; Dibner *et al.*, 2010). Disruption of daily rhythmicity is associated with health problems, reduced life expectancy and altered well-being (Vitaterna *et al.*, 2001; Froy, 2011). Thus, the study of behavioural and physiological daily rhythmicity in animals provides knowledge of their daily organization. The resulting findings are useful to ensure animals are managed in such a way as to meet their requirement of daily rhythms, safeguarding their welfare (Berger, 2011). This chapter focuses on the daily rhythms of behaviour in horses and on how real-time monitoring with modern smart technologies can be used to aid early identification of shifts in behaviour and, consequently, poor health and welfare.

Time Budget

Time budget means the amount of time horses spend in their various activities during a 24-hour period. Two main phases of circadian rhythms have been described: photo phase, or daylight, and scotophase, or dark period. Diurnal animals tend to be more active during the photophase (daylight) and nocturnal animals tend to be more active during the scotophase (dark period). Horses are diurnal animals with a circadian rhythm of both active and inactive behaviours. Horses are awake and alert for about 80% of daylight time.

During daylight, horses focus their time on foraging. Horses distribute their time between activities that allow them to satisfy their basic demands for food, water, movement and rest. The amount of time changes with the features of the environment, the time of year, gender and age. Horses spend about 90% of their time eating and resting, with considerable variation in the total time spent grazing. This is influenced by the environment: horses that have more availability of forage spend about 16–17 hours a day grazing, but, when forage is limited, this may extend to 19 hours (Mills and McDonnell, 2005).

Seasons also affect the amount of time for activities. For example, in winter, horses graze 79% of the time while, in summer, this reduces to 61%. At night they spend 54% of the time grazing and 40% resting. Time budgets for feral horses differ from those of domestic horses at grass. Feral horses spend 60% of their time eating, while domesticated horses in a single-box stall may spend only 16%, paying more attention to standing. Night feeding accounts for 23% of total feeding time in pastured fillies.

Resting time can be classified into stand-resting and lying. Lying occupies a small percentage of time; 10% for feral horses and 16% for the domesticated ones. Standing differs between feral horses, which stand for 20% of their time, and domesticated horses, which stand for 60%. Horses sleep mostly at night. They spend 30–40% of the dark period sleeping, but most of the sleep is slow-wave sleep with the horse standing. With the evolution of the horse from wild to domesticated, changes in their time budget have occurred. Horses average 2.5 hours sleep per 24-hour period; for most of the day they stand in boxes (Figs 4.1a and 4.1b) (Kiley-Worthington, 1999).

Relative to the natural grazing time, modern nutritional management is correlated with tangible

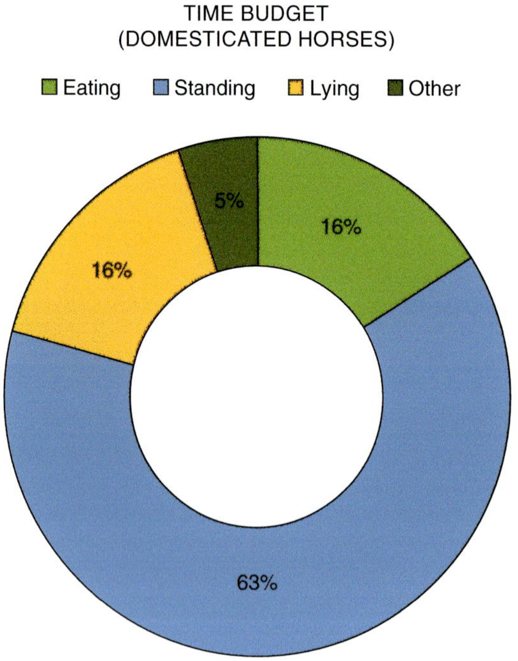

Figs. 4.1a. Time budget for domesticated horses. Adapted from Kiley-Worthington (1999).

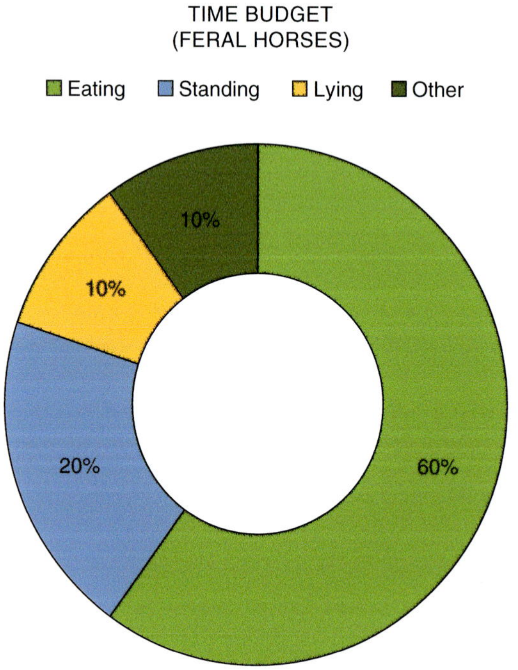

Figs. 4.1b. Time budget for feral horses. Adapted from Kiley-Worthington (1999).

differences in the nature, quantity and frequency of feed consumption in horses, and it can be hard to separate diet from other aspects of management (Hothersall and Nicol, 2009). The temporal distribution of feeding behaviour is of primary importance in horses; locomotor activity and the daily routine of maintenance behaviour depend on it. Changes in the diet reinforce the suggestion that diet is implicated in cribbing behaviour and could have important behavioural and physiological effects. Locomotory and oral stereotypes have been frequently observed among intensively managed horses as a result of unnatural management systems. Comparing horses housed in standard stalls with those kept in stalls with access to paddocks, locomotor activity shows that a diurnal pattern and the acrophase (i.e the cycle crest) always occurs in the middle of the photophase of the experimental photoperiod. In horses housed in stalls, locomotor activity is prevalent during the diurnal period. On the other hand, in horses kept in stalls with paddocks, the intensity of locomotor activity observed is lower but constant in its daily rhythm (Piccione and Giannetto, 2011).

Different stabling conditions influence time budgets in horses. Horses kept under natural temperatures and photoperiods in individual stalls with or without paddock access have different time budgets. After monitoring behaviours like feeding, drinking, walking, grooming and locomotor activity, it has been observed that, in both of these groups, activity during the light phase is significantly greater than that occurring during the dark phase. Activity in groups with paddock access is significantly lower than in the stall-housed-only groups during light and dark phases. Furthermore, in the group with paddock access, minor activity occurs between the 23rd hour and 2nd hour with major activity at the 8th hour. In the stall-only group, minor activity occurs between the 1st and 2nd hour and the major activity between the 7th and 14th hour. These findings outline a diurnal pattern of locomotor activity in horses, establishing that, for horses kept in different stabling conditions, the activity rhythm reaches its peak in the middle of the day, emphasizing stabling conditions' effects on locomotor activity rhythms (Piccione *et al.*, 2008).

To ensure a positive welfare status, housing and management practices must meet the daily behavioural needs of horses. The following section offers useful information for managing horses according to their circadian rhythms, allowing them to maintain homeostasis with minimum effort.

Inactive Behaviour

Inactive behaviour is defined as resting or sleeping. Sleep is a condition of decreased awareness of environmental stimuli that is distinguished from states such as coma or hibernation. It is also inversely related to the danger of predation for some species. For that reason, horses, which are prey animals, sleep less than predators, but more than smaller animals. They spend anywhere from 4 to 15 hours a day in standing rest and from minutes to several hours lying down. They are also known for drowsing and sleeping while standing (Chung *et al.*, 2018).

Sleep is a periodical and recurring state affecting the mind and body. It is divided into 'sleep of the mind', or slow-wave sleep (SWS), and 'sleep of the body', or rapid eye movement (REM). For the horse, this phenomenon alternates between stages of wakefulness and drowsiness. The four different states of vigilance have been studied using electroencephalogram technology for neural activity evaluation, recording electromyograms to measure skeletal muscular activity, electrooculograms to monitor eye responses, and electrocardiograms to track heart activity. From this work, wakefulness has been identified as the state in which horses stand and support their weight on all limbs unless actively moving around the stall. Drowsiness is defined as the state in which the weight of horses is supported on both thoracic limbs and one pelvic limb, with the head held above the withers. SWS is the state in which horses tend to lower their head and rotate their ears caudally or laterally. REM sleep occurs when the brainwaves paradoxically resemble normal wakefulness with the body completely relaxed. The latter only happens when horses lay down.

In another study, three different stable groups of horses were monitored (Chung *et al.*, 2018). They were fed concentrate and alfalfa hay either two, three or four times daily, but with the same daily activities. Horses were let into the paddock, groomed, and went for morning riding classes every day from 8 am to noon. They were observed over 12 hours a day for 6 days. Using body position as an indicator of sleeping state, equine sleeping behaviour was recorded. All horses rested when there were no stable activities, and the environment was quiet. Furthermore, during the day, they tended to stand, rest and forage in bedding materials. They slept on average for two hours after every feeding. At night they drowsed, foraged in bedding materials, and exhibited a recumbent position. The horses on different feeding regimens exhibited a different total sleeping time. Horses spent more time recumbent in larger enclosures than in smaller ones and feeding frequency and bedding affected horse resting behaviour.

Sleep frequency is affected by physiological variables, like hormones, by housing systems and horse management. If any of these factors are inadequate, sleep deprivation may occur. As previously stated, sleep is a behavioural state, homeostatically controlled and characterized by reduced movement and sensory responsiveness. A slight change in the physiological homeostatic state of the organism, induced by stress factors like an inadequate housing system, poor feeding techniques or aggressive behaviours within the herd, may lead to circadian rhythm sleep disorders (Fullagar *et al.*, 2015).

Sleep deficiency is linked to immune system dysfunction caused by increases in pro-inflammatory cytokines (Besedovsky *et al.*, 2019). Extreme cases of sleep loss can manifest with collapsing episodes (Aleman *et al.*, 2008). These tend to occur at night, matching the period of REM sleep (Fuchs *et al.*, 2018). The frequency of collapses is influenced by lying down behaviour, and horses that do not lie down while sleeping show a more frequent occurrence. Horses with this problem have altered sleeping behaviour, spending most of the time in light sleep and less time in SWS and REM sleep. Related injuries vary from fetlock abrasions to scars and swollen synovial bursae at the carpal and tarsal joints to head and tail fractures. These episodes are the result of a REM-sleep deficiency associated with recurrent sleep deprivation. Unfortunately, few data are available on cases and causes of collapsing episodes; a better understanding is needed.

Narcolepsy, a neurological sleep disorder that differs from sleep deprivation, is characterized by excessive daytime sleepiness, hypnagogic hallucinations, sleep paralysis and cataplexy. In adults, episodes occur only during rest periods (Fuchs *et al.*, 2015).

Sleep is fundamental for overall animal welfare. Possible causes of sleep disorders include environmental and housing conditions, isolation, dietary changes, and exhausting exercise activity. Therefore, providing appropriate housing, using proper feeding techniques, and preventing environmental stress are critical to ensure the horses' overall health.

Active Behaviour

Feeding behaviour

Feeding behaviours and feed intake are controlled by multiple homeostatic signals like hormones and somatosensory stimuli such as odour, taste and nutrients, and also by environmental parameters. An examination of feeding behaviours and food preferences provides some interesting insights (see Chapter 5). Preference testing has shown that nutrient content is a driver for diet selection and feed intake, as are taste and odour (van den Berg *et al.*, 2016). As large solid-hoofed herbivorous ungulate mammals, horses spend a significant amount of time feeding. The temporal distribution of feeding behaviour is of primary importance. The continuous feeding of hay has been shown to improve welfare, with an enriched behavioural repertoire characterized by more occurrence of relaxed behaviours and more positive social interactions. An optimal and appropriate feeding strategy is required to improve horses' welfare (Rochais *et al.*, 2018a).

Food intake shows a rhythmicity that is regulated by the circadian system and depends on the nature and availability of forage, the level of nutrient demand, and consumption behaviour. Although the diet of feral horses is fibre based because it consists of grass, in domesticated horses, the total ration is often not distributed *ad libitum*. Here different feed management conditions influence behaviour. For example, horses fed a concentrated diet spend only 3% of their time eating (Giannetto *et al.*, 2015). In comparison, the same researchers found that searching behaviour occupies 12% of the horse's time when the horses were fed with a pelleted diet and 1% when they fed on a hay-based diet.

It is important to highlight that feeding behaviours and feed intake are controlled not only by multiple homeostatic signals like hormones and somatosensory stimuli such as odour, taste and nutrients but also by environmental parameters. Grazing time and feeding behaviour are also influenced by ambient temperature

Explorative behaviour

The natural behaviours of horses include the necessity to investigate the environment. These behaviours include elements of exploration, hunting or foraging and other explorative interactions driven by curiosity, facilitating the learning of skills. Explorative behaviours are immediately present in foals, which are playful and curious. These include experiences of desire and appreciation accompanied by increased activity that is manifested as energized investigation and interaction with the environment (Mellor, 2015). The environment has a noteworthy effect on the health status and performance of animals, so providing a good environment for the young foal is essential for preserving their health throughout their adulthood (Šišková *et al.*, 2006). In particular, for feral horses, the exploration of their territory is vital for their survival since it allows them to acquire geographic information, the locations of water sources, and the distribution and types of vegetation and of other animals (Edwards, 2010). It also allows them to choose preferred sites to feed, rest and hide. The horse's harmony with its environment is partially dependent on adequate exploratory activities. The inability to explore (as frequently occurs with confinement in single stalls) may lead horses to display signs of apathy, boredom, low responsiveness and abnormal stereotypical behaviours (Mellor, 2015). As suggested throughout this chapter, to prevent such abnormalities and to maintain the welfare of the domesticated horses, group housing and pasture systems are preferred.

Social behaviour

Horses are social animals that are more secure with others and tend to live in bands. They follow a hierarchy that promotes stability and sets some rules that affect behaviour; higher ranks have priority access to resources. Therefore, the social order determines the order in feeding, defecation, sleeping and mating. The oldest mare guides the natal band; frequently, it is she that is the group leader. The stallion is normally the group coordinator, spending his time keeping the group together, and when the group moves, he tends to escort at the tail (McGreevy, 2012). Apart from the natal band, small bachelor groups may be formed by young stallions. Solitary animals are usually young females who have left the natal band to avoid inbreeding, a stallion who has lost his harem, or a stallion who has left the bachelor group to build a new natal band. As previously mentioned, social stability has a pivotal role in the welfare of horses. To establish social stability dominance behaviour may occur until the achievement of a stable social order. Giles *et al.* (2015) suggest a correlation between dominance rank and body weight, while in other studies, an association of age with rank is implied. Dominance relies upon leadership and may be viewed as a social impact in which prominent leaders seem to guide the actions of group members (Smith *et al.*, 2016; Hartmann *et al.*, 2017). Within social behaviour, there are other vital behaviours such as grooming and play.

Paddock size and housing conditions may lessen stereotypic behaviours and positively affect social relationships in domesticated horses. Social behaviour can be influenced by paddock size. The number of aggressive interactions is significantly reduced when horses are kept in paddocks, and the number of friendly interactions (including play) are significantly fewer in larger pastures or grass paddocks (Majecka and Klawe, 2018). Large paddocks make it possible for submissive horses to avoid the company of aggressive individuals, which prevent injuries (Majecka and Klawe, 2018). There are also significant differences between the stable systems. In active barns, where an automatic concentrate feeder was available, the activity level is much higher than in the open barns; increasing space results in increasing movement behaviour per hour (Rose-Meierhofer *et al.*, 2010). In conclusion, to prevent abnormal or aggressive behaviour, the choice of housing system is important. The frequent availability of a paddock of necessary size and the provision of food in several places in the paddock will improve horses' welfare. Having to move from one feed spot to another, and the freedom to ambulate at will, decreases physical and psychological stress and thus increases homeostaosis.

Grooming

Grooming occupies an important part of the daily time budget of horses. In feral horses, it expresses itself prevalently as rolling, but nibbling, rubbing and scratching also occur. For allogrooming, one horse approaches another and begins sniffing or nuzzling the approached horse along the dorsal surface of the body from the neck, over the withers and the back, to the rump. In some feral horses grooming behaviour has been observed at least once an hour, but others in the group may only participate with much lower frequency or not at all. The frequency of grooming changes during the seasons, peaking during spring (Wolter *et al.*, 2018). Since grooming is considered a behavioural need, horses must budget time for this behaviour. When this is not possible, owners should spend time grooming their horses every day (see Chapter 5).

Play

Play by young horses optimizes their coordination of movement and allows them to practise social behaviour. The drive to play is particularly dominant in foals since it provides for learning, enhanced social relationships, and the practice of the motor skills involved in these interactions (Cameron *et al.*, 2008). Play is especially important during early life because of its role in the development of the musculoskeletal system. Horses seem to be keen on playing with social partners, allowing them to form tight relationships (Keeling and Gonyou, 2001).

Locomotory behaviour and exercise

Locomotion is the preeminent factor that allows feral horses the ability to satisfy hunger and thirst. In contrast, domesticated horses often suffer limited movement because they are housed in single stalls. Limited movement can result in a series of problems associated with the locomotor system itself. The main locomotor activity is provided by physical exercise (Padalino *et al.*, 2014). Different exercise intensity affects body temperature, heart rate, arterial pressure, and other biological variables. Piccione *et al.* (2009) observed a change of these parameters during the morning and the afternoon hours, with all variables being greater in the afternoon at rest and in response to the same exercise.

Padalino *et al.* (2014), investigated the effect of two types of exercise and racing on behavioural patterns of horses housed in single stalls. Their experiment showed an increase in heart rate with daily training (40 min at a slow trot) that was lower than that induced by maximal exercise and racing over 1600 m. Moreover, time spent on drinking is higher in horses after racing, while explorative behaviour is not affected by exercise.

The time spent in the stable, and consequently the time spent on locomotory activities, may affect the occurrence of abnormal behaviours. Stereotypies that involve locomotory movements where the animals repeatedly walk from one point to another include pawing, weaving and stall walking (Hanis *et al.*, 2020). Locomotion stereotypies are predominantly observed in a confined stable environment in association with inadequate physical exercise. It is clear that adequate stabling conditions and adequate exercise are critical to prevent abnormal locomotory behaviours that frequently happens because housing conditions do not often meet the natural needs of horses (Ransom and Cade, 2009). Locomotor activity, in particular of feral horses, should occupy the third largest amount of the daily time budget of horses. To guarantee and provide equivalent welfare to domesticated horses, a transfer to group housing systems or pasture shows positive effects on the activity of horses with increasing movement behaviours (Rose-Meierhofer *et al.*, 2010).

Technological Advances for Monitoring Behaviour and its Rhythms

With the increasing emphasis on animal welfare and the necessity to monitor health and well-being, precision livestock farming (PLF) supported by new 'smart' technologies is gaining acceptance. These allow the continuous acquisition, processing and analysis of data relative to the animal and its environment. PLF is aimed at the optimum management of the animal through access to new services such as animal localization, individual feeding and health monitoring. The results allow more efficient management by combining an animals' welfare and time productivity (Terrasson *et al.*, 2017).

In contrast to previous approaches, PLF systems offer real-time monitoring 24 hours a day through cameras or sensors applied on the animal's body. Over the last decade, various technologies have been developed to monitor the welfare of animals, improve health and traceability and ensure good performance. Technological development and progress have advanced to such an extent that accurate, powerful and affordable tools are now available (Berckmans, 2014). These include cameras, microphones, sensors (such as 3D accelerometers, temperature sensors, skin conductivity sensors and glucose sensors), wireless communication tools, internet connections and cloud storage.

Slow and automatic feeders

Feeding techniques are important to prevent or reduce the frequency of stereotypies. Controlling and managing the quantity and speed at which horses eat has become important. To address these needs, slow and automatic feeders have been introduced. Slow-feeders present special grates or nets (hay bags) to the horse, and are designed to hold better the hay, or balls that release small doses of food (Turner, 2010). This helps to avoid episodes of choke and overeating. The positive effect of slow feeders on the general well-being of the horse and on its mental state has recently been highlighted (Mazzola *et al.*, 2016; Rochais *et al.*, 2018a). Horses spend more time eating when their ration is placed in hay bags or slow feeders to distribute pellets than when the hay is simply distributed on the ground in the stable. However, stereotypies and stress-related behaviours are more frequent when the horses are fed from hay bags rather than slow feeders. Evidence suggests that slow-feeders reduce stereotypies and enhance horse–horse as well as horse–human interactions. More relaxed behaviours have been observed, highlighting that the temporal distribution of feeding behaviour is important. These findings emphasize the need to identify optimal feeding strategies and ways to improve the well-being of horses in confined housing. Slow feeders have recently been shown to have positive health benefits for horses housed in stalls. When compared to commonly practised twice daily feeding, horses fed via a slow feeder had fewer and less severe gastric ulcers (Bass *et al.*, 2018). Automatic feeding shortens fasting time between feeds, leading to a reduction in the presence of gastric ulceration. Their use can help prevent the beginning of serious diseases, especially in young horses. For the horse carer and breeder, behavioural management of the animal becomes easier.

Wearable heart rate monitors

Heart rate (HR) and heart rate variability (HRV) provide estimates of responses to the autonomic nervous system regulation of cardiovascular function. HRV is useful to determine the neurophysiological response to stressful situations. In horses, HRV fluctuates in response to foaling, weaning, road transport and stabling system changes (Ille *et al.*, 2014). Analysis of these data provides physiological parameters on which to base interventions to improve animal health and welfare. An innovative approach, using smart textile electrodes, has been tested to monitor cardiac activity in horses under various conditions, providing better quality electrocardiogram (ECG) traces for monitoring HR and HRV (Guidi *et al.*, 2017).

One type, Smartex® srl electrodes, collect fewer corrupted ECG segments than standard silver (Ag/AgCl) electrodes. This crucial advance allows better quality ECG collection while eliminating the need for glue or cohesive bandages. Therefore Smartex® srl electrodes provide a more versatile wearable tool for investigations of equine behaviour, emotion and welfare. This monitoring system could provide reliable information on the mood and state of arousal of horses (Guidi *et al.*, 2017).

Even if less accurate than ECG, Polar® heart rate monitors have been used in many behavioural studies. For example, the HR, heartbeat-to-beat (RR) times, and HRV of warmblood horses have been investigated over 24 hours (Janczarek *et al.*, 2020). Using this approach substantial differences between the time and frequency of HRV parameters were found in older horses compared with younger ones. Significant decreases in HR and an increase in the time interval between HR peaks were noticed in old horses during the night, while this interval decreased during the day, suggesting a need for special care in handling older horses to ensure their relaxation.

Wearable electroencephalography

Electroencephalography (EEG) is a diagnostic tool that detects electrical problems associated with brain activity, identifying neurological diseases and attentional states (Williams *et al.*, 2008). It is a non-invasive method for measuring the bioelectric activity of the central nervous system, most often used to diagnose neurological disorders. Introduced to veterinary anaesthesiology, EEG has resulted in a drastic and positive change in anaesthetic management and in the study of sleep patterns in animals (Drewnowska *et al.*, 2019). EEG is a precise tool, but it requires the absence of movement, which is impossible to achieve in conscious animals. A growing welfare awareness has pushed researchers to study and develop non-invasive EEG systems that consider the well-being of the animal (Cousillas *et al.*, 2017).

Interest in equine behaviour has resulted in recent studies that seek to understand how the lateralization of the brain affects the expression of social interactions and intense emotional states such as aggression, escape behaviour and fear (Farmer *et al.*, 2018; Rochais *et al.*, 2018a). Using observational methods, Farmer *et al.* (2018) reported uniform and meaningful bias to the left that was affected by herd rank, age, sociability or sex. For example, grooming behaviours are lateralized to the left. A pivotal role of the right hemisphere on social interactions and emotions was suggested, but further research on the role of sensory laterality in affiliative behaviour is required. Contemporaneously Rochais *et al.* (2018b) explored the role of laterality on the attentional state of horses. Using an attention test to measure the visual attentional responses of horses towards standardized stimuli, and a portable EEG telemetric tool to measure brain responses, beta and the gamma waves that showed higher awareness states were obtained. The sight of an unknown but not frightening element caused an increase in gamma wave activity in the right hemisphere. At the same time, lack of interest was associated with the alpha and beta waves in the left hemisphere.

D'Ingeo *et al.* (2019) tested brain lateralization and emotional processing in the human–animal relationship. To better understand the reaction of horses to the human voice, they submitted 21 horses to a positive or negative experience during which they were hearing one of two different human voices. When an associative memory of the experience was established, a test condition was conducted and horses' lateralized responses to the acoustic stimuli were examined through EEG technique. Results showed that horses can distinguish different human voices and react to them positively or negatively based on their previous experience. This was also confirmed by EEG results that highlighted an increase in gamma activity in the right hemisphere in response to the positive voices associated with palatable food. Opposite changes in wave power were observed when horses interpreted as 'negative' voices associated with the provision of unpalatable food soaked in vinegar.

The direct role of humans in the welfare of horses in some respects is a new frontier of research. Further investigation of the lateralization of brain responses accompanied by EEG measurements are needed to highlight the valence of interactions on sensory memories and the potential in predicting affective states, acute emotions and long-lasting moods. EEG recordings will be a vital tool for future studies aiming to introduce further the EEG technique in precision livestock farming (PLF). The approach will improve the ability to evaluate vigilance states, especially sleep, and to diagnose sleep disorders such as narcolepsy, determining a possible REM phase deficit.

Equiwatch system

The EquiWatch System® (EWS) records the frequency and duration of grazing activity, bite and chew acts. It allows the study of the feeding behaviour of horses by accurately counting the amount of prehension by the animal. Behavioural variables like feeding time and other nonfeeding jaw movements are also recorded. For example, using this technology, it has been shown that horses spend more time in motion on pasture than when fed only hay, and more time feeding on pasture than on hay (Weinert *et al.*, 2020). Therefore, forage type affects natural equine feeding behaviours, highlighting the potential of EWS to monitor horse nutrition, health and management. Not only can EWS be used to document feeding patterns, but it may provide an alert to anorexia or other feeding anomalies, colic, fever, pain or sickness.

Pedometers, accelerometers and wearable GPS

Monitoring horse activity is helpful to improve animal welfare, using technologies such as pedometers, accelerometers and wearable GPS. Since 2016 a wearable GPS monitoring device, HoofStep®, has been available. It is designed to map the perimeter of the farm allocated to the horse, allowing carers to obtain and interpret the horse's movements and behaviours and inform them of any abnormal behaviour. Burla *et al.* (2014) tested the suitability of an MSR145 accelerometer for automatic gait determination comparing the results with those obtained with an ALT-Pedometer. The accelerometer was more useful because of increased sampling ability, identifying gaits despite the exercise type, ground speed and direction of movement.

Equisense® is another device to monitor horse activity that permits the recognition and recording of gait. However, it necessitates the purchase of extra hardware that connects to the saddle girth. Equisense® provides riders with feedback of their training by recording and transferring data in real-time to an app that analyses their entire training performance, including the distance, speed and time at each gait (Brauch, 2020). Motor activity can also be tracked by Seaver®. This device consists of a girth strap with embedded sensors and records the efforts of the horse, monitors and anticipates anomalies (Seaver, 2018). Other devices include Equilab, a free smartphone app that gives riders feedback concerning their training session, and Estride, a platform that uses sensors located on the legs of the horse embedded into protective boots (Estride Media, 2019).

In contrast to the above devices, Orscana® analyses movement using sensors that lie underneath the horse's blanket by the hollow of the hip. It allows riders to better understand the type of rug to put on horses, taking into account the weather and the well-being of the animals. It has demonstrated its utility in analysing day and night activity, providing handlers with instant information on the horse's comfort according to the temperature and humidity of its environment (Arioneo, 2019).

Welfare Implications

Meeting the daily behavioural needs of horses is essential to safeguard their physical and psychological well-being. Housing, feeding and overall management should be synchronized as closely as possible to the innate circadian rhythms of horses. New technologies are available to continuously monitor the behavioural and physiological parameters of domesticated horses. They may be useful for the early detection of shifts from normality, health and behavioural issues. However, to date, only a few technologies have been validated. Many of them are complex and require a connection to the internet or power. Although their use is not yet common, they may be critical tools for the future of enhanced equine management and welfare.

References

Aleman, M., Williams, D.C. and Holliday, T. (2008) Sleep and sleep disorders in horses. *Neurology* 54, 180–185.

Arioneo (2019) How to monitor the temperature of your horse with Orscana? Available at: https://training.arioneo.com/en/orscana-horses-connected-sensor/ (accessed 21 January 2022).

Bass, L., Swain, E., Santos, H., Hess, T. and Black, J. (2018) Effects of feeding frequency using a commercial automated feeding device on gastric ulceration in exercised Quarter Horses. *Equine Veterinary Science* 64, 96–100.

Berckmans, D. (2014) Precision livestock farming technologies for welfare management in intensive livestock systems. *Revue Scientifique et Technique* 33, 189–196.

Berger, A. (2011) Activity patterns, chronobiology and the assessment of stress and welfare in zoo and wild animals. *International Zoo Yearbook* 45, 80–90.

Besedovsky, L., Lange, T. and Haack, M. (2019) Sleep-immune crosstalk in health and disease. *Physiological Reviews* 99, 1325–1380.
Brauch, S. (2020) Equisense; Sensor or coach - Why choose? Available at: https://blog.equisense.com/en/sensor-or-coach/ (accessed 21 September 2021).
Burla, J.B., Ostertag, A., Westerath, H.S. and Hillmann, E. (2014) Gait determination and activity measurement in horses using an accelerometer. *Computers and Electronics in Agriculture* 102, 127–133.
Cameron, E.Z., Linklater, W.L., Stafford, K.J. and Minot, E.O. (2008) Maternal investment results in better foal condition through increased play behaviour in horses. *Animal Behaviour* 76, 1511–1518.
Chung, E.L.T., Khairuddin, N.H., Azizan, T.R.P.T. and Adamu, L. (2018) Sleeping patterns of horses in selected local horse stables in Malaysia. *Journal of Veterinary Behaviour* 26, 1–4.
Cousillas, H., Oger, M., Rochais, C., Pettoello, C., Menoret, M. *et al.* (2017) An ambulatory electroencephalography system for freely moving horses: An innovating approach. *Frontiers Veterinary Science* 4, 57.
Dibner, C., Schibler, U. and Albrecht, U. (2010) The mammalian circadian timing system: organisation and coordination of central and peripheral clocks. *Annual Review of Physiology* 72, 517–549.
D'Ingeo, S., Quaranta, A., Siniscalchi, M., Stomp, M., Coste, C., *et al.* (2019) Horses associate individual human voices with the valence of past interactions: a behavioural and electrophysiological study. *Scientific Report* 9, 11568.
Drewnowska, O., Lisowska, B. and Turek, B. (2019) What do we know about the use of EEG monitoring during equine anesthesia: A review. *Applied Science* 9, 3678.
Edwards, L.N. (2010) Animal wellbeing and behavioural needs on the farm. *Improving Animal Welfare: A Practical Approach*. CAB International, Wallingford, UK.
Estride Media (2019) Estride trackers. Available at: www.estride.store/trackers (accessed 21 September 2021).
Farmer, K., Krüger, K., Byrne, R.W. and Marr, I. (2018) Sensory laterality in affiliative interactions in domestic horses and ponies (*Equus caballus*). *Animal Cognition* 21, 631–637.
Froy, O. (2011) Circadian rhythms, aging, and life span in mammals. *Physiology* 26, 225–235.
Fuchs, C., Kiefner, L.C., Reese, S., Erhard, M.H. and Wöhr, A.C. (2015) Narcolepsy - or REM-deficient? In: Krüger, K. (ed.) *International Equine Science Meeting 2015*. Wald, Germany, pp. 6–17.
Fuchs, C., Kiefner, L.C., Kalus, M., Reese, S., Erhard, M. *et al.* (2018) Polysomnography as a tool to assess equine welfare. *11th International Conference on Methods and Techniques in Behavioral Research.* Manchester, UK.
Fullagar, H.H.K., Skorski, S., Duffield, R., Hammes, D., Coutts, A.J. *et al.* (2015) Sleep and athletic performance: The effects of sleep loss on exercise performance, and physiological and cognitive responses to exercise. *Sports Medicine* 45, 161–186.
Giannetto, C., Fazio, F., Alberghina, D., Panzera, M. and Piccione, G. (2015) Meal size and feeding management strategies influence the daily rhythm of total locomotor activity in horses (*Equus caballus*). *Biological Rhythm Research* 46, 537–543.
Giles, S.L., Nicol, C.J., Harris, P.A. and Rands, S.A. (2015) Dominance rank is associated with body condition in outdoor-living domestic horses (*Equus caballus*). *Applied Animal Behaviour Science* 166, 71–79.
Guidi, A., Lanata, A., Valenza, G., Scilingo, E.P. and Baragli, P. (2017) Validation of smart textile electrodes for electrocardiogram monitoring in free-moving horses. *Journal of Veterinary Behavior* 17, 19–23.
Hanis, F., Chung, E.L.T., Kamalludin, M.H. and Idrus, Z. (2020) Discovering the relationship between dietary nutrients on cortisol and ghrelin hormones in horses exhibiting oral stereotypic behaviour: A review. *Journal of Veterinary Behavior* 1–33.
Hartmann, E., Christensen, J.W. and McGreevy, P.D. (2017) Dominance and leadership: Useful concepts in human–horse interactions? *Journal of Equine Veterinary Science* 52, 1–9.
Heidemann, S.R. (2007) The cell. In: Cunningham, J.G. (ed.) *Veterinary Physiology*. Saunders Elsevier, Amsterdam.
Hothersall, B. and Nicol, C. (2009) Role of diet and feeding in normal and stereotypic behaviors in horses. *The Veterinary Clinics of North America* 25, 167–181.
Ille, N., Erber, R., Aurich, C. and Aurich, J.E. (2014) Comparison of heart rate and heart rate variability obtained by heart rate monitors and simultaneously recorded electrocardiogram signals in non-exercising horses. *Journal of Veterinary Behavior Clinical Applications and Research* 9, 341–346.
Janczarek, I., Kedzierski, W., Wilk, I., Pawlak, E.W. and Rakowska, A. (2020) Comparison of daily heart rate variability in old and young horses: A preliminary study. *Journal of Veterinary Behavior Clinical Applications and Research* 38, 1–7.
Keeling, L.J. and Gonyou, H.W. (2001) *Social Behavior in Farm Animals*. CABI International, Wallingford, UK.
Kiley-Worthington, M. (1999) *The Behaviour of Horses in Relation to Management and Training*. Trafalgar Square Books, North Pomfret, Vermont, pp. 284.
Majecka, K. and Klawe, A. (2018) Influence of paddock size on social relationships in domestic horses. *Journal of Applied Animal Welfare Science* 21,1, 8–16.
Mazzola, S., Palestrini, C., Cannas, S., Fè, E., Bagnato, G.L. *et al.* (2016) Efficacy of a feed dispenser for horses in decreasing cribbing behaviour. *Veterinary Medicine International* 1–6.
McGreevy, P. (2012) *Equine Behavior: A Guide for Veterinarians and Equine Scientists*. Elsevier-Saunders, St. Louis, MO, pp. 119–150.

Mellor, D.J. (2015) Positive animal welfare states and encouraging environment-focused and animal-to-animal interactive behaviours. *New Zealand Veterinary Journal* 63, 9–16.

Mills, D. and McDonnell, S.M. (2005) *The Domestic Horse: The Origins, Development and Management of its Behaviour*. Cambridge University Press, Cambridge.

Padalino, B., Zaccagnino, P. and Celi, P. (2014) Effect of different types of physical exercise on the behavioural and physiological parameters of standardbred horses housed in single stalls. *Veterinary Medicine International* 2014, 1–8.

Palmer, J.D. (2002) *The Living Clock: The Orchestrator of Biology Rhythms*. Oxford University Press, Oxford.

Piccione, G. and Caola, G. (2002) Biological rhythm in livestock. *Journal of Veterinary Science* 3, 145–157.

Piccione, G. and Giannetto, C. (2011) State of the art on daily rhythms of physiology and behaviour in horses. *Biological Rhythm Research* 42, 67–88.

Piccione, G., Costa, A., Giannetto, C. and Caola, G. (2008) Daily rhythms of activity in horses housed in different stabling conditions. *Biological Rhythm Research* 39, 79–84

Piccione, G., Giannetto, C., Assenza, A., Casella, S. and Caola, G. (2009) Influence of time of day on body temperature, heart rate, arterial pressure, and other biological variables in horses during incremental exercise. *Chronobiology International* 26, 47–60.

Ransom, J.I. and Cade, B.S. (2009) Quantifying equid behavior - A research ethogram for free-roaming feral horses. *Geological Survey Techniques and Methods 2-A9* 23, 1–21.

Refinetti, R., Cornélissen, G. and Halberg, F. (2007) Procedures for numerical analysis of circadian rhythms. *Biological Rhythm Research* 38, 275–325.

Rochais, C., Henrya, S. and Hausberger, M. (2018a) “Hay-bags” and “Slow feeders”: Testing their impact on horse behaviour and welfare. *Applied Animal Behaviour Science* 198, 52–59.

Rochais, C., Sébilleau, M., Menoret, M., Oger, M., Henry, S. *et al.* (2018b) Attentional state and brain processes: state-dependent lateralisation of EEG profiles in horses. *Scientific Report* 8, 10153.

Rose-Meierhofer, S., Klaer, S., Ammon, C., Brunsch, R. and Hoffmann, G. (2010) Activity behavior of horses housed in different open barn systems. *Journal of Equine Veterinary Science* 30, 624–634.

Seaver (2018) Understanding Seaver's “Heart Rate” Feature. Availableat:www.seaverhorse.com/en/understanding-seavers-heart-rate-feature/ (accessed 21 September 2021).

Šišková, P., Jiskrová, I. and Mikule, V. (2006) An ethological study of young horses. *Acta Universitatis Agriculturae Et Silviculturae* 5, 129–136.

Smith, J.E., Gavrilets, S., Mulder, M.B., Hooper, P.L., El Mouden, C. *et al.*, (2016) Leadership in mammalian societies: emergence, distribution, power, and payoff. *Trends in Ecology & Evolution* 31, 54–66.

Terrasson, G., Villeneuve, E., Pilnière, V. and Llaria, A. (2017) Precision livestock farming: A multidisciplinary paradigm. *The Sixth International Conference on Smart Cities, Systems, Devices and Technologies* 55–59.

Turner, J. (2010) Controlled hay feeder. Available at: https://patents.justia.com/inventor/julie-turner (accessed 21 January 2022).

van den Berg, M., Giagos, V., Lee, C., Brown, W.Y., Cawdell-Smith, A.J. *et al.* (2016) Influence of odour, taste and nutrients on feeding behaviour and food preferences in horses. *Applied Animal Behaviour Science* 184, 41–50.

Vitaterna, M.H., Takahashi, J.S. and Turek, F.W. (2001) Overview of circadian rhythms. *Alcohol Research and Health* 25, 85–93.

Weinert, J.R., Werner, J. and Williams, C.A. (2020) Validation and implementation of an automated chew sensor–based remote monitoring device as tool for equine grazing research. *Equine Veterinary Science* 88, 102971.

Williams, D.C., Aleman, M., Holliday, T.A., Fletcher, D.J., Tharp, B. *et al.* (2008) Qualitative and quantitative characteristics of the electroencephalogram in normal horses during spontaneous drowsiness and sleep. *Journal of Veterinary Internal Medicine* 22, 630–638.

Wolter, R., Stefanski, V. and Krueger, K. (2018) Parameters for the analysis of social bonds in horses. *Animals* 8, 191.

5 Ingestion, Elimination and Comfort

Christopher B. Riley BVSc(Hons), PhD, Diplomate ACVS*

Massey University, Palmerston North, New Zealand

Introduction 61
Food Ingestion 62
  Behaviour and motivation 62
  Grazing 63
  Concentrates 68
  Welfare 69
Drinking 70
  Behaviour 70
  Welfare 70
Elimination 70
  Behaviour 70
  Defecation 71
  Urination 71
  Welfare 72
Comfort 72
  Grooming 72
    Behaviour 72
    Welfare 73
  Pandiculation 74
  Thermoregulation and shelter 75
    Behaviour 75
    Welfare 77
References 77

Introduction

Body maintenance behaviours rely upon a range of adaptations that confer specific evolutionary advantages for equine survival and well-being. In terms of neurophysiology, these behaviours may be viewed as fixed, heritable responses to stimuli. However, this does not preclude the ability to respond to novel stimuli. Learning and memory contribute to modifications that reinforce the motivations underpinning behaviours and the fulfilment of emotional needs (Peters *et al.*, 2012). This chapter focuses on behaviours that maintain physiological homeostasis, including ingestion, elimination and comfort. The latter includes grooming (hair and skincare) and sheltering behaviours that support thermoregulation and provide refuge from biting insects (Keiper and Berger, 1982; Hartmann *et al.*, 2015a). The maintenance behaviours of foals, including suckling, transitional eating and pandiculation, are discussed in Chapter 11.

*Corresponding author: c.b.riley@massey.ac.nz

DOI: 10.1079/9781789242133.0005

Food Ingestion

Behaviour and motivation

The eating behaviours of horses are the most heavily researched of the maintenance behaviours (Beaver, 2019). Past research has been heavily weighted towards evaluating the nutrient or management value of pasture species and feedstuffs. Now, feed preference testing and choice evaluation (e.g. social interaction versus food availability) uses food motivation to study equine behaviour (Müller and Udén, 2006). Ingestive behaviours and associated actions include suckling, grazing and browsing, intake of pasture or grain-based processed feeds, exploration of novel feedstuffs, salt licking, drinking, and chewing and swallowing.

Anatomic structures provide for energetically efficient and safe grazing for long periods. For example, the long nuchal ligament extending from the withers to the skull base allows suspension of the head in a low grazing position without fatigue. The placement of the eyes distant from the muzzle provides for surveillance for predators while grazing. The stay apparatus of the hind limbs facilitates energy conservation by allowing the stifle to be locked while standing. These adaptations bear witness to the evolution of the horse as a grazing species.

The centre for motivation and the regulation of hunger is located within the hypothalamus, with input from other centres within the brain (see Chapter 3). Feeding behaviour is strongly influenced by reinforcement, positive and negative, food palatability, environmental and social associations (Giraldeau and Caraco, 2000). For example, young foals learn much about grazing from their mothers, optimizing reward-seeking and reinforcing behaviours (Fig. 5.1). Concepts of motivation, learning

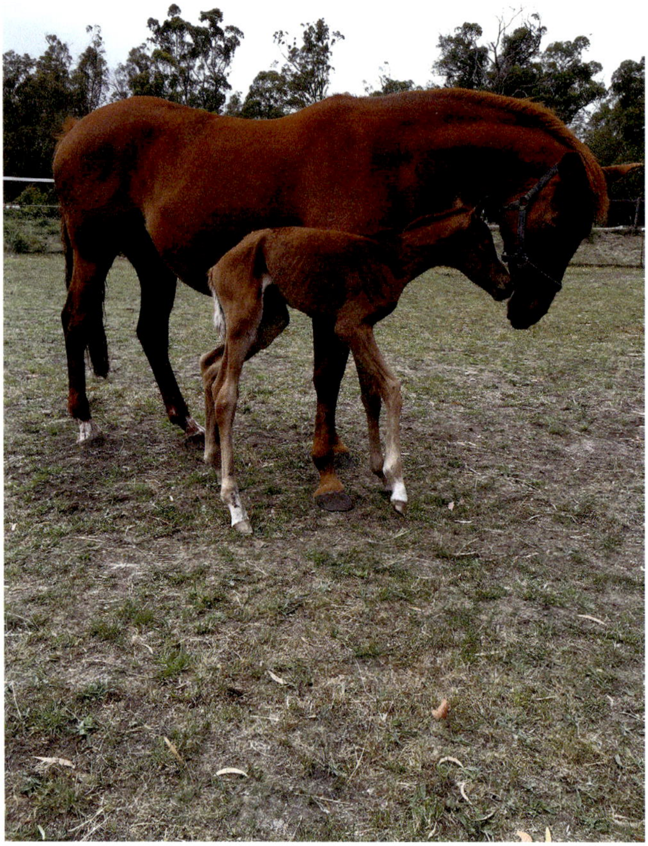

Fig. 5.1. Foals learn much about grazing from their mothers. Photo: author.

and reinforcement must be considered with food intake (Toates, 2002; Hogan, 2005). When feed motivation is combined with learning and reinforcement, horses develop anticipatory behaviour associated with auditory and visual cues before presenting the food (Peters *et al.*, 2012). This anticipatory behaviour is also influenced by the horse's internal circadian clock (Giannetto *et al.*, 2019). Nutritional deficiencies, in general, do not appear to have specific homeostatic methods of self-correction, and generalized food deprivation causes behaviours that may or may not appropriately address the deficiency (e.g. pica). Except for salt, the ability of the horse to correct specific mineral deficiencies is generally poor (Fraser, 2010).

Neurohormonal responses drive homeostatic mechanisms that preserve blood volume and tissue perfusion (see Chapter 3). Stable concentrations of solutes within the circulation maintain a constant plasma osmolality and sufficient fluid volume for tissue perfusion. The solutes include salts, notably sodium chloride. When depleted, serum osmolality is lowered, stimulating a physiologically driven desire by the horse to ingest salt. For this reason, freely available salt licks are well used by domestic horses. Other trace elements (e.g. selenium) that might not otherwise be ingested are incorporated into these licks. In free-ranging horses, the appetite for salt leads to active searches over considerable distances to known salt lick locations. Grazing horses with access to the seashore forage below the high tide line frequently ingest seaweeds or lick other salted materials (Fig. 5.2). Thirst, on the other hand, is driven by an increase in plasma osmolality. A rise of 3% or more stimulates drinking (Sufit *et al.*, 1985).

Grazing

Grazing is the primary ingestive behaviour of horses at pasture. It provides all the required nutrients for feral or wild equids and many pasture-managed domestic horses (Hoskin and Gee, 2004). This activity is performed with the head down, extending from the neck (Fig. 5.3). Depending on the pasture length, the lips and incisors are used to tear off the grass as close to the base as possible. The grass is moved between the cheek teeth where

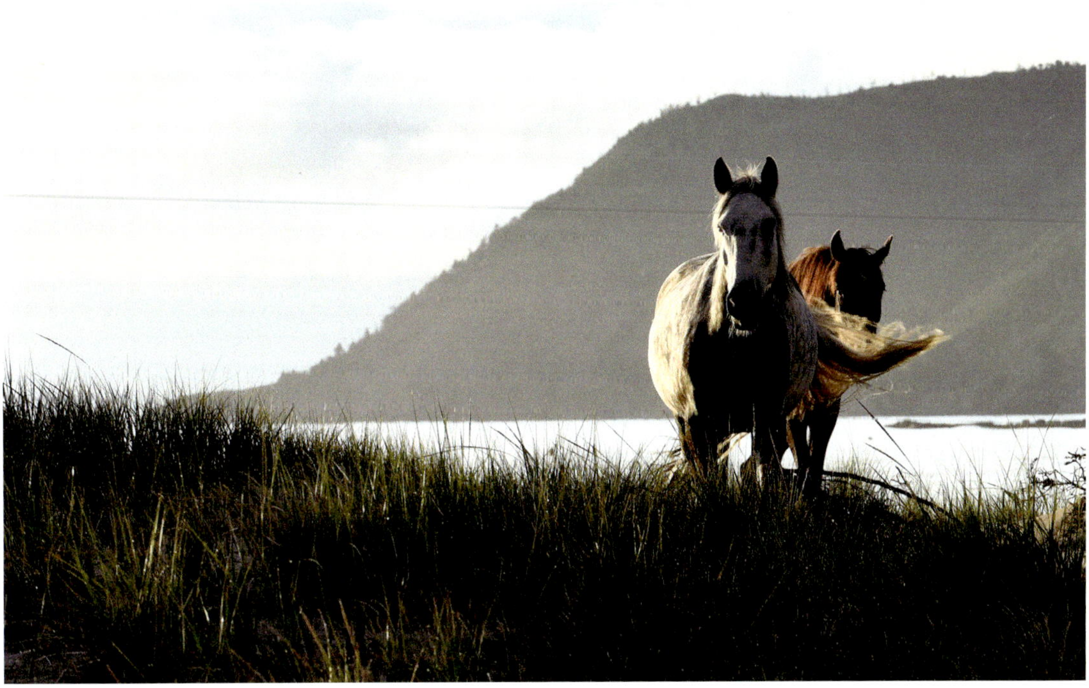

Fig. 5.2. The semi-feral horses of the islands of Saint-Pierre and Miquelon forage among salt-covered grasses in the sand dunes. Photo: Pascale Carrère.

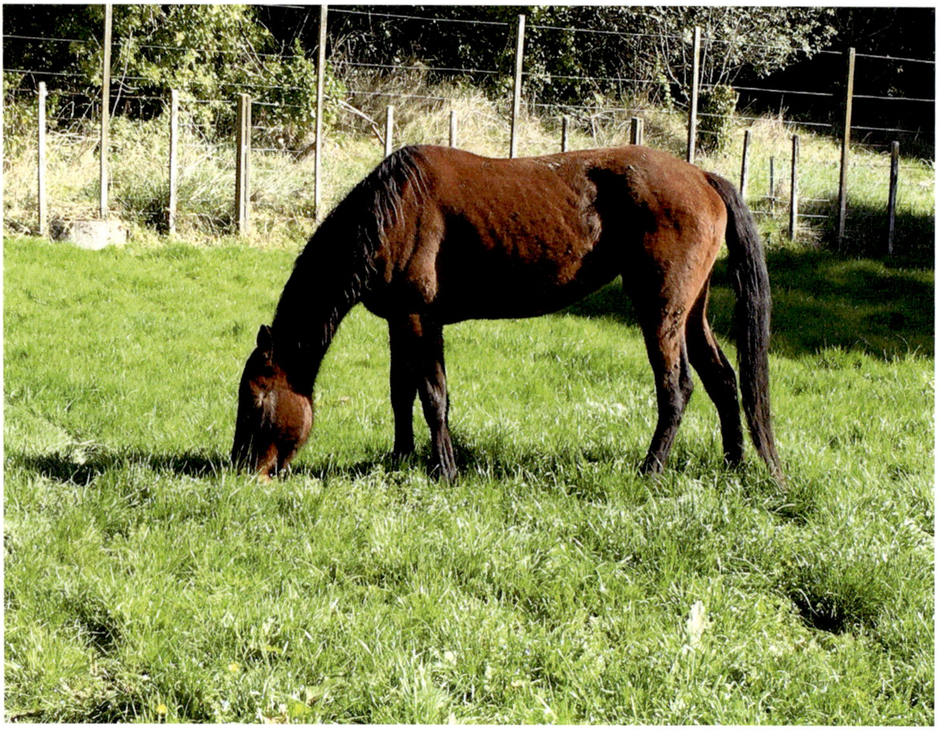

Fig. 5.3. Grazing is the primary ingestive behaviour of the horse. Photo: author.

it is mechanically broken down, mixed and buffered with saliva. The tongue is then used to form a food bolus that is swallowed. The horse steps forward to continue grazing with the head moving left or right depending upon which forelimb is advanced. Monitoring for predators is facilitated by moving into the wind. The grazing rate is influenced by the density and quality of vegetation and the observation of other horses grazing (Sweeting *et al.*, 1985). Appropriate management of horses at pasture provides for maintenance while creating a suitable environment for locomotory activity and social interactions.

Horses are discriminatory grazers and selective in their choice of pasture species, with preferred grasses grazed until they are no longer available. Grass species vary among geographic regions. In the Southern Hemisphere, there is a preference for tetraploid ryegrass over Yorkshire fog and cocksfoot. The ryegrasses contain a higher percentage of soluble carbohydrates and a greater percentage of digestible organic matter; these are well correlated with the grazing preferences of the horse (Randall *et al.*, 2014). In North America, alfalfa, timothy, and coastal bermudagrass are commonly grown, with horses preferring alfalfa to other grasses as a more digestible and palatable food (La Casha *et al.*, 1999).

Another driver for moving on to less preferred grazing is displacement by a high-ranking herd mate. Horses with the highest social rank have more opportunity to graze preferred areas than those ranked lower (Ingolfsdottir and Sigurjonsdottir, 2008). When moved on to the less preferable grasses, horses tend to consume higher fibre foods, increasing grazing time. In situations of drought where there may be no preferred grass species, horses consume pasture species of lower nutritional value or those with possible toxicity. Plant-related toxicities are more commonly encountered in drought conditions, posing a welfare concern for horses and ponies with no alternative sources of nutrition.

Selectivity in grazing is also influenced by faecal contamination. If there is sufficient grazing area, horses will not eat within a metre of faeces, guided by their sense of smell (Rogers *et al.*, 2018). This results in under-grazed areas known as 'roughs' and more heavily grazed areas called 'lawns', giving the pasture an uneven appearance. If the stocking density on the pasture is high, horses are forced to feed closer to the faeces (Fig. 5.4). This increases the risk of ingesting the larvae or eggs of intestinal parasites associated with the faeces. For foals, such infections markedly compromise their welfare. When assessing the suitability of pasture, the presence of roughs must not be included as available pasture, and stocking densities must be adjusted accordingly.

Horses, and particularly ponies, show a preferential selection of alternative sources of fibrous matter. They can eat hedges, dead nettles and fallen leaves, particularly in autumn and winter. In situations of restricted grazing, they also eat tree bark, de-barking them to a height of 2 m or more. Poplar bark is a top choice, and ash, oak and rowan are also favoured. Occasionally, horses nibble off small branches of trees. The seeds, leaves, or bark of yew, oak, black walnut, red maple and sycamore are toxic to horses and may result in death.

In summer, horses spend approximately 50–60% of their time grazing during the day; less at night (40–50% of the time) (Boyd *et al.*, 1988; Maisonpierre *et al.*, 2019). The ratio of day-to-night grazing is affected by hot weather, and heat and fly attacks adversely affect summer grazing activity. During hot days, horses will focus on grazing earlier in the morning, and less during the afternoon, particularly if seeking shelter from biting insects. More frequent night grazing occurs in summer than in other seasons, while cold and wet spells of winter weather reduce grazing activity. In the latter case, this may be due to a lack of food availability or increased time seeking the comfort of shelter.

In temperate climates, pasture growth peaks in the late spring with a smaller peak in autumn, whereas in cooler climates, there may only be one peak in the spring. After the peak, there is a steady decline in the quality and nutritional value of pasture. In temperate climates, more than 75% of horses are kept at pasture or provided access year-round (Thompson *et al.*, 2017). Nevertheless, 70% of these horses receive supplementary feed, including concentrates and hay, particularly during times of poorer pasture quality or availability. In stabled horses or cooler climates without year-round access to the pasture, there is a reliance upon processed or stored grasses (hay, haylage or silage) and concentrate feeding (Müller and Udén, 2006). The harvesting of hay for storage and later feeding is the most common form of pasture conservation. Depending upon species and climate, one or two cuts are taken from the same pasture. Sun drying in the field is the most economical processing method, but it is dried in a barn

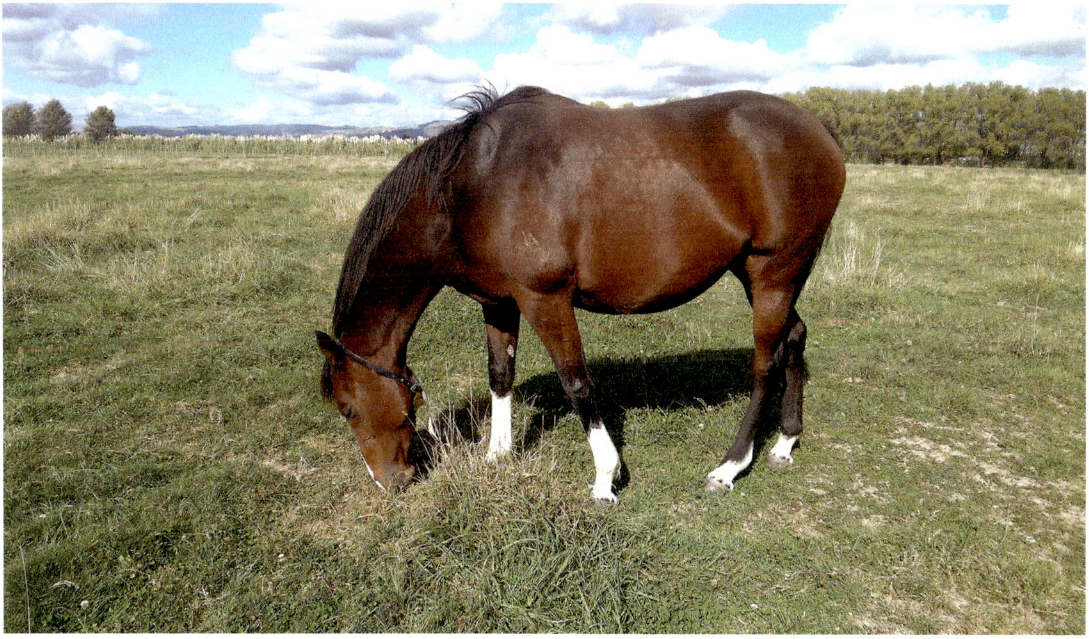

Fig. 5.4. A horse grazes next to a rough because of overgrazing of the lawns. Photo: C. Rogers.

in some countries. Once dry, the hay is packaged into a small or large square or large round bales. Bales are protected from sunlight and moisture to minimize deterioration and mould growth, slowing the decline in nutritional value. Correct storage reduces the oxidation of beta carotenes and the decline of other essential nutrients. For a healthy 500 kg horse, hay is fed at 8–12 kg per day depending on the nutrient concentration and digestibility of the hay and its physical activity level (Table 5.1) (Geor, 2013). The balance of the ration includes mineral or trace element supplements, vitamin A, and vitamin E.

Hay contaminated with noxious weeds during harvesting creates a welfare concern. Additionally,

Table 5.1. Examples of diets based on hay as the source of forage with additional supplementation depending upon the physiological status of the horse. All diets except for the weanling diet are based on a horse bodyweight of 500 kg, per day. Adapted from Geor, 2013.

Adult maintenance	
Grass hay based maintenance diet	Legume (clover or alfalfa/lucerne) based maintenance diet
12 kg good meadow hay containing 8% crude protein 30 g salt (NaCl) 100 g trace element/vitamin supplement (copper, zinc, selenium, vitamins A and E No grain or other concentrates	12 kg mature legume hay 30 g salt 80 g mineral supplement
Adult with heavy exercise or work schedule	
Grass hay plus grain option	Grass hay plus concentrate option
10 kg good meadow hay 2 kg oats 0.5 kg vegetable oil (e.g. corn oil) 120 g trace element/vitamin supplement 60 g salt	10 kg good meadow hay 4 kg commercial concentrate 60 g salt
Pregnant mare during the last month of gestation	
Grass hay plus grain option	Grass hay plus concentrate option
8 kg good meadow hay (minimum) 1 kg barley 0.5 kg linseed meal 150 g trace element/vitamin supplement 60 g salt	8 kg good meadow hay (minimum) 2.5 kg concentrate containing 18% crude protein
Lactating mare (two months postpartum)	
Grass hay plus grain option	Grass hay plus concentrate option
12 kg good meadow hay 4 kg corn (flaked) 1 kg linseed meal 150 g trace element/vitamin supplement	8 kg good meadow hay (minimum) 5 kg concentrate containing 16% crude protein
Weanling (six-month-old and approximately 250 kg)	
Grass hay plus concentrate option	Alfalfa hay plus grain option
4 kg good meadow hay 2.5 kg concentrate	4 kg alfalfa hay (first cut) 1.5 kg oats 0.5 kg sugar beet pulp 0.1 kg vegetable oil 0.2 kg soybean meal 80 g trace element/vitamin supplement

if it is incorrectly stored and becomes mouldy, there are risks of toxicity if ingested and chronic respiratory disease if inhaled. The country of origin and the pasture species greatly influence the nutritional value of forages. Therefore, if only hay is fed to the horse, feed analysis is performed to ensure that the hay can safely meet the horse's nutrient requirements. If it is not, then supplementation to meet the nutrient deficits is required.

Ensiling is another forage conservation practice widely used for livestock and, increasingly, horses (Müller and Udén, 2006). Cut pasture is fermented under anaerobic conditions, during which the soluble carbohydrates undergo microbial conversion to organic acids such as lactic acid. Bales of harvested pasture, usually round, are plastic wrapped for the process (Fig. 5.5). This process takes about 21 days, at which point microbial growth stops, and the forage is preserved. Haylage has a moisture content of between 15 and 40% (60–85% dry matter [DM]). Silage has a moisture content of greater than 40% (DM < 60%). These forages are fed more commonly during the winter months when pasture is unavailable and if horses are stabled without pasture access. Of the conserved forages, horses have a taste preference for silage over haylage and hay. Once horses learn to recognize the smell and taste of silage, they are preferentially motivated to consume it. In common with hay, feed analysis is recommended to ensure its nutritional value. A welfare risk is posed by ensiled forage when it contains rotten or poorly fermented areas. This occurs when contaminants, including soil, faeces or dead rodents, are harvested with the forage. These areas are then more likely to contain clostridial organisms, including botulism, that may be fatal to the horse.

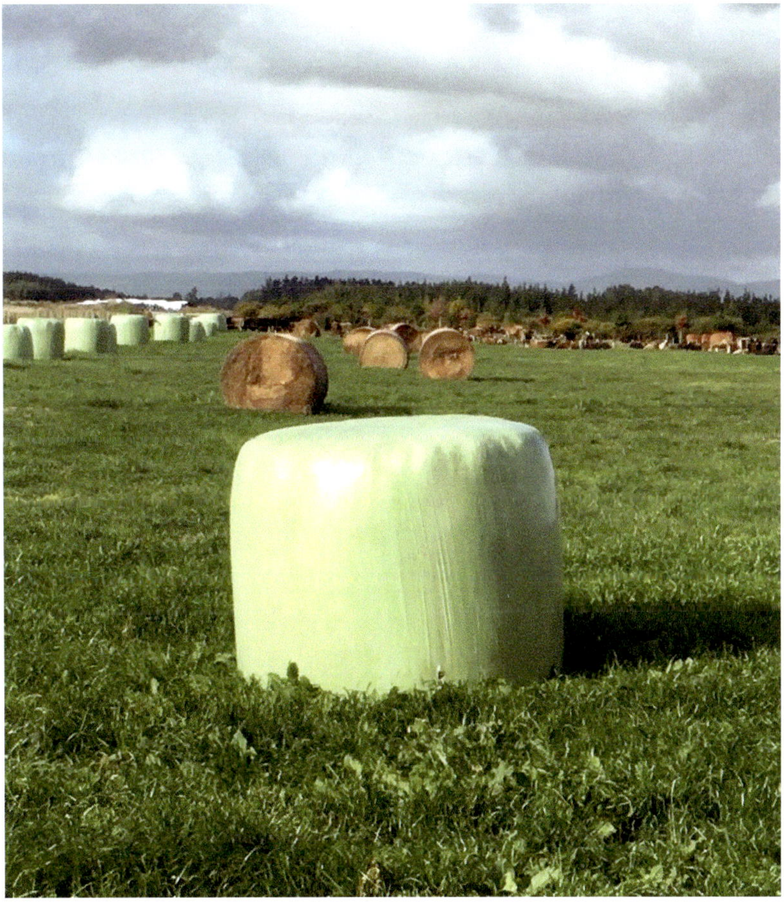

Fig. 5.5. Round bales of plastic packaged haylage (foreground) and unpackaged hay (background). Photo: author.

Concentrates

Cereal grains, their byproducts, and commercial feeds produced from grains (concentrates) provide concentrated sources of energy, protein and other nutrients. Although they may be consumed in their natural state when grazing summer pastures, their provision in harvested form has developed with the domestication of the horse. Differences in nutritional properties are related to differences in grain species or varieties and climate (Table 5.2) (Lindberg, 2013). The feeding of concentrates allows for control of the feeding regimen and nutrition of the horse, particularly when they do not have access to good-quality pasture or have higher nutritional needs for performance, growth or lactation. They provide a concentrated energy source in support of thermal homeostasis during winter. When cereal grains are included within a formulated commercial concentrate, vitamin and mineral needs are also added. A smaller feed storage area and ease of distribution are additional benefits. However, in most situations where grains or concentrates are relied upon as the main source of nutrients, stabled horses cannot express normal foraging behaviours.

Most horses fed a mixed forage with oats, barley or rice as a cereal source have a sufficient source of high-quality protein. Table 5.2 provides a summary of the concentration of major nutrients available in commonly fed grains. Caregivers seeking more information about the appropriate feeding and nutrition of horses should consult one of the reference books available (e.g., Geor, 2013). Wheat has the highest protein content, followed by oats and barley and is lowest in rice and maize. However, the percentage of lysine relative to crude protein means that the quality of the protein is highest in oats, followed by barley and rice (Table 5.2). Diets based on wheat or maize may require supplementation with lysine. For lactating mares, a mixed forage with cereal grains is likely to require an additional source of protein (e.g. lupin seeds). Oats and maize have higher fat content than the other grains, which is helpful when reducing carbohydrate as a source of energy. Cereal grains may be rolled, crushed, dehulled, cooked, germinated or otherwise processed to increase digestibility, nutrient availability and for their inclusion in concentrate products. The byproducts of grain used in distilleries have also been used to supplement feeds. These additives are characterized by high crude protein concentrations, fat and fibre, with low levels of starch and sugars.

There are significant risks to the welfare of horses with feeding grain-based feeds, and their ingestion is recognized as an important cause of gastrointestinal disease in the horse (Lopes, 2008). The gastrointestinal tract of the horse has evolved to digest the high-fibre plant materials found in pastures. The enzymes secreted by the salivary glands, stomach, pancreas and small intestine hydrolyse the nutrients in grasses to make them available for absorption. Grains and concentrates require less mastication, and are therefore less buffered by saliva, and leave large amounts of hydrolysed nutrients that are readily fermented in the large intestine, producing gas. This can lead to

Table 5.2. Dry matter nutrient composition of grains commonly fed to horses. Adapted from Sauvant *et al.*, 2004.

		Barley	Maize		Oats		Rice		Wheat	
Component	Units	Grain	Grain	Bran	Grain	No hull	Grain	Bran	Grain	Bran
Starch	g/kg	602	742	340	411	614	882	304	697	227
Sugars	g/kg	24	18	25	12	14	5	32	28	77
Crude protein	g/kg	116	94	123	111	124	153	160	121	170
Lysine	% CP	3.8	3.0	3.7	4.2	4.2	3.7	4.4	3.1	3.9
Crude fat	g/kg	21	43	41	55	29	14	182	17	39
Crude fibre	g/kg	53	25	146	138	47	13	87	25	106
Neutral detergent fibre	g/kg	216	120	594	372	135	59	227	143	455
Digestible energy	Kcal/kg	3511	3798	2627	3129	3511	3750	3392	3678	2794
	MJ/kg	14.7	15.9	11.0	13.1	14.7	15.7	14.2	15.4	11.7
Metabolizable energy	Kcal/kg	3272	3630	2365	2842	3272	3678	2938	3463	2412
	MJ/kg	13.7	15.2	9.9	11.9	13.7	15.4	12.3	14.5	10.1

CP = crude protein; Kcal = kilocalories; MJ = megajoules.

gastric dilation or tympany of the large intestine, causing colic (abdominal pain), impairing gastrointestinal blood perfusion, and inducing respiratory distress. Motility of the gut may also be altered and result in displacement or volvulus (twisting) of the large intestine. The horse's gastrointestinal tract has a unique ecosystem of microorganisms that aid in digestion and gut health. Feeding concentrates has a profound effect on these organisms due to the lactic acid produced and other changes associated with ingestion of large amounts of digestible carbohydrates (Table 5.3). These negative effects are proportional to the amount of grain fed, and the abruptness with which it is introduced to the horse's diet. For that reason, the introduction of grain or concentrates should occur slowly over a minimum of 2–3 weeks to allow adaptation of the gut and its microflora. The direst consequences occur when horses accidentally access large amounts of grain or other forms of highly digestible carbohydrate (e.g. bakery waste). These horses can become profoundly depressed with severe colic, laminitis and diarrhoea. All are life-threatening conditions requiring emergency veterinary treatment.

Welfare

Feeding practices have raised several welfare challenges. Grazing pasture allows for the normal ingestive behaviours that have evolved with the horse. However, it may increase their exposure to infection with parasites compared to stabled horses and to ingestion of pasture-associated toxins in some regions (Hoskin and Gee, 2004). Horses that are stabled or in yards without access to pasture spend considerably less time foraging and consuming roughage. As described above, negative effects may be compounded by a diet rich in concentrates. Even when fed hay in the stable, a considerably lower percentage of the horse's time is spent eating because there is less scope to explore its preferences. Concentrates require less time for consumption and result in substantial changes to the microflora of the gut (Table 5.3). In addition to the gastrointestinal changes, the combination of stabling and reduced foraging increases the risk of developing stereotypical behaviours. Some issues are moderated by more frequent feeding, but the total time taken to consume the feedstuffs is unlikely to be impacted, and there is a risk of overnutrition. Consumption can be significantly slowed, and the time spent on this activity increased when the hay is placed within overlapping hay nets (Ellis *et al.,* 2015). Straw bedding has been suggested to engage horses in foraging, but horses that consume significant amounts of bedding have a higher risk of small colon impaction. Draught horses and American Miniature Horses are at a higher risk in this regard.

In both Northern and Southern Hemispheres, horses and ponies receive supplementation with concentrates despite having access to adequate hay or pasture (Hoffman *et al.*, 2009; Thompson *et al.*, 2017). In parallel with the human population, overfeeding has resulted in increased obesity in horses and ponies (McCue *et al.*, 2015). Obesity is a risk factor for pasture-associated laminitis in ponies. The fat deposits associated with obesity in areas

Table 5.3. The effects of grain ingestion on the microflora and biochemistry of ingesta in the large intestine. Modified from Lopes and Johnson, 2017.

Acute or chronic	Numerical decrease	Numerical increase
Hours after the sudden ingestion of grain	Gram-negative rods	Bacterial population
	Enterobacteriaceae species	*Lactobacillus* species
	Streptococcus species (aerobic)	Microbial population associated with starch digestion
	Streptococcus species (anaerobic)	Concentrations of volatile fatty acids
	Microbial population associated with fibre digestion	Concentration of lactate
	Protozoa	Concentration of endotoxin[a]
	Acetate	
	pH	
	Organic matter digestibility	
On a diet with chronic ingestion	Digestibility of organic matter	Lactate processing bacteria
		Digestibility of fibre (forage)

[a]Increases the risk of colic, diarrhoea, laminitis.

such as the crest of the neck, behind the shoulder and around the tail head are risk factors for equine metabolic syndrome. This syndrome refers to a cluster of abnormalities associated with an increased risk of laminitis. Laminitis is a life-threatening disease in which the laminae of the hooves become markedly inflamed and painful, resulting in acute or chronic lameness. Although obesity is only one risk factor for equine metabolic syndrome, it is one that can be managed by the caretaker providing appropriate exercise and avoiding overfeeding. For ponies and some horse breeds, it may mean limiting the duration of grazing at pasture. Grazing muzzles allow for foraging while reducing intake by at least 30%. Exercise in situations where horses are paddock managed can be encouraged by locating the water and feed sources distant from each other.

Drinking

Behaviour

Water consumption is essential for body maintenance. Although the horse has substantial homeostatic mechanisms to conserve water, losses associated with elimination, sweat and exhalation must be replaced. A small amount of water is absorbed from plants, depending on the species and season, but most comes from natural or human-supplied water sources.

With an open water source, horses contact the water with a partially closed mouth and suck it in (Schöning, 2008). The horse extends its neck slightly, the tongue presses on the top of the mouth, and the horse swallows. Horses usually drink 15–20 swallows per drinking bout at two second intervals, 5–7 times a day in the warmer months, and 2–3 times in winter. Foals rarely drink water, obtaining most of their fluid intake from the dam's milk. In arid or free-ranging environments, horses may have access to water only once or twice a day, usually in the early morning or evening. The frequency of drinking is determined by the distances between grazing, shelter and water sources. These horses may spend up to 30 minutes at the water source and consume most of their daily water intake at these times. The maintenance water requirement of adult horses is 50–60 mL/kg of body weight (25–30 L per day for a 500 kg horse), whereas foals require 100–120 mL/kg. Physiologic conditions requiring an increased water intake include high workloads and lactation. Environmental conditions increasing water intake include high ambient temperature and high humidity.

Interestingly, water consumption in summer weather is not improved if the water is chilled (McDonnell and Kristula, 1996). In contrast, the consumption of continuously heated water is 40% greater in sub-zero temperatures (Kristula and McDonnell, 1994). Fluid losses significantly increase when horses have an illness that increases the respiratory rate or sweating and medical conditions such as diarrhoea. The latter situation requires urgent veterinary attention to address fluid and electrolyte losses. Ill horses are often too depressed to increase their water intake to meet the faecal losses.

Welfare

The source of water has significant welfare implications for the horse. Horses relying upon natural water bodies risk encountering pollutants in waterways that course through urban areas. In rural areas relying upon dams and water troughs, dead animals in the water pose a risk of exposure to botulism, salmonellosis and other disease-causing organisms. There is a risk of algal blooms in the dams or water pools in some geographic regions, which are extremely toxic. Therefore, water sources should be checked daily, and any pollutants removed. Where water is provided via tanks or other containers with the flow regulated by a floating stopcock, their function must be checked daily to ensure that they fill these reservoirs. In stables or stalls, water is provided either through an automatic drinker or in buckets or similar containers. Some horses have difficulty with automatic drinkers. When introducing them to horses, it is wise to offer water in a bucket at the same time until they are seen to use the drinker. The volume of the bucket should be sufficient to contain the water required for the period between replenishing. Buckets should be cleaned and disinfected between feedings. Water provided should be potable; where this is not possible, regular water quality testing is suggested. Tethered horses are frequently provided with inadequate free access to clean water (Mullan *et al.*, 2014).

Elimination

Behaviour

The behaviours associated with elimination rid the body of the waste products of digestion and metabolism.

Urination and defecation also have social functions related to marking and communication through odour. Faeces also provide the microbiota foals require as their digestive tract matures and adapts to the ingestion of pasture.

Some behaviours occur with the elimination of both faeces and urine. Domesticated horses kept in paddocks use latrine areas and, unless pasture is scarce, do not graze within a metre of the area (Rogers et al., 2018). Adult horses usually interrupt grazing to defecate in a latrine area (rough) but less frequently leave the grazing area to urinate (Ödberg and Frances-Smith, 1977). Geldings and mares walk to the latrine and stop just as they enter and eliminate at the periphery, slowly enlarging the diameter of the area (Beaver, 2019). Stallions are more likely to urinate or defecate within the latrine. The translation of this behaviour to housed environments means that many horses eliminate in the corner of the stall or box. A more random elimination pattern occurs if the horses are under stress, depressed or ill. Free-ranging or feral horses are less likely to interrupt grazing to defecate and urinate (Lamoot *et al.*, 2004).

Purposeful elimination is performed for scent marking, preceded by olfaction. Stallions smell the faeces and urine of mares for longer but do not preferentially defecate on the deposits of other stallions or mares within their herd (Jezierski *et al.*, 2018). However, stallions do observe, investigate, and exclusively mark mares' faeces with urine (McDonnell, 1986). They show a similar response to the excretions of oestrus mares compared with those in dioestrus and are more responsive during breeding seasons (Marinier *et al.*, 1988). Mares preferentially mark the faeces or urine of other mares and foals within their herd. This behaviour is more focused on mares within the herd that have close social bonds and increases in the absence of the stallion (Tučková *et al.*, 2018). The faecal deposits of geldings are often more randomly deposited in the long grass. In the foals of wild equids, olfaction is associated with marking behaviour (Pluháček *et al.*, 2019). They are more likely to smell and eliminate on the faeces or urine of their dam. In novel social environments, horses spend more time sniffing the faeces of horses that have displayed aggressive behaviours towards them (Krueger and Flauger, 2011). Horses do not normally lay down where they have excreted.

Defecation

Horses defecate an average of 6–12 times per day, depending on the nature of the feedstuff consumed. Faeces are passed without posturing, apart from tail elevation, normally without straining. In the case of stallions and mares, the muscles of the perineum contract following defecation and the tail is lashed several times downwards. Horses with obstruction of the rectum, rectal trauma or diarrhoea may strain. In normal health, the faeces are passed in the form of substantial accumulations of compacted balls that are mid-brown to olive green in colour, according to the type and quality of material eaten. The faecal mass is dry to semi-moist within and often breaks up when it falls to the ground. Small amounts of fluid may be observed with the faeces when the horse defecates in response to stress (e.g. road transport) or as an early sign of colonic impaction. Faecal balls coated with small stringy fibrinous material occur with a delayed intestinal passage, as seen with colon impactions.

Urination

Normally, urination occurs 3–6 times per day. Stallions and geldings adopt a characteristic stance while urinating; the hind legs are abducted and extended so that the back becomes hollowed (Fig. 5.6). Urination takes place with the penis released from the sheath. Afterwards, the stallion usually smells the area before walking away. The mare does not show the same marked straddling posture; nevertheless, the posture is similar. Following urination, the vulva of the mare contracts (winks). Broodmares with young foals and mares in oestrus show more elaborate patterns of urination. Mares in oestrus urinate in limited quantities frequently. They straddle and eject mucoid urine in an oestrous display, including tail arching with the toe of one hind hoof touching the ground as that leg is abducted. Each ejection causes splashing of the clear fluid. This eliminative behaviour continues for the 4–10 days of oestrus. Late pregnant mares periodically straddle, strain and pass small quantities of urine in the first stage of labour.

Most urination occurs during rest periods in the hours of darkness. Normal urine production for adult horses is 15–30 mL/kg per day (1.5–3% of body weight). However, the urinary output varies with the physiological state of the horse. When

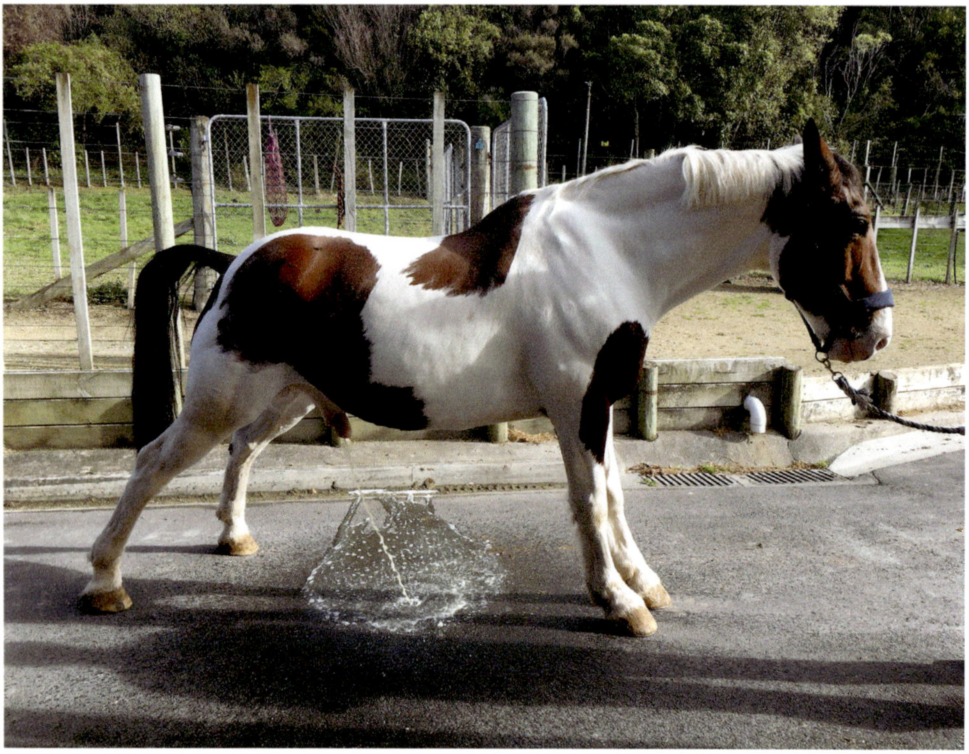

Fig. 5.6. A gelding posturing during urination. Photo: author.

dehydrated, urine volume is reduced, and the concentration of waste products within increased. Domesticated horses can usually be induced to urinate when they are led into a stall deeply bedded in fresh straw. Signs of abnormal urination include dribbling blood during or at the end of the stream, small volume, frequent urination episodes, straining and vocalization when urinating. Each of these signs warrants a veterinary examination.

Welfare

The welfare issues associated with elimination are largely associated with difficulties imposed by human management. Increased contact with faeces facilitates greater infection with the eggs and larvae of gastrointestinal parasites (Fleurance *et al.*, 2007). This is more likely to occur in situations of overstocking or overgrazing. Effective manure management in pastures requires the removal or dispersal of manure and exposure to sunlight. Stall bedding should be changed regularly to prevent the build-up of noxious odours.

Comfort

Grooming

Behaviour

Grooming behaviour is a comfort behaviour that also facilitates social interaction. There are three horse-initiated techniques: self-grooming, grooming using inanimate objects and allogrooming. Horses spend approximately 4% of their daily time in self or mutual grooming (Boyd *et al.*, 1988). Human grooming of horses provides comfort in situations when horses cannot interact with others or achieve fulfilment through their own efforts. The functions of grooming behaviours include responses to itching, the maintenance of skin health and social interaction through allogrooming. It removes sloughing skin and hair, distributes skin oils, including those containing pheromones, and removes biting and blood-sucking ectoparasites. Evidence for the latter function of grooming is lacking for the horse, and rubbing is more often due to itching resulting from an immune response after bites (Wilson, 2014).

Self-grooming, especially around the hip and flank, is commonly practised using the teeth, tongue, and upper lip. Horses do not use their tongues to clean out their nostrils as do cattle; instead, they snort to do so. Self-grooming is done by turning the neck, extending the head, and repeatedly nibbling at the skin in these regions. Horses occasionally groom their limbs, fore and hind, by nibbling or snapping. Foals self-groom more frequently than their dams, 6–8 times more often during the second month of life, and 3–4 times more during 5–6 months of age (Crowell-Davis, 1987). Foals are more likely to scratch their head and neck with a hind limb or bite and stretch the trunk and hindlimbs with the teeth. Mares are more likely to use inanimate objects or other herd mates and spend more time rolling.

The use of inanimate objects occurs when horses have access to suitable locations. Horses can groom their crest, top line and rump by rubbing them to and fro beneath a manger or tree branch. Rolling is related to coat care and drying to remove sweat or other moisture, utilizing the ground to rub the dorsal surface of its own body (Fraser, 1980). A layer of dust forms on the back, providing some protection from the sun and insects. Rolling also plays a role in stretching the muscles of the spine, neck, thorax, flanks and buttocks (Matsui *et al.*, 2009). The horse often rolls before rising from a lying position, flexing its limbs against the body and rolling about on the topline as it does so. When the rolling ceases, the horse rises, stands squarely and performs the 'wet-dog shake'. A wave of rippling skin passes from the head to the hindquarters, legs and tail, dislodging matter from the hide and hair in this manoeuvre. Loose soil or bare ground is preferred, usually in a specific location in the paddock to which they return. In insect-ridden areas or hot weather, this may be a mud wallow. Free-ranging herds may engage in a mutual rolling session, with the dominant stallion going last, leaving his scent. Horses frequently rub against trees, fences, water and feed troughs. An inverted U-shaped structure with broom heads with stiff bristles attached to the underside of the upper beam can be built for horses. Horses and cattle soon learn to use this manufactured scratching post. Horses scratch the buttocks and tail head against inanimate objects. However, excessive scratching of this area may be associated with irritation from pinworm eggs deposited by the parasite on the perineum.

Allogrooming is mutual grooming between horses that share a close association or bond. This practice is demonstrated early in life and is of evolutionary significance. In terms of neurophysiology, mutual grooming initiates the release of endorphins, resulting in reward and reinforcement of the motivational pathways that initiate allogrooming (VanDierendonck and Spruijt, 2012). In free-ranging horses, allogrooming reduces individual stress and herd tension and injury from conflict within the herd. It is practised by two horses standing alongside each other, facing head to tail. The tail swishing across the face of the other helps to keep insects at bay. Horses engage in active nibbling, with a focus on the mane, neck and withers. This form of grooming provides the benefits of self-grooming. More importantly, it facilitates social cohesion and companionship. Surprisingly, this form of grooming is not influenced by social rank within the herd (Kimura, 1998). Foals commence allogrooming within weeks of birth. Fillies are more likely to interact with their dam when allogrooming, whereas colts predominately focus on yearling fillies (Rho *et al.*, 2007). Groups of mostly young horses and small herds practise more frequent allogrooming (Sigurjónsdóttir and Haraldsson, 2019). Mutual grooming is more common in summer than in winter. Fences do not overcome the drive for allogrooming (Fig. 5.7).

Welfare

If grooming has individual comfort and herd benefits, then it follows that individually housed horses without access to allogrooming are more likely to suffer from stress. Similarly, if horses are aged or debilitated, they may not perform or complete self-grooming activities that benefit their welfare. Therefore, the human caregiver must assume responsibility for assisting the horse in obtaining the benefits of grooming. The objectives in human-provided grooming are hygienic, physiological and aesthetic, with the probable provision of some sensory satisfaction to the horse. Human-delivered massage decreases stress-related behaviour and the equine heart rate when delivered in preferred and nonpreferred areas (McBride *et al.*, 2004). Additional welfare benefits to the horse of human-assisted grooming include deepening the human–animal bond and improved handling as a horse becomes accustomed to the routine procedure. It also provides the opportunity for the careful observation of injury or

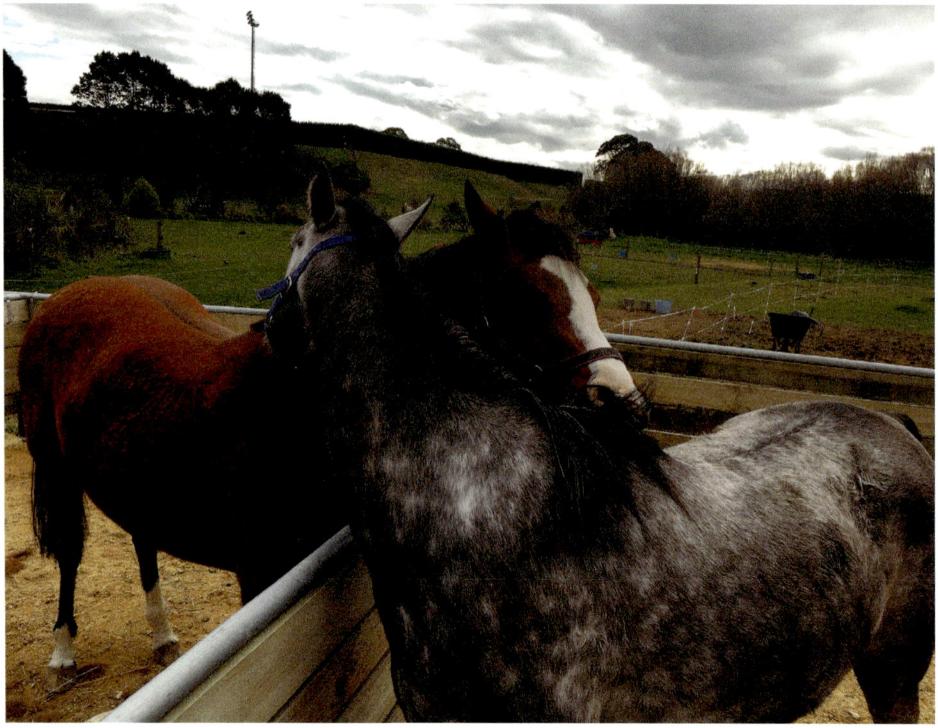

Fig. 5.7. Allogrooming mare and gelding. Photo: author.

ectoparasites and their management, removal of loose hair and skin debris, and circulation of the oils secreted by sebaceous glands. Grooming tasks include: picking debris out of the feet; brushing the coat with firm and soft brushes depending on the horse's comfort level and the amount of skin debris, and brushing tangles and debris out of the mane, forelock and tail. Readers less familiar with routine grooming protocols are directed to the many books available on basic horse care.

Pandiculation

Pandiculation is a somatic form of body care referring to systematic stretching associated with transitions between cyclic biological behaviours, most commonly the sleep-wake rhythm (Bertolucci, 2011). The general way horses stretch themselves in a stationary position shows that equine stretching actions have much consistency. In its various forms, pandiculation appears to function as an expression of well-being, especially in foals. The stimulus to pandiculation is assumed to be feedback from stiffness. Stretching and then relaxing muscles allows for them to be more rapidly responsive. The phenomenon at times may be in response to a period of asymmetry in position.

As a comparative phenomenon, pandiculation has a core of common actions that characterize the behaviour (Table 5.4). These include extending the forelimbs, extending the hindlimbs, extending the head and neck upwards or forward, flexing the vertebral column by arching it regionally, stiffening the trunk and periodic yawning. These behaviours generally have a high degree of consistency. Variations such as the absence of yawning or exertion at only one pole of the body occur (i.e. anterior or posterior). Equine pandiculation can have symmetry in the simultaneous or alternating extension of limb pairs. All four limbs cannot easily be fully extended simultaneously in the standing position, but this is possible in lateral recumbency. In this latter situation, the tensile form of the phenomenon is most evident (Fraser, 1989). During pandiculation, the musculature is stretched, and the connective tissues surrounding the joints are placed under tension. Considerable articulation extension and/or flexion of the atlantooccipital joint occurs. Other

Table 5.4. Features associated with pandiculation in the horse. From Fraser, 1989.

Feature	Interpretation
Polarity	The action pattern has direction relative to the body's long axis with recognition of the horse as outstretched, upraised, anterior or posterior
Position	Pandiculation can occur in an upright stance or lateral recumbency
Totality	Pandiculation may encompass all the activities described (complete) or some of the activities (partial)
Periodicity	Pandiculation is associated with cyclic activity, including sleep–wake cycles; it frequently occurs after rising from sternal recumbency
Illness and recovery	Horses, especially the young, are less likely to display pandiculation when ill. Restoration of normal pandiculation is expected on recovery
Age	Young animals more completely and frequently demonstrate pandiculation
Confinement	Recovery from confinement, where there is insufficient space for full extension of body and limbs, often manifests as pandiculation on release
Comfort	After pandiculation, the state of relaxation and awareness suggests some degree of comfort. A neurohormonal response is yet to be confirmed

major joints involved in fully extended articulations are the shoulder, elbow, carpus, stifle and tarsus. Stretching also stiffens the extremities and trunk. In such patterns of stretching, the musculature, tendons and articulations involved are, in general, used in equine locomotion.

Yawning occurs with body-stretching episodes, or it may occur alone. When it happens with generalized pandiculation, it is called the stretch-yawning syndrome (Bertolucci, 2011). It affects the muscles of the mouth, respiratory system, and upper spine. Its form is slow and displays maximal extension of the temporomandibular joints, critical for ingestive behaviours. An interesting minor feature in this stretching is eye closure during the activity. The eyes are closed for saccadic suppression to allow the activity without opposing visual signals interrupting the process. Slow movement also overcomes any influence from optomotor feedback, which functions to correct the body's position. The centre of gravity and body angles change during bodily stretching. Finally, the body-based (somatic) character of pandiculation emphasizes the need for sufficient space for basic kinetic output and general comfort; this must be considered in horse stall design.

Thermoregulation and shelter

Behaviour

The thermoregulatory pathway controls metabolic activity to maintain the horse's core temperature within a narrow range of 37.2–38.3 °C. The capacity of the body to regulate its internal temperature is affected by health, ambient temperature, wind and precipitation. Horses seek shelter for relief from extremes of heat or cold. In the absence of wind or moisture, temperatures down to −20 °C are well tolerated by horses in winter coat (down to −40 °C if sheltered). Horses in summer coat are most comfortable in mild temperatures in the range of 10–20 °C. Shade from direct sunlight is typically sought in temperatures over 25 °C if there is no air movement. In addition to moderating weather exposure, a shelter may provide refuge from biting insects (Hartmann *et al.*, 2015a). In temperate climatic conditions, unless it is hot and dry, donkeys spend less time outdoors than horses, preferring the sanctuary of a shelter. Donkeys are three times more likely than horses to stay indoors when it rains and it is less than 14 °C, and 12 times more likely to seek shelter in a light-to-moderate breeze (Proops *et al.*, 2019).

Horses and ponies have evolved with adaptations that improve their cold tolerance. In severe cold, horses group closely together to afford mutual shelter and conserve body heat. In winter, they have been observed galloping in the snow to generate heat and warm their extremities. Coat length and density play a role in protection from the cold. Its length depends on breed, husbandry conditions and season (Bocian *et al.*, 2017; Jørgensen *et al.*, 2019). Cold-blooded breeds such as the Shetland pony have a heavier winter coat than warm-blooded breeds, improving their cold tolerance (Autio *et al.*, 2006). Horses shed their winter coat with increasing day length. Donkeys do not have a winter coat and are less cold tolerant than horses (Proops *et al.*, 2019).

There are behavioural adaptations to adverse weather. In severe, stormy weather, horses cease to graze. A combination of cold and wind, especially combined with rain or snow, can inflict great stress. The effects of frost in severely cold weather are worse in a saturated horse. The tail is held close to the dock in adverse weather, allowing the free end to be blown between its hind legs. In this way, the tail hair then shields the hairless area of its perineum, its inguinal region and the inner thighs. In a strong wind, horses usually graze with the wind at their backs, especially if no windbreak exists in the paddock. In the contrasting conditions of hot, sunny weather, horses seek shaded or partly shaded areas. They put their heads, rather than hindquarters, into the limited shade.

The provision of shelter for domesticated horses includes natural features such as trees, solid fence lines and shelterbelts of vegetation. Supplementary shelter is provided either through the provision of blankets or by readily accessible constructed shelters. Shelter protects horses from extremes of cold, rain (especially when windy), extremes of heat and biting insects (Keiper and Berger, 1982). Natural features provide shelter for wild horses and are heavily relied upon by owners that keep domesticated horses at pasture (Fig. 5.8) (Thompson *et al.*, 2017). Depending on the time of year and geographic location, these include sand dunes, coastal shores, snowbanks, trees, hedges, gullies and valleys (Fig. 5.9). Domesticated horses have a preference for artificial shelters compared to natural shelters, particularly at temperatures >25 °C, and <7 °C, and on rainy days when the wind speed is >2.8 m/s (Snoeks *et al.*, 2015).

Blankets (horse rugs) and neck rugs are commonly used for horses to provide weather and insect protection for horses kept in pasture and additional warmth for housed equids (Azarpeycan *et al.*, 2016; Hammer and Gunkleman, 2019). Heavier blanket weights provide a greater degree of thermal comfort in cold climates, but blankets are not a replacement for human-made shelters under these conditions (Jørgensen *et al.*, 2019). Horses prefer blankets 80–90% of the time at temperatures of less than −10 °C and display a preference for blanket removal at temperatures >20 °C (Mejdell *et al.*, 2019). The clipping of horses to prevent body temperature increases during performance activities is practised widely (Morgan *et al.*, 2002). In the case of winter clipping, >90% of owners blanket

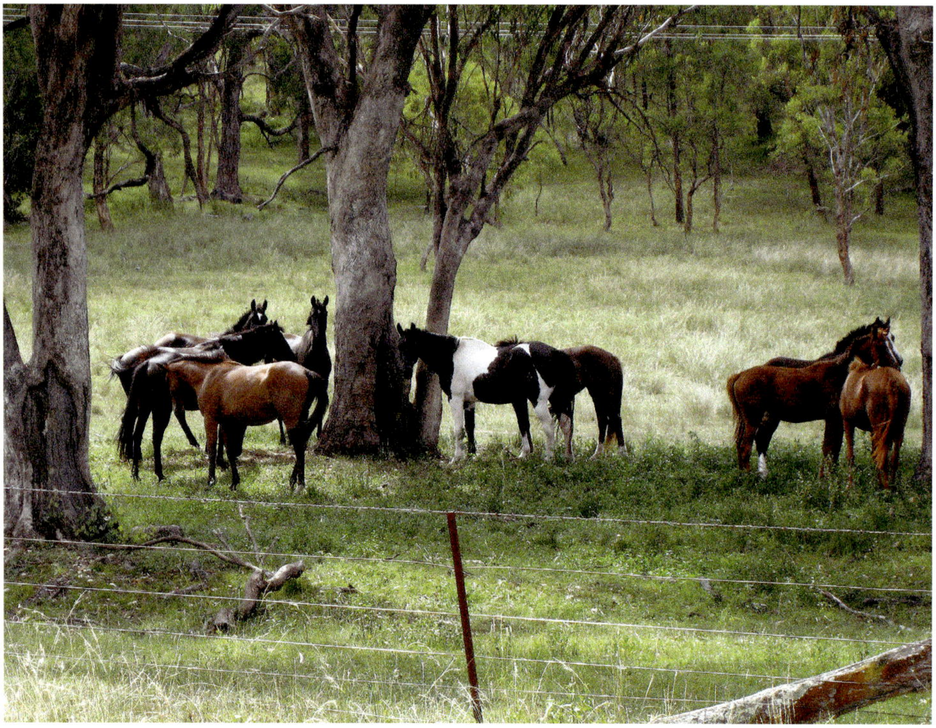

Fig. 5.8. A group of young mares seek shelter from the summer sun. Photo: author.

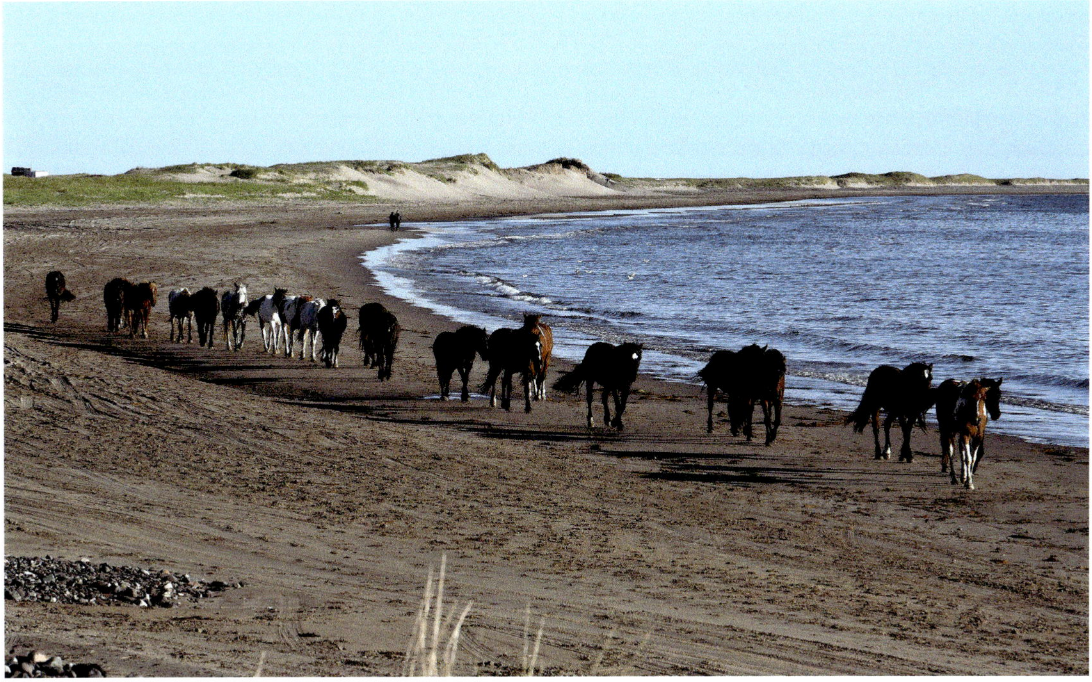

Fig. 5.9. The semi-feral horses of the islands of Saint Pierre and Miquelon seek shelter from wind, protected by the sand dunes along the shoreline. Photo: Pascale Carrére.

their horse day and night (Steinhoff-Wagner, 2019). Application of repellent to the blanket aids in protection from insects.

Constructed shelters are used by compatible horses during temperature extremes as described above and may also be designed to exclude insects. Shelter design should encompass considerations of equine behaviour and the social dynamics of the herd, as well as the likely directions of prevailing winds. Surprisingly, there is little published objective research on this topic. Insect defensive behaviours are less common when horses seek a fully enclosed shelter. Nevertheless, horses in a herd require separate ingress and egress to enclosed shelters to facilitate movements associated with social hierarchy (Hartmann *et al.*, 2015b).

Welfare

The welfare consequences of clipping horses seasonally or year-round are unknown. From the available evidence, it appears that greater monitoring of the thermal state of the horse and the ambient temperature is warranted to ensure that blankets are removed or replaced accordingly. Possible risks associated with the use of blankets include harbouring dust mites that affect the skin of hypersensitive horses (Wallace and Vogelnest, 2010) and design features that increase the risk of pressure sores over the withers (Clayton *et al.*, 2010). Blankets and human-made shelters require maintenance, and injuries associated with them are frequently encountered. The magnitude of this risk is currently unknown. Equine welfare assessment should include evaluating the availability and quality of natural and constructed shelters for the number of horses within the group, their compatibility, the climatic conditions likely to be encountered and the environmental risks for the horses.

References

Autio, E., Neste, R., Airaksinen, S. and Heiskanen, M.-L. (2006) Measuring the heat loss in horses in different seasons by infrared thermography. *Journal of Applied Animal Welfare Science* 9, 211–221.

Azarpeycan, S., Dittmer, K.E., Gee, E.K., Marshall, J.C., Wallace, J. *et al.* (2016) Influence of blanketing and season on vitamin D and parathyroid hormone, calcium, phosphorus, and magnesium concentrations in

horses in New Zealand. *Domestic Animal Endocrinology* 56, 75–84.
Beaver B.V. (2019) *Equine Behavioral Medicine.* Academic Press, London.
Bertolucci, L.F. (2011) Pandiculation: Nature's way of maintaining the functional integrity of the myofascial system? *Journal of Bodywork and Movement Therapies* 15, 268–280.
Bocian, K., Strezelec, K., Janczarek, I., Jabłecki, Z. and Kolstrung, R. (2017) Length of winter coat in horses depending on husbandry conditions. *Animal Science Journal* 88, 339–346.
Boyd, L.E., Carbonaro, D.A. and Houpt, K.A. (1988) The 24-hour time budget of Przewalski horses. *Applied Animal Behaviour Science* 21, 5–17.
Clayton, H.M., Kaiser, L.J. and Nauwelaerts, S. (2010) Pressure on the horse's withers with three styles of blanket. *The Veterinary Journal* 184, 52–55.
Crowell-Davis, S.L. (1987) Self-grooming by mares and foals of the Welsh pony (*Equus caballus*). *Applied Animal Behavioural Science* 17, 197–208.
Ellis, A.D, Redgate, S., Zinchenko, S., Owen, H., Barfoot, C. *et al.* (2015) The effect of presenting forage in multi-layered haynets and at multiple sites on night-time budgets of stabled horses. *Applied Animal Behavioural Science* 171, 108–116.
Fleurance, G., Duncan, P., Fritz, H., Cabaret, J., Cortet, J. *et al.* (2007) Selection of feeding sites by horses at pasture: Testing the anti-parasite theory. *Applied Animal Behaviour Science* 108, 288–301.
Fraser, A.F. (1980) *Farm Animal Behaviour*. Bailliere Tindall, London.
Fraser, A.F. (1989) Pandiculation: The comparative phenomenon of systematic stretching. *Applied Animal Behaviour Science* 23, 263–268.
Fraser, A.F. (2010) *The Behaviour and Welfare of the Horse*. 2nd edn. CAB International, Wallingford, UK.
Geor, R.J. (2013) Appendix: Nutritional requirements, recommendations and example diets In: Geor, R.J. (ed.) *Equine Applied Clinical Nutrition: Health, Welfare and Performance*. Saunders, Philadelphia, Pennsylvania, pp. 639–658.
Giannetto, C., Cannallla, V., Guidice, E., Guerico, A. and Piccione, G. (2019) Behavioral and physiological processes in horses and their linkage with peripheral clock gene expression: A preliminary study. *Journal of Veterinary Behaviour* 34, 37–41.
Giraldeau, L.-A. and Caraco, T. (2000) *Social Foraging Theory*. Princeton University Press, Princeton, NJ.
Hammer, C. and Gunklemam, M. (2019) Effect of different blanket weights on surface temperature of horses in cold climates. *Journal of Equine Veterinary Science* 85, 102848.
Hartmann, E., Hopkins, R.J., von Brömssen, C. and Dahlborn, K. (2015a) 24-h sheltering behaviour of individually kept horses during Swedish summer weather. *Acta Veterinaria Scandinavica* 57, 45.
Hartmann, E., Hopkins, R.J., Blomgren, E., Ventorp, M., von Brömssen, C. and Dahlborn, K. (2015b) Daytime shelter use of individually kept horses during Swedish summer. *Journal of Animal Science* 93, 802–810.
Hoffman, C.J., Costa, L.R. and Freeman, L.M. (2009) Survey of feeding practices, supplement use, and knowledge of equine nutrition among a subpopulation of horse owners in New England. *Journal of Equine Veterinary Science* 29, 719–726.
Hogan, J.A. (2005) Motivation. In: Bolhuis, J.J. and Giraldeau, L.A. (eds) *The Behaviour of Animals.* Blackwell, Malden, Maryland, pp. 41–70.
Hoskin, S.O. and Gee, E.K. (2004) Feeding value of pastures for horses. *New Zealand Veterinary Journal* 6, 332–341.
Ingolfsdottir, H.B. and Sigurjonsdottir, H. (2008) The benefits of high rank in the wintertime – a study of the Icelandic horse. *Applied Animal Behaviour Science* 114, 485–491.
Jezierski, T., Jaworski, Z., Sobcyńska, M., Ensminger, J. and Górecka-Bruzda, A. (2018) Do olfactory behaviour and marking responses of Konik polski stallions to faeces from conspecifics of either sex differ? *Behavioural Processes* 155, 38–42.
Jørgensen, G.H.M., Medjell, C.M. and Bøe, K.N. (2019) The effect of blankets on horse behaviour and preference for shelter in Nordic winter conditions. *Applied Animal Behaviour Science* 218, 104822.
Keiper, R.R. and Berger, J. (1982) Refuge-seeking and pest avoidance by feral horses in desert and island environments. *Applied Animal Ethology* 90, 111–120.
Kimura, R. (1998) Mutual grooming and preferred associate relationships in a band of free-ranging horses. *Applied Animal Behaviour Science* 59, 265–276.
Kristula, M.A. and McDonnell, S.M. (1994) Drinking water temperature affects consumption of water during cold weather in ponies. *Applied Animal Behaviour Science* 41, 155–160.
Krueger, K. and Flauger, B. (2011) Olfactory recognition of individual competitors by means of faeces in horse (*Equus caballus*). *Animal Cognition* 14, 245–257.
La Casha, P.A., Brady, H.A., Allen, V.G., Richardson, C.R. and Pond, K.R. (1999) Voluntary intake, digestibility, and subsequent selection of Matua bromegrass, coastal bermudagrass, and alfalfa hays by yearling horses. *Journal of Animal Science* 77, 2766–2773.
Lamoot, I., Callebaut, J., Degazelle, T., Demeulenaere, E., Laquiére, J. *et al.* (2004) Eliminative behaviour of free-ranging horses: Do they show latrine behaviour or do they defecate where they graze? *Applied Animal Behaviour Science* 86, 105–121.
Lindberg, J.E. (2013) Feedstuffs for horses. In: Geor, R.J. (ed.) *Equine Applied Clinical Nutrition: Health, Welfare and Performance*. Saunders, Philadelphia, Pennsylvania, pp. 319–331.

Lopes, M.A.F. (2008) Effects of feeding on equine gastrointestinal function or physiology. In: White, N.A., Moore, J.N. and Mair, T.S. (eds). *The Equine Acute Abdomen*. Teton NewMedia, Jackson, Wyoming.
Lopes, M.A.F. and Johnson, P.J. (2017) Effects of feeding on equine gastrointestinal function or physiology. In: Blikslager, A.T, White II, N.A., Moore, J.N. and Mair, T.S. (eds). *The Equine Acute Abdomen*, 3rd edn. John Wiley and Sons Inc., Hoboken, New Jersey.
Maisonpierre, I.N., Sutton, M.A., Harris, P., Menzies-Gow, N., Weller, R. *et al.* (2019) Accelerometer activity tracking in horses and the effect of pasture management on time budget. *Equine Veterinary Journal* 51, 840–845.
Marinier, S.L., Alexander, A.J. and Waring, G.H. (1988) Flehmen behavior in the domestic horse: discrimination of conspecific odours. *Applied Animal Behaviour Science* 19, 227–237.
Matsui, K., Kahlil, A.M. and Takeda, K. (2009) Do horses prefer certain substrates for rolling in grazing pasture? *Journal of Equine Veterinary Science* 29, 590–594.
McBride, S.D., Hemmings, A. and Robinson, K. (2004) A preliminary study on the effect of massage to reduce stress in the horse. *Journal of Equine Veterinary Science* 24, 76–81.
McCue, M.E., Geor, R.J. and Schultz, N. (2015) Equine metabolic syndrome: a complex disease influenced by genetics and the environment. *Journal of Equine Veterinary Science* 35, 367–375.
McDonnell, S. (1986) Reproductive behavior of the stallion. *Veterinary Clinics of North America: Equine Practice* 2, 535–555.
McDonnell, S.M. and Kristula, M.A. (1996) No effect of drinking water temperature (ambient vs. chilled) on consumption of water during hot summer weather in ponies. *Applied Animal Behaviour Science* 49, 159–153.
Mejdell, C.M., Jørgensen, G.H.M., Buvik, T., Torp, T. and Bøe, K.E. (2019) The effect of weather conditions on the preference in horses for wearing blankets. *Applied Animal Behaviour Science* 212, 52–57.
Morgan, K., Funkquist, P. and Nyman, G. (2002) The effect of coat clipping on thermoregulation during intense exercise in trotters. *Equine Veterinary Journal Supplement* 34, 564–569.
Mullan, S., Szmaragd, C., Hotchkiss, J. and Whay, H.R. (2014) The welfare of long-line tethered and free-ranging horses kept on public grazing land in South Wales. *Animal Welfare* 23, 25–37.
Müller, C.E. and Udén, P. (2006) Preference of horses for grass conserved as hay, haylage or silage. *Animal Feed Science and Technology* 132, 66–70.
Ödberg, F.O. and Frances-Smith, K. (1977) Studies on the formation of ungrazed eliminative areas in the field used by horses. *Applied Animal Ethology* 3, 27–34.
Peters, S.M., Bleijenberg, E.H. van Dierendonck, M.C., van der Harst, J.E. and Spruijt, B.M. (2012) Characterization of anticipatory behaviour in domesticated horses (*Equus caballus*). *Applied Animal Behaviour Science* 138, 60–69.
Pluháček, J., Tučková, V., King, S.R.B., and Šárová, R. (2019) Test of four hypotheses to explain the function of overmarking in foals of four equids species. *Animal Cognition* 22, 231–241.
Proops, L., Osthaus, B., Bell, N., Long, S., Hayday, K. *et al.* (2019) Shelter-seeking behavior of donkeys and horses in a temperate climate. *Journal of Veterinary Behavior* 32, 16–23.
Randall, L., Rogers, C.W., Hoskin, S.O., Morel, P.C. and Swainson, N.M. (2014) Preference for different pasture grasses by horses in New Zealand. *Proceedings of the New Zealand Society of Animal Production* 74, 79–84.
Rho, J.R., Srygley, R.B. and Choe, J.C. (2007) Sex preferences in Jeju pony foals (*Equus caballus*) for mutual grooming and play fighting behaviours. *Zoological Science* 24, 769–773.
Rogers, C.W., Gee, K.E., Back, P., van Zon, S., Hirst, R.L. *et al.* (2018) Pasture use and management in commercial equine production systems. *New Zealand Journal of Animal Science and Production* 78, 40–44.
Sauvant, D., Perez, J.M. and Tran, G. (2004). *Tables of Composition and Nutritional Value of Feed Materials*. Wageningen Academic Publishers, The Netherlands.
Schöning, B. (2008) *Horse Behaviour*. 5M Publishing, Sheffield, UK.
Sigurjónsdóttir, H. and Haraldsson, H. (2019) Significance of group composition for the welfare of pastured horses. *Animals* 9, 14.
Snoeks, M.G., Moons, C.P.H., Ödberg, F.O., Aviron, M. and Geers, R. (2015) Behavior of horses on pasture in relation to weather and shelter - A field study in a temperate climate. *Journal of Veterinary Behavior* 10, 561–568.
Steinhoff-Wagner, J. (2019) Coat clipping of horses: A survey. *Journal of Applied Animal Welfare Science* 22, 171–187.
Sufit, E., Houpt, K.A. and Sweeting, M. (1985) Physiological stimuli of thirst and drinking patterns in ponies. *Equine Veterinary Journal* 17, 12–16.
Sweeting, M.P., Houpt, C.E. and Houpt, K.A. (1985) Social facilitation of feeding and time budgets in stabled ponies. *Journal of Animal Science* 60, 369–374.
Thompson, K.R., Clarkson, L., Riley, C.B. and van den Berg, M. (2017) Horse-keeping practices in Australia: findings from a national online survey of horse owners. *Australian Veterinary Journal* 95, 437–443.
Toates, F. (2002) Physiology, motivation and the organization of behaviour. In: Jensen, P. (ed.) *Ethology of*

Domestic Animals: An Introduction. CAB International, Wallingford, UK.
Tučková, V., Šárová, R., Bartšová, J., King, S.R.B. and Pluháček, J. (2018) Overmarking by adult females in four equids species: social bonds and group cohesion. *Journal of Zoology* 306, 180–188.
VanDierendonck, M.C. and Spruijt, B.M. (2012) Coping in groups of domestic horses - Review from a social and neurobiological perspective. *Applied Animal Behaviour Science* 138, 194–202.
Wallace, J.C. and Vogelnest, L.J. (2010) Evaluation of the presence of house dust mites in horse rugs. *Veterinary Dermatology* 21, 602–607.
Wilson, A.D. (2014) Immune responses to ectoparasites of horses, with a focus on insect bite hypersensitivity. *Parasite Immunology* 36, 560–572.

6 Kinetic Behaviour and Athletic Performance

Chris W. Rogers MAgrSc, PhD*

Massey University, Palmerston North, New Zealand

Introduction	81
Evolution, Morphology and Gait	81
The Gaits of Locomotion	83
The walk	85
The trot	86
The canter	87
The gallop	87
Other gaits	88
Jumping	88
Racing Behaviour and Welfare	89
Racing	89
Use of the whip	91
Swimming	91
Need for Daily Exercise	92
Lungeing	93
Riding	93
Summary	94
References	94

Introduction

The horse is cursorial, that is, an animal adapted to run. This definition was initially applied to describe ungulates capable of running on open plains. It now has a broader definition based on functional morphology and describes animals with a structure that facilitates running at high speed. The concept of a cursorial browser describes the functional anatomy of the horse, the ecological niche it occupies, and some of the requirements for movement that need to be considered within modern intensive management systems and by those using horses for athletic performance activities.

The ecological niche occupied by the horse has driven the evolution of a musculoskeletal system that is highly efficient for low speed movement (walking) and short bursts of high speed to escape predation. However, this selection pressure has resulted in a trade-off between reduced limb mass and the efficiency of gait versus tissue safety limits and increased susceptibility for injury at maximal speed.

Evolution, Morphology and Gait

A horse's velocity is limited by how fast it can move its legs and the relative length of its stride. Evolution has driven changes in morphology to maximize both these variables to produce an animal capable of high-speed locomotion with relatively low energetic cost. Indeed, many of the physiological processes in the horse, including locomotion, can be viewed as evolving to minimize energy expenditure.

*Corresponding author: c.w.rogers@massey.ac.nz

DOI: 10.1079/9781789242133.0006

The basic structure of the horse can be described colloquially as a 'sausage with toothpicks for legs'. While this is a slightly 'tongue in cheek' and perhaps comical descriptor of the horse's body shape, it emphasizes the two significant evolutionary changes in horse morphology that have permitted an efficiency of gait. These include the combination of localization of the large muscle mass around the pivot points of the limbs and the reduction in the mass of the distal limbs to reduce weight, both of which provide mechanisms to reduce the energetic cost of limb movement.

The distal limb of the horse is an elegant piece of biological engineering. Muscle and limb masses are reduced to a functional unit that maximizes locomotion while reducing the energetic requirement (muscular effort) to maintain rigidity, preventing or restricting mediolateral deviation and rotation of the limb. This reduction in muscular effort is achieved by reducing the vestigial digits (pastern and hoof) and the use of joints that restrict movement to the craniocaudal direction (i.e. the sagittal plane). In conjunction, the wrapping of tendons and ligaments around and about the joints has evolved to confine movements predominantly to the sagittal plane. This reduction in mass and consolidation of muscles around the pivot points of the limbs (shoulder and hip) makes the equine limb appear like a pendulum. The lighter the end of the pendulum, the faster it can move through the swing phase. This refinement has led to the horse having no muscle mass below either the carpus or the tarsus.

The second analogue for the equine limb is that of movement generated using a whip-like action. A muscular effort is required to initiate protraction, but early in the swing phase, there is a reduction in muscular effort and at mid-swing. Then, when the hoof is directly under the pivot point (i.e. point of shoulder), the muscular restriction is responsible for braking. This muscular braking action is analogous to the flick used when cracking a whip and propels the hoof forward with minimal muscular effort. Muscular contraction is once again initiated at the end of protraction as the limb enters retraction and then the start of the stance phase.

The distal limb structure consisting of long flexor tendons, particularly the superficial and deep digital flexor tendons, provides an opportunity for energy conservation by utilizing elastic recall when the tendons stretch during the stance phase. This ability to utilize stored elastic energy from the tendons provides another analogue akin to the horse running on pogo sticks. The transitions between trot and canter are, in part, governed by this concept of maximization of elastic recoil and minimization of the metabolic cost of locomotion, with gait transitions taking place over a narrow velocity range. The speed at which gait transitions occur is reinforced by a feedback system referred to as the mechanostat in bone. This term describes how mechanical loading influences bone structure by changing its mass and architecture to provide a structure that resists habitual loads with an economical amount of material. Therefore, this system stimulates the appropriate bone response to load (speed) and strains outside the normal physiological range that stimulate a change in gait. Simplistically this is observed with horses trotting on hard non-compliant surfaces taking shorter but faster strides to achieve the same speed within a gait and a lowering of speed at which they will change gait.

This anatomical structure of the equine forelimb is shown in Fig. 6.1. The key points of interest are the long flexor tendons at the back of the distal limb (below and palmar to the carpus) and the large range of motion possible in the fetlock (metacarpophalangeal joint). This structural arrangement permits the limb to function as a damped mass spring. Most limb loading is attenuated by the distal spring (the distal limb from carpus below the tendons and the fetlock joint) and, to a lesser extent, the proximal spring (the elbow joint).

The evolutionary adaptations for gait efficiency have been achieved with trade-offs in the mechanical safety limits of the tissue in the limb. Examples are seen in the small margin of error calculated for the maximal strain of the superficial digital flexor tendon (SDFT) of the horse at a gallop. When galloping, the SDFT is within 12% of the strain required for rupture (disruption) (Riemersma and Schamhardt, 1985). Thus, when galloping, incorrect placement of the hoof in a divot may be sufficient to provide an increase in strain high enough to induce a tendon injury. The bones in the distal limb have rapid dynamic responses to load (as is observed with shin soreness) in racehorses (Firth *et al.*, 2005). Data obtained with implanted strain gauges have demonstrated that the horse changes its gait and loading of the limb to maintain the strain within a relatively narrow physiological range. Strains outside this range prompt rapid changes in the material properties of the bone (bone mineral density) and its architecture. Repetitive loads outside the physiological range applied with insufficient

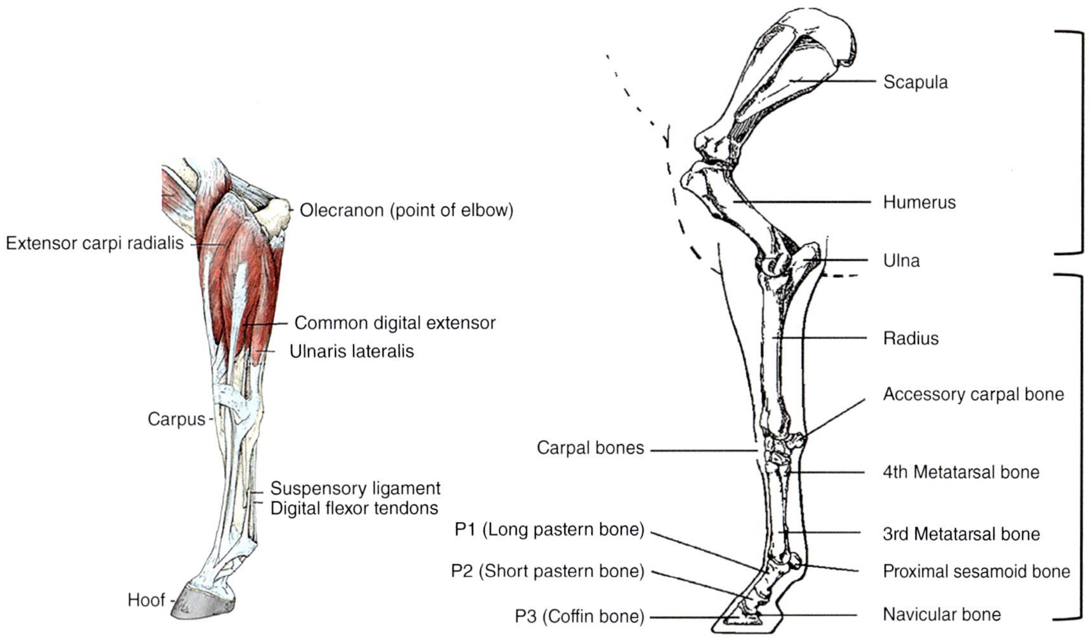

Fig. 6.1. Diagrams of the equine forelimb joints, tendons and bones. The brackets on the right represent the two major sections of the horse's limb that act as springs to absorb loading. Illustration: author.

rest periods between are implicated in cyclic overload injuries (fracture) in racehorses and endurance competition horses (Morrice-West *et al*., 2020).

The Gaits of Locomotion

Within mammalian quadrupeds, the gaits (the unique sequence of footfalls) are remarkably similar. The genetic regulation of gait is similar among species as diverse as the mouse and the horse (Andersson *et al*., 2012). Hildebrand (1965) provided the earliest description of the different gaits in quadruped locomotion, identifying symmetrical and asymmetrical gaits. The definitions or descriptors supplied by him form the basis of how we describe the horse's gaits today (Figs. 6.2 and 6.3).

In symmetrical gaits, the movements of limbs on one side repeat those of the other side but half a stride later. In asymmetrical gaits, the movements of limbs on one side do not repeat those of the other. Symmetrical gaits include the walk, the pace and the diagonal trot. Asymmetrical gaits include the various forms of the canter and gallop, including the lope and the rotary gallop.

A stride is a full cycle of movement of all four limbs. A stride cycle has two main components: the stance phase (limb is on the ground) and suspension (limb is off the ground). The stance phase is subdivided into a braking component (when the limb first contacts the ground and decelerates), mid stance (the point when the limb is perpendicular to the ground and the ground reaction force is orientated vertically), and propulsion (the time from midstance until break-over and loss of contact with the ground) (Fig. 6.4). The swing phase is divided into protraction (bringing the limb forward) and retraction (the time from maximal protraction until ground contact).

Each individual horse has its own harmonic frequency, which describes the optimal stride frequency for that horse given its structure (conformation). This value has a relatively narrow range between horses at different gaits. The stride frequency at the walk is approximately 1 hertz (1 stride/second or a stride duration of 1 second), and that of the trot and canter approximately 1.6 hertz (1.6 strides/second or a stride duration of about 0.6 seconds). This consistency of stride duration is also observed when looking at the gait of horses when they are foals and then later, adults. The conservation of stride frequency within horses may explain why increases in the gait speed are due to increases in stride length rather than changes in stride frequency.

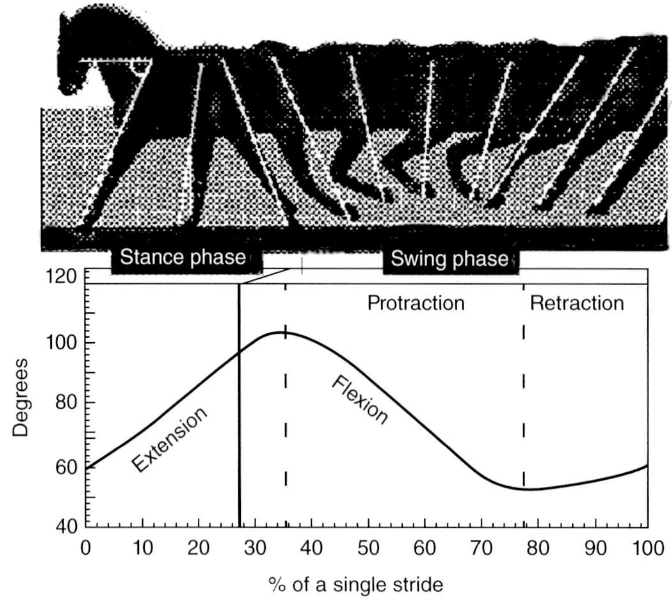

Fig. 6.2. Representation of the phases of gait, stance and swing. (Modified from Holmström *et al.*, 1993.)

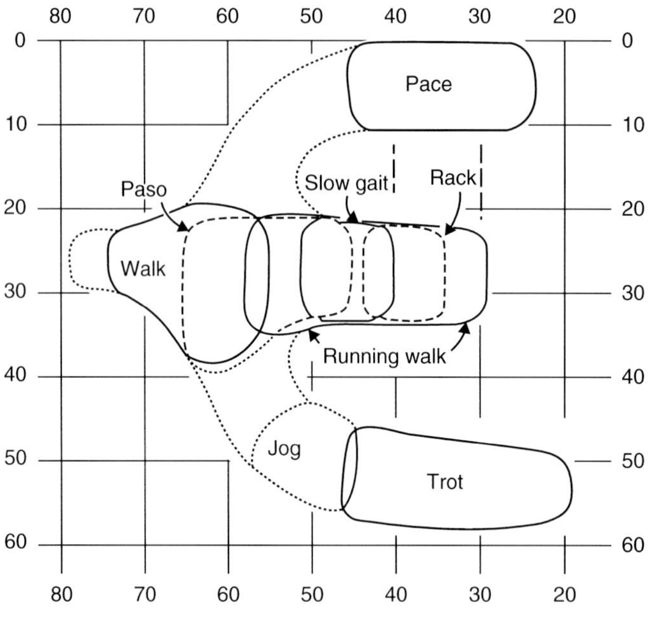

Fig. 6.3. Milton Hildebrand's diagram of the classification of symmetrical gaits in the horse. (Modified from Hildebrand, 1965.)

Stride length is the distance covered between successive imprints of the same hoof. The sound produced when a hoof strikes the ground is the beat. If each limb strikes the ground separately, the gait will be a four-beat gait. If diagonal limb pairs are placed down simultaneously, such as in the diagonal trot, the gait is two-beat since only two sounds are heard per stride. The canter is a three-beat gait

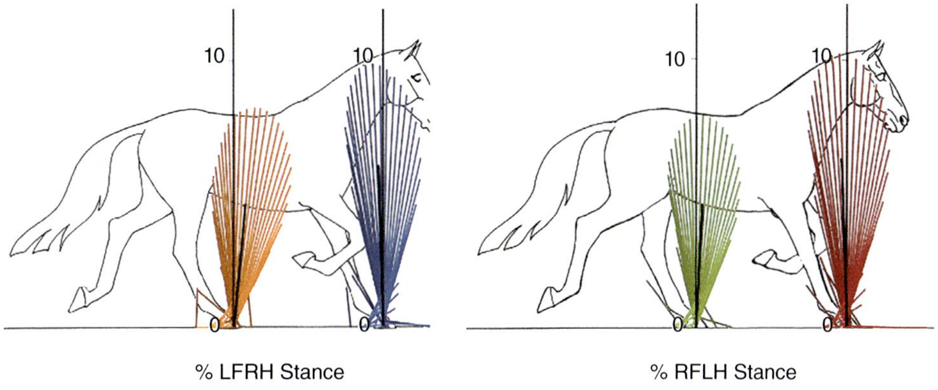

Fig. 6.4. The magnitude and direction of the ground reaction forces (at 10% of stance time intervals) in the forelimb and hindlimb of a horse trotting. (Modified from Hobbs *et al.*, 2018.)

(e.g., right hind, left hind and right fore forming a diagonal pair, and then the left fore and a suspension period). The lead leg leaves the ground last during the canter or gallop (such as the left fore in the example above). The gallop resembles the canter but has a four-beat gait due to the disassociation of the diagonal pair. Within every stride, each limb for a time acts in a support phase and a non-supportive or swing phase. The primary role of the forelimbs during stance is to support the body. The primary role of the hindlimbs during the stance phase is to generate propulsive force (Back *et al.*, 1994).

The full gallop common to racing can only be sustained for a limited time, usually a few minutes. In addition to muscular physiology, one reason for this is that respiratory rate is synchronized with limb movement, also referred to as locomotor respiratory coupling. When the forelimbs at a gallop contact the ground, the horse must exhale, and inspiration can only be achieved when the horse propels itself forward into the suspension phase. At maximal speed, this greatly restricts the horse to short rapid breaths, generating an oxygen debt, rapid accumulation of lactic acid and muscle fatigue.

Observations of feral (wild) horses indicate that most of the locomotor activity is at the walk with short periods of canter. The walk is the primary gait used (on a time basis) by all horses, and this is because horses spend ~16 hours per day grazing or browsing (Kurvers *et al.*, 2006). The preference for using a canter when faster locomotion is required may be due to the greater energy efficiency of this gait over the trot.

The walk

The walk is the gait most used by the horse and, in its slowest form, is used in conjunction with grazing/browsing. At this time, most of the duration of each stride is spent with all four feet on the ground simultaneously, each leg only moving singly forward during the remainder of the stride. The speed of the walk ranges up to 5 km/h (3 mph). It is a four-beat gait with the footfall sequence left hind, left fore, right hind, right fore gait that can be very brisk, steady or slow. Its slowest form occurs when the animal is grazing. At this time, most of the duration of each stride is spent with all four feet on the ground simultaneously, each leg only moving singly forward during the remainder of the stride. In the slower walking stride, the horse always has three of its hooves in contact with the ground while one leg is advancing.

At the faster walking rate, the horse already has the hoof of the flexing leg raised as the advancing hoof hits the ground while the next leg starts flexing. The animal's full weight is then borne for a moment by a diagonal pair, with the other pair in the motions of advancing and flexing. Although the two latter leg actions are not exactly simultaneous, they bear less weight than the other two, with their hooves flat on the ground in the continuum of the stride.

The amble is a specific type of walk; essentially, it is accelerated walking. In the amble, the increase in walking speed is achieved by quicker swinging action. The following leg starts its flexion while the preceding leg is lifted. This is a more demanding gait than the normal walk since only two legs are fully weight-bearing at one time.

The trot

The major difference between the walk and the trot is that the latter has a moment of suspension where all limbs are off the ground, making this gait appear more energetic, active and elevated in its manner and speed. The horse trots by lifting two diagonally opposite legs at exactly the same time (Fig. 6.5a). Thus, the right foreleg moves with the left hindlimb in synchrony. There are only two supportive beats during the trot because the horse raises and sets down two diagonal feet simultaneously, giving the typical two-beat tempo of this gait. The moment of suspension between diagonal pairs means an increase in the relative loading of the limbs with typical ground reaction forces of around 1.0–1.2 times the horse's body weight in each limb (Back *et al.*, 2007). This increased loading of the limbs permits the horse to engage the elastic recoil in the tendinous structures to reduce the energetic cost of locomotion.

In equestrian sports, the trot is classified from slowest to fastest as collected trot, working trot, medium trot and extended trot. In theory, the horse should maintain the same stride frequency but should have a longer stride length (maximal limb protraction) as we move from collected to extended trot. In contrast to the extended trot, the collected trot is characterized by flexion and high carriage of the knees and hocks in a generally elevated way-of-going. This appearance is achieved by increasing the stance time, increasing the braking phase of stance in the forelimbs, and greater flexion in the hindlimbs during the stance, providing an appearance of collection and increased weight-bearing of the stance hind limbs.

At the other end of the spectrum is the racing trot, as demonstrated by trotting Standardbred racehorses. At maximal speeds in this breed (up to 50 km/h), there is often disassociation of the limb pairs and significant diagonal advanced placement (the hindlimb of the pair contacting the ground before the forelimb of the pair) and a reduction in the stance phase as a percentage of total stride time (Drevemo *et al.*, 1980). Selective breeding of Standardbreds for maximal trotting speed has increased the speed threshold for the trot to canter transition. Some conformation changes like mild outward rotation of the hind limbs helps to facilitate the dramatic diagonal advanced placement seen at racing speeds.

The pace is a symmetrical gait similar to the trot, but paired legs move together on the same side. This gait allows slightly greater extension of the hindlimb, and less vertical displacement of body mass, since the paired forelimb (on the same side) is also extended at the same time. The gait is most commonly known in the Standardbred, but forms of pacing are well recognized in the Icelandic horse (the skeið) and the Peruvian Paso (the Sobreandando). There is a strong genetic component to the ability to pace that was first localized to a specific genetic mutation on chromosome 23, but more recently has been associated with multiple loci in the equine genome (McCoy *et al.*, 2019). Pacers typically have a longer suspension time than stance time in their gait. Pacing is symmetrical and similar to the trot, which permits full respiration at a faster rate as there is no or limited locomotor respiratory coupling. The pacing horse can turn its body slightly to the side of the extending pair of legs and away from the two supporting legs to increase its reach

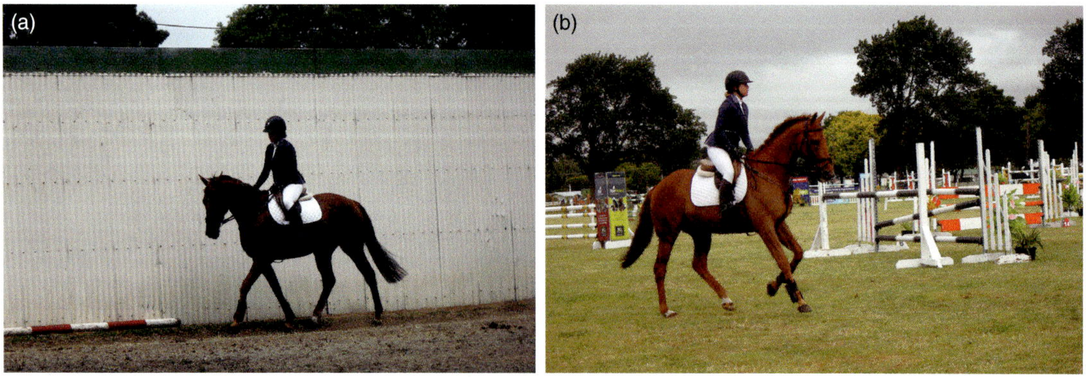

Fig. 6.5. A ridden horse trotting (a) and cantering (b). Photos: author.

and speed. Standardbred pacers have a higher maximum speed than trotters and are capable of speeds up to 56 km/h (35 mph).

The canter

The canter is an asymmetric three-beat bounding gait (Fig. 6.5b). The gallop is the faster four-beat version of the same gait. There is no separation of terms in continental Europe, and both the three and four-beat versions of the gait are commonly called a gallop. In this form of locomotion, the horse has only one pair of limbs in synchrony, namely one foreleg and the opposite hind leg. Convention describes the canter as either a left lead, or right lead, and this relates to the last forelimb to contact the ground before suspension. Therefore, a left lead canter would be right hind, left hind and right forelimbs forming a diagonal pair, and then the left fore and a period of suspension. The footfall sequence of this asymmetric bounding gait results in the trunk of the horse rotating around the transverse axis and significant flexion–extension around the lumbosacral joint. During the stride sequence, there is a raising and lowering of the head and neck; elevation during suspension and lowering the head as the forelimbs begin the stance phase.

When turning to the left, a left lead canter is preferred and *vice versa* when turning to the right. Possibly, due to natural asymmetry, observational data indicate that horses prefer a left lead canter. Horses will naturally switch leads (using a flying change) to minimize load and fatigue. These lead changes are reported in Thoroughbred racehorses during races, and canter lead changes are often employed by endurance riders during competition to reduce fatigue during a competition ride. To change leads the horse brings its lead leg down on the ground quicker than the other foreleg, which then becomes the lead leg. The leading leg performs more muscular effort by stiffening the shoulder and the elbow, throwing the body upwards, and by taking the final impact of landing on a firmly fixed leg. The horse effectively vaults itself over this leg in this diagonal gait.

Speed in the canter is dependent on the stride length, with stride frequency remaining relatively consistent. However, there are some subtle changes in limb timing sequences with increasing speed, notably the decrease in the timing between the hind limb footfall sequences. As speed increases, there is an increase in the relative contribution of the suspension phase from ~5 mS of total stride time during the working canter to 54 mS in the medium canter (Clayton, 1994).

During the canter (and gallop), there is locomotor–respiratory coupling. The horse inspires (inhales) during the bounding with hind limbs and then expires when the forelimbs contact the ground at the start of the stance phase. This efficient mechanism synchronizes the movement of the viscera against the diaphragm so that the forward movement of the viscera during stance is synchronized with exhalation, and removal of pressure on the diaphragm is associated with inhalation.

The gallop

In the English nomenclature, the gallop is the four-beat version of the canter (Fig. 6.6). The gallop is faster than the canter, resulting in disassociation of the diagonal pair of limbs with the hind limb of the diagonal pair contacting the ground first. This disassociation results in the distinct four-beat sound to the gallop. We consider horses to be galloping in a racing context once they are covering 14 m/s (50 km/hr). At a gallop, horses are capable of speeds up to 88 km/hr (55 mph).

Like the canter, increases in speed at a gallop are achieved through increases in stride length. During the gallop, there is significant flexion–extension around the lumbosacral joint, permitting an increase in stride length of ~6m. Some elite performance horses are capable of stride lengths up to 8 m. Quarter horses achieve greater maximal speeds over the shorter racing distance (400 m) with a higher stride frequency than that observed with Thoroughbred racehorses (average race distance 1600 m (one mile); range 1200–3200 m for flat racing). Differences in the relationship between stride length and stride frequency also occur among Thoroughbreds, with sprinters having a faster stride frequency than staying horses (Morrice-West *et al.*, 2021).

The majority of the energy demands for a Thoroughbred during a race requires aerobic metabolism. During the start and the end of the race, the horse functions in oxygen debt. The ability to cope with the oxygen debt differentiates the performance of horses at the end of the race and their subsequent recovery rates. The oxygen debt creates air hunger as exhaustion occurs. This is revealed by the horse extending its bobbing head and neck to the fullest extent while running. Horses breathe only through the nose, so the nostrils are now dilated to their limit. There is a relative

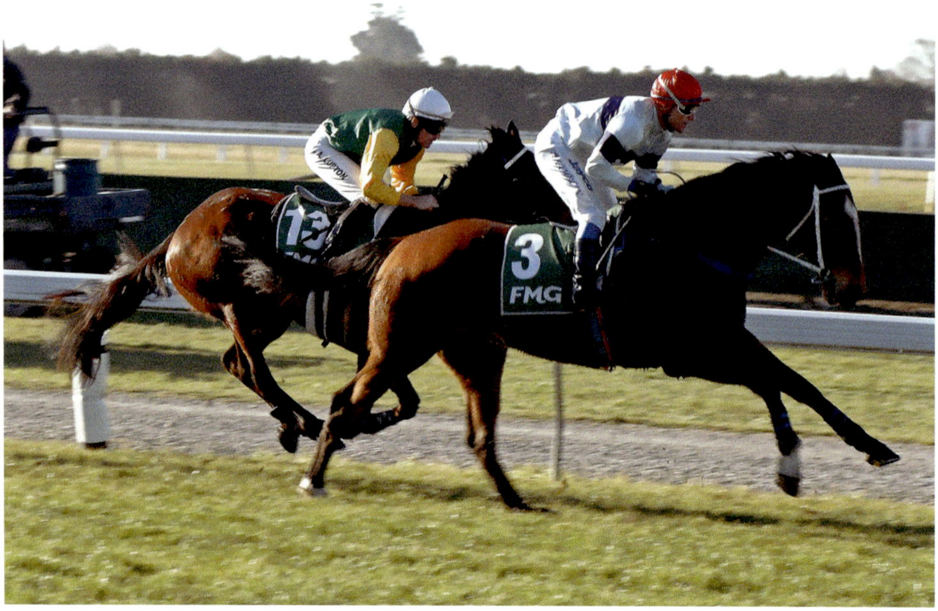

Fig. 6.6. Pair of thoroughbred racehorses galloping during a race. Both horses are using a left lead gallop. The horse closest to the camera is in the stance phase, and the horse away from the camera is nearing the end of the suspension phase. Photo: Kylie Legg.

increase in the stance time as a percentage of total stride time with fatigue. The increase in stance time percentage may be due to muscular fatigue and a mechanism to provide greater opportunity for respiration (longer and deeper breaths).

A variation in leg use in galloping sometimes occurs in a pattern called the rotary gallop. During this version of the gallop, the feet are placed down in a circular order (e.g., right hind, left hind, left fore, right fore) as the horse lands from suspension. Some species of herbivores use the rotary gallop, but apart from some early comments within the literature, based on observational data, the current consensus appears to be that horses rarely use the rotary gallop (Cully *et al.*, 2018).

Other gaits

In addition to these natural gaits of the horse, some other ways of going exist. These are classified as 'running' gaits, such as a very brisk 'stepping pace', 'slow rack' or the tölt. With such gaits there is no bouncing of the back or bobbing of the head, due to a lack of a suspension phase. These running gaits also include the 'paso' and the 'rack', which characterize the Latin American and Tennessee Walking horses, respectively. Other 'gaited horses' include the American Saddlebred and the Missouri Fox-Trotter, which have the easy 'gliding' gaits as do the Paso breeds of South America. In Europe, the Icelandic horse also displays these variations in gait and is becoming an increasingly popular breed for recreational riding. The toelt gait of the Icelandic horse is a four-beat gait with the sequence of footfalls left hind left fore, right hind and right fore. The time between footfalls should be even and there should be no moment of suspension. At faster speeds, a minor level of suspension (up to 10% of total stride time) is tolerated. The double support phases of fore and hind limbs are either diagonal or ipsilateral and of approximately similar duration. The Icelandic horse and the other breeds mentioned have an innate aptitude for such special ambulatory gaits, that appear to have a common genetic origin across the different breeds (Andersson *et al.*, 2012).

Jumping

Feral horses are rarely observed jumping an obstacle and will make an effort to go around, rather than over, even small obstacles. With training, horses with sufficient talent can consistently jump 1.6 m high fences (with oxers up to 1.8 m wide) during top-level show jumping competitions.

Horses can leap over gaps in terrain in any normal gait. However, a jump is considered as a special, upward, symmetrical stride (Figs 6.7a and b). The jump consists of three phases – the approach stride, take-off and landing. In sport (e.g., jumping, show jumping or stadium jumping) the horse typically approaches the jump at a canter. Immediately before the obstacle the horse usually makes a shorter, strutting stride and lowers the forehand (head, neck and shoulders) in preparation to then prop the forehand off the ground with significant braking action of the forelimbs (an action very similar to that of a pole vaulter). During take-off, the forehand is propped up, and the horse brings its hind legs under it to the take-off point about 1.5–2 m in front of the jump. At the same time, the knees are fully flexed, with the hooves coming close to the elbows. The lightened weight of the forequarters with the hindquarters under the body allows the forelegs to be fully flexed to clear the jump. The forearms are raised so that the carpus leads over the jump. At mid-jump, the horse starts to extend the forelegs as it then descends, the hind legs trailing over the jump.

On landing from a jump, both forefeet hit the ground almost at the same time, with one slightly ahead of the other, to become the lead leg when the canter is resumed. At the time of impact on the forefeet, the fetlocks go into hyperextension. At the high-level competition, up to 22% of these sport horses may sustain orthopaedic injuries (Egenvall *et al.*, 2013), and a greater prevalence of injuries to the forelimb superficial digital flexor tendon and deep digital flexor tendon (Murray *et al.*, 2006). These injuries may be acute or non-acute and have been associated with jumping course design (particularly in eventing and steeplechase), fatigue during competition, and poor footing on landing over jumps.

Racing Behaviour and Welfare

Racing

It is natural for horses to run and compete against each other. Based on this observation, galloping and racing may be considered an inherent behaviour in the horse, and possibly the equestrian sport most closely aligned with the ecological niche occupied by the horse. The difference between horses galloping freely and racing is the rider. The rider dictates the galloping duration and intensity, and their weight provides a greater load on the distal limbs. However, in the racehorse's favour, they are usually competed against horses of a similar age or ability (race class or group), are physically fit, and conditioned by selection, training, feeding and general care. The racehorse is an athlete. Every aspect of the horse's training and management is focused on optimizing its finite genetic potential.

The preparation of the horse for racing usually starts with foundation training ('breaking-in') when the horse is a 'long' yearling (~18 months old). Once habituated to saddle and able to be ridden out in company, the horse will then have a break of a couple of weeks to months before beginning

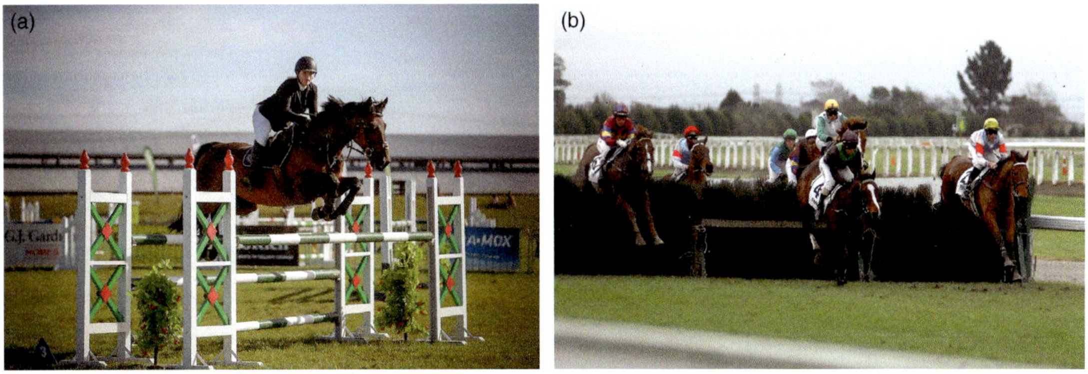

Fig. 6.7. A horse jumping a fence during a competition (a), and steeplechase horses jump a brush fence during a steeplechase race (b). Photos: author.

race training as a 2-year-old (Rogers *et al.*, 2020). Most horses enter race training as 2-year-olds, but not all will have a race start. Many will only complete the training up to the stage of being ready to race. Many trainers start horses at this age. There is now an abundance of scientific literature that supports this practice from a physiological point of view (i.e. promotion of tissue development when the horse's musculoskeletal system is most receptive (Rogers and Dittmer, 2019). Early race training is also associated with longer and more successful racing careers (Tanner *et al.*, 2013).

Most horses race as a 3-year-old, and the duration of the racing career is dependent on its ability and the avoidance of injury. Voluntary retirements are the major reason for retirement from racing, generally due to a horse's inability to remain competitive as it progresses up racing grades. Lameness and musculoskeletal injury are the primary reasons for the retirement of horses for involuntary reasons. Because of this, much management of the horse revolves around avoidance of training or management practices that place the horse at risk of injury.

A horse galloping at full speed is very close to its mechanical limits. This is in part due to how evolution, and to a lesser extent selective breeding, has shaped the racehorse to be a fast and athletic animal with minimal mass in the distal limb. At the racing gallop, the equivalent load of up to 2.5 times the horse's body weight is placed on a single leg. This provides significant strain on the bones in the limb and the soft tissue structure, specifically the superficial digital flexor tendon, which is the main tendon involved in the attenuation of strain. At a gallop, it has been estimated that the maximal strain in the superficial digital flexor tendon is within 6% of the safety limit for that tissue. Thus, even a small misstep in a divot is sufficient to induce an injury. Epidemiology studies have identified that older horses, fast tracks and fatigue are risk factors. For the bones in the distal limb, the main cause of injury is associated with cyclic overload and an imbalance between exercise and recovery. The art of race training is the possession of sufficient skill to recognize subtle changes in gait and behaviour in the horse that indicate this may be occurring, as the horse as a prey species has evolved to minimize outward displays of discomfort or lameness.

The racing and recovery pattern depends on the horse, age, race distance, and, to some extent, the racing jurisdiction. Thoroughbreds can race every two weeks though most trainers will start a horse in a pattern closer to once every three weeks. Each horse may have an optimal pattern to the frequency of racing, which relates to the physiological need for tissue recovery and the mental challenges of racing and training (Morrice-West, 2020).

Horse racing is both a sport and an industry. It is controlled by its own authorized organizations, at an international and national, regional or state level, which establish rules and regulations for every aspect of racing. These exist to ensure that racing operates properly, humanely, honestly and fairly in the interests of the horses and the race attendees. Both the international and national/state regulatory bodies have their own code of horse welfare, by which all participants must abide. Since events are under public observation, horse racing, as an acceptable activity, has the further guarantee of general scrutiny as a monitoring force. Individual horses that excel in this sport are of great commercial value, and this underpins the racing and breeding aspects of the industry. The gambling aspect draws wider massive public support. However, some people are simply attracted to the sight of fine horses in motion.

Opponents of racing (animal rights lobby groups and others) often portray the horse as a subservient or slave to the rider, forced to gallop to fatigue and whipped to respond (see the section to follow). In contrast, supporters of racing portray the horse as a willing partner in a natural aspect of horse behaviour (Legg *et al.*, 2019). There are invariably aspects of truth in both arguments. There is little advantage in running in a race for the horse when it appears that its primary behavioural motivations are access to forage feed and the company of other horses. Conversely, those who have owned and worked with horses appreciate that it is impossible to motivate a horse to successfully race if it does not have the innate desire to run and compete. The disparity in views represents very different philosophical perspectives; one that any use of an animal is unacceptable, and the other that the racing sport represents the involvement of humans in a natural behaviour of the horse. As society changes, the social licence, or acceptability, of different activities evolves. An increasingly urban society that does not regularly interact with horses provides a real challenge for the appeal and viability of horse racing and, to a limited extent, other equestrian sport.

Standardbred horses generally race in harness at the trot or the pace, though they sometimes race under saddle in France. Standardbred racing on a global scale is less popular than Thoroughbred racing and is concentrated in North America, Northern Europe, Australia and New Zealand. The racing gait of the Standardbred is either the diagonal trot (most common in Europe and North America) or the pace (most common in Australia and New Zealand). In the pace, the pair of legs on the same side move in unison. Since this type of running permits some side-to-side bending of the spine, a slightly longer stride length can be attained per stride in the pace than in the diagonal trot. Horses that race as pacers usually race in harnesses called hobbles that encourage the pace rather than the trotting action. Unlike galloping, which has locomotor–respiratory coupling, the coupling does not appear strongly enforced or necessary in trotting and pacing. Thus, Standardbreds, when racing, range from one breath per stride to one breath every second stride. Possibly, due to pulling a driver in a racing cart, rather than having a jockey on top, we see subtly different patterns of injury in Standardbred racehorses compared to Thoroughbreds. Standardbred horses also generally have a training regimen of greater duration and frequency than practiced with Thoroughbred racehorses.

Use of the whip

The use of the whip, particularly in racing, has been the focus of media attention and significant lobbying by animal rights groups. In the United Kingdom, the debate has been elevated to the level of a ministerial enquiry into the use of the whip in racing. Whip use in equestrian sport is a barometer of the social licence of the equestrian sport and changing public attitudes as to what is acceptable 'best practice'. In response to these challenges, many racing jurisdictions have clear guidelines on the restricted use of the whip in racing and the introduction of the padded whip. However, industry administrators recognize that whip use may not be a common part of racing in the future.

The type of whip used varies with the equestrian sport. In racing, as mentioned previously, all racing jurisdictions have switched to a padded racing crop. Most racing jurisdictions have regulations on how the whip may be used and the frequency of times a horse may be hit. Regulation of this is under the control of the racing stewards, who enforce the rules and impose a punishment (usually in the form of a fine or being prohibited from riding on a number of race days). In equestrian sport, a whip, sometimes called a crop, can be carried by the rider. Within a sport, there are restrictions on the length of the whip, the dimensions of the leather loop, and when and how it may be used. The International Equestrian Federation publishes the rules around whip use in equestrian sport for most countries. The whip used in harness racing is much longer and very flexible, with a small flap on the end. When applied to the horse, it could cause sharp pain, but most drivers usually apply it to the cart's side harness or shaft to urge the horse. Some harness racing tracks and jurisdictions (Sweden and Australia) have introduced a 'no-whipping' rule.

Part of the public ill-feeling towards using the whip in sport and racing is focused on its use for punishment rather than as an aid or tool to reinforce the leg. Work by scientists and practitioners with the International Society for Equitation Science has increased the understanding of applying learning theory to equestrian sport and horse management (Doherty *et al.*, 2017). Based on classical conditioning during foundation training, the horse is taught to move forward, or then later in training, forward and sideways, from applying leg pressure. This use of pressure and release (negative reinforcement) forms the basis of much training with horses. In this context, if the appropriate response is not achieved with the leg, the use of a whip may reinforce this action. At all times, the horse must have the opportunity to move away or forward in response to the use of the whip. Failure to permit this negates the learning experience and constitutes unacceptable punishment and abuse.

Swimming

As a rule, horses are not thought of as naturally swimming animals even though most can swim for limited periods, even without previous experience. The gait adopted by the horse during swimming is best described as a modified doggie paddle with horses either adopting a trot- or pace-like gait when swimming. There does not appear to be a uniform pattern to the swimming gait adopted by horses. While the body does provide some buoyancy, the thin distal limbs and relatively small surface area of the hoof mean the horse must work hard to achieve forward momentum. Horses often appear to invert the top line when swimming, and there are reports in the literature indicating a decrease in respiration rate when swimming (Jones *et al.*, 2020).

Swimming is often used as a non-weight bearing exercise for racehorses, with ~80% of Victoria (Australia) Thoroughbred trainers and ~40% of Australian Standardbred racehorse trainers using swimming in their training programme (Steel and Morrice-West, 2019). However, despite the frequency of use, there is limited published data on the horse's physiological response to swimming. Bouts of swimming exercise by Thoroughbred racehorse trainers generally relatively short, lasting 45 s to 1.5 min which equates to 50–90 m, assuming a horse swims at 0.95–1.05 m/s (Figs 6.8a and b). The same authors report that Australian Standardbred trainers will swim their horses for up to 7 min in a session. Current data indicates that swimming is strenuous, but not at the intensity of overground work. Therefore it is classified as submaximal exercise based on peak heart rate and several other physiological parameters; see Steel and Morrice-West (2019) for a summary table of the physiological response of horses to swimming. There are reports of adverse events after swimming, including post-swim colic and epistaxis (exercise-induced pulmonary haemorrhage). There are also anecdotal accounts of back soreness, upper pelvic limb lameness and drowning.

Need for Daily Exercise

The horse, as a cursorial browser, appears to have an innate drive for movement. The evolutionary design of the horse, particularly the distal limb, is orientated around constant movement. Evidence for this is seen in the lymphatic system and the structural design of the blood vessels in the lower leg, which effectively utilizes every step for assistance with blood flow in the distal limb. There is limited data on how much exercise a horse needs or seeks during a day. Behaviour trials have indicated that access to feed and company override any seeking for self-selected exercise. When at pasture or in feral environments, the horse spends most of its time walking and browsing (rather than grazing behaviour). It appears that ~7 km/day is the typical or upper range of movement when the horse has access to adequate feed resources. In wild environments, horses may travel up to 45 km/day; this is usually associated with the need to cover considerable distances between the limited feed supply and the closest water supply (Hampson *et al.*, 2010).

When provided with adequate resources and an opportunity to exercise freely at pasture, there is considerable variation in an individual horse's desire for locomotor activity. Unpublished data by the author and collaborators have found persistent self-selected pasture activity levels between individuals, remaining consistent even with confinement to loose boxes for part of the day.

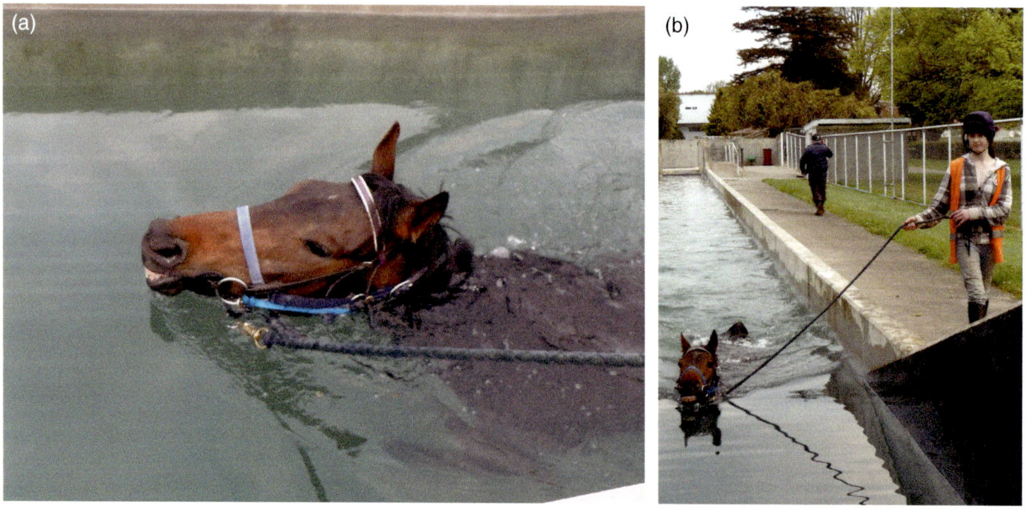

Fig. 6.8. Close up of the head of a racehorse while swimming (a) and a groom walking with the horse while in a swimming pool (b). Photos: author.

Loose exercise or turning horses out of their stables into paddocks or yards can provide them with mild exercise and relief from an enclosure. In such circumstances, the released horses may need several hours to move adequately. If this is a regular practice, a windbreak or shelter should be provided so the horses can deal with hot or cold weather during their release. The self-exercise period may need to be curtailed in very severe weather. Nevertheless, even in poor weather, intensively managed horses should have some exercise daily.

Most countries' welfare codes indicate that appropriate horse management includes some ability for exercise, either ridden, or as free exercise at liberty in a yard or paddock, dependent on climatic conditions. None of the welfare codes appears to specify how much exercise meets the minimum requirement or what may be considered ideal. The lack of a tight definition or prescription of how much is required is due to a current lack of data on what is necessary for physiological and psychological well-being. In many countries where climate, or space, restricts the ability to provide free exercise at pasture, mechanical walkers offer the opportunity to increase the exercise level of intensively managed (stabled) horses.

Lungeing

Lungeing can be used as a riderless (usually) means of controlled exercise within a limited space or aid in the diagnoses of musculoskeletal, neurologic or respiratory conditions in the horse. For the lungeing of any horse, a lungeing head collar should be used with a lungeing line about 8–10 m (25–30ft) in length. A cavesson with a ring on the noseband is preferred to a head collar. The horse should be lunged in a proper location. A smooth, sand-covered area or an indoor riding arena would be most suitable, but an area of pasture can be converted for this use. With the aid of a driving whip, the horse is directed around a circular route. The person lungeing the horse occupies a central position and turns continuously to face the horse to urge it in its progress while holding the long lungeing rein.

The best gaits of the horse in lungeing are alternately the walk and the trot. The horse must be driven for equal amounts of exercise in both directions. At times, a lunged horse will engage in a canter. If cantering is included in the exercise, the horse must exercise in each direction long enough to adopt the proper lead for the direction. In the clockwise direction, the right foreleg should lead. In the counter-clockwise direction, the exercise should continue until there is a left lead to prevent one-sidedness (McGreevy and Thomson, 2006).

Riding

Riding is an efficient way to exercise a horse. However, the horse did not evolve for riding. This consideration needs to be accounted for when riding, including the selection of the terrain/ground surface over which it is exercised, the horse's age and fitness and the temperature and relative humidity. In equestrian sport, the duration and the intensity of exercise during training and competition appear highly repeatable between countries (Lönnell *et al.*, 2014; Verhaar *et al.*, 2014). Show jumping and dressage horses are generally ridden ~5 days per week for ~45 min duration. The workload for these horses is relatively low, with most covering only 3–4 km per session with a heart rate of ~140 bpm.

Lameness is the single largest reason for the involuntary days off or wastage within most equestrian sports or activities. Many equestrian activities also include turning or repetitive movements at a much greater frequency or intensity observed in feral horses. As described earlier, the horse has evolved to have an elegant limb structure to restrict movement of the limb to the sagittal plane (mostly forwards and backwards). Feral horses spend little time at gaits faster than walking or turning in small diameter circles. Analysis strain on the distal limb during turns on 20 m diameter circles provides an example of how such a simple exercise, when ridden, can provide a significant increase in the strain that exceeds that expected, based on just the addition of rider weight (Chateau *et al.*, 2013).

In recent years consideration of rider weight in relation to horse size (bodyweight) has come under some scientific investigation (Dyson *et al.*, 2020). Some obvious examples are now included in the rules of many equestrian bodies (i.e. preventing adults from riding children's small ponies), but refinement of the data to provide an optimal or ideal ratio has not yet been achieved. The implications of rider weight are also further compounded by rider ability. Advanced riders can synchronize their movement in phase with the horse and thus minimize the impact of their weight. In contrast, beginner riders often find this difficult, increasing the fatigue effects of carrying a rider for the horse.

The ground surface upon which the horse moves has major implications on the intensity and duration of the ridden exercise. The ideal ground surface should provide sufficient yield to minimize the concussion of hoof impact at loading but enough resistance to permit the horse to utilize the elastic recoil potential of the flexor tendons. The ideal ground surface has been the focus of much research and is dependent on the activity (i.e. racing versus dressage), the frequency of use and the duration of the activity.

Heat is a by-product of muscular work. Even at a low level compared to the resting metabolic rate, there can be a 10–20-fold increase in heat production. To increase gait efficiency, the horse has concentrated muscle mass around the hip and shoulder pivot points. An unfortunate side effect of this is a reduction in the surface area to volume ratio. To counteract this, the horse has two adaptations. The first is the ability to tolerate a high core temperature during exercise and the redirection of blood flow. At rest, ~15 % of equine cardiac output is directed toward muscles. However, during strenuous exercise, ~80% of cardiac output is directed to the muscles. The second major adaptation in the horse is the prolific capability to sweat and lose heat via evaporation. At high intensities, a horse can produce between 10–15 L of sweat per hour. This must be replenished with water and electrolytes. Horses may also maintain a high respiration rate after exercise in hot conditions, as the lungs also provide a large surface area over which to dissipate heat.

Summary

The horse has evolved as a cursorial herbivore. As such, much of its behaviour and physiology had adapted to be capable of large periods of low-level activity (walking and browsing) interspersed with short bouts of high-speed activity. These evolutionary adaptions have suited the horse firstly as a work or draft animal and, in more recent years, use in equestrian sport. They need to be considered when managing the horse and using it in sport.

References

Andersson, L.S., Larhammar, M., Memic, F., Wootz, H., Schwochow, D. *et al.* (2012) Mutations in DMRT3 affect locomotion in horses and spinal circuit function in mice. *Nature* 488, 642–646.

Back, W., Barneveld, A., Bruin, G., Schamhardt, H.C. and Hartman, W. (1994) Kinematic detection of superior gait quality in young trotting Warmbloods. *Veterinary Quarterly* 16, 91–96.

Back, W., MacAllister, C.G., van Heel, M.C.V., Pollmeier, M. and Hanson, P.D. (2007) Vertical frontlimb ground reaction forces of sound and lame warmbloods differ from those in quarter horses. *Journal of Equine Veterinary Science* 27, 123–129.

Chateau, H., Camus, M., Holden-Douilly, L., Falala, S., Ravary, B. *et al.* (2013) Kinetics of the forelimb in horses circling on different ground surfaces at the trot. *Veterinary Journal* 198, E20–E26.

Clayton, H.M. (1994) Comparison of the collected, working, medium and extended canters. *Equine Veterinary Journal Suppl.* 17, 16–19.

Cully, P., Nielsen, B., Lancaster, B., Martin, J. and McGreevy, P. (2018). The laterality of the gallop gait in Thoroughbred racehorses. *Plos ONE* 13, e0198545.

Doherty, O., McGreevy, P.D. and Pearson, G. (2017) The importance of learning theory and equitation science to the veterinarian. *Applied Animal Behaviour Science* 190, 111–122.

Drevemo, S., Fredricson, I., Dalin, G. and Bjorne, K. (1980) Equine locomotion. 2. The analysis of coordination between limbs of trotting standardbreds. *Equine Veterinary Journal* 12, 66–70.

Dyson, S., Ellis, A.D., Mackechnie-Guire, R., Douglas, J., Bondi, A. *et al.* (2020) The influence of rider:horse bodyweight ratio and rider-horse-saddle fit on equine gait and behaviour: A pilot study. *Equine Veterinary Education* 32, 527–539.

Egenvall, A., Tranquille, C.A., Lonnell, A.C., Bitschnau, C., Oomen, A. *et al.* (2013). Days-lost to training and competition in relation to workload in 263 elite show-jumping horses in four European countries. *Preventive Veterinary Medicine* 112, 387–400.

Firth, E.C., Rogers, C.W., Doube, M. and Jopson, N.B. (2005) Musculoskeletal responses of 2-year-old Thoroughbred horses to early training. 6. Bone parameters in the third metacarpal and third metatarsal bones. *New Zealand Veterinary Journal* 53, 101–112.

Hampson, B.A., Morton, J.M., Mills, P.C., Trotter, M.G., Lamb, D.W. *et al.* (2010). Monitoring distances travelled by horses using GPS tracking collars. *Australian Veterinary Journal* 88, 176–181.

Hildebrand, M. (1965) Symmetrical gaits of horses. *Science* 150, 701–708.

Hobbs, S.J., Robinson, M.A. and Clayton, H.M. (2018) A simple method of equine limb force vector analysis and its potential applications. *PeerJ* 6, e4399

Holmström, M., Fredricson, I. and Drevemo, S. (1993) Biokinematic analysis of the Swedish Warmblood riding horse at trot. *Equine Veterinary Journal* 26, 235–240.

Jones, S., Franklin, S., Martin, C. and Steel, C. (2020). Complete upper airway collapse and apnoea during tethered swimming in horses. *Equine Veterinary Journal* 52, 352–358.

Kurvers, C.M.H.C., van Weeren, P.R., Rogers, C.W. and van Dierendonck, M.C. (2006) Quantification of spontaneous locomotion activity in foals kept in pastures under various management conditions. *American Journal of Veterinary Research* 67, 1212–1217.

Legg, K.A., Breheny, M., Gee, E.K. and Rogers, C.W. (2019). Responding to risk: regulation or prohibition? New Zealand media reporting of Thoroughbred jumps racing 2016–2018. *Animals* 9, 276.

Lönnell, A., Bröjer, J., Nostell, K., Hernlund, E., Roepstorff, L. *et al.* (2014) Variation in training regimens in professional showjumping yards. *Equine Veterinary Journal* 46, 233–238.

McCoy, A.M., Beeson, S.K., Rubin, C.J., Andersson, L., Caputo, P. *et al.* (2019) Identification and validation of genetic variants predictive of gait in standardbred horses. *Plos Genetics* 15, 16.

McGreevy, P.D. and Thomson, P.C. (2006) Differences in motor laterality between breeds of performance horse. *Applied Animal Behaviour Science* 99, 183–190.

Morrice-West, A. (2020) An investigation of training and racing workloads in thoroughbred racehorses in Australia and their relationship to performance and bone fatigue. PhD Thesis. University of Melbourne, Melbourne, Australia

Morrice-West, A.V., Hitchens, P.L., Walmsley, E.A., Stevenson, M.A. and Whitton, R.C. (2020) Training practices, speed and distances undertaken by Thoroughbred racehorses in Victoria, Australia. *Equine Veterinary Journal* 52, 273–280.

Morrice-West, A., Hitchens, P., Walmsley, E.A. and Whitton, R.C. (2021) Variation in GPS and accelerometer recorded velocity and stride parameters of galloping horses. *Equine Veterinary Journal* 53, 1063–1074.

Murray, R.C., Dyson, S.J., Tranquille, C. and Adams, V. (2006). Association of type of sport and performance level with anatomical site of orthopaedic injury diagnosis. *Equine Veterinary Journal Supplement* 36, 411–416.

Riemersma, D.J. and Schamhardt, H.C. (1985) In vitro mechanical properties of equine tendons in relation to cross-sectional area and collagen content. *Research in Veterinary Science* 39, 263–270.

Rogers, C.W. and Dittmer, K. (2019) Does juvenile play programme the equine musculoskeletal system? *Animals* 9, 646.

Rogers, C.W., Bolwell, C.F., Gee, E.K. and Rosanowski, S.M. (2020) Equine musculoskeletal development and performance: impact of the production system and early training. *Animal Production Science* 60, 2069–2079.

Steel, C. and Morrice-West, A. (2019) A survey of trainers on the use of swimming and other water-based exercise for Thoroughbred racehorses in Australia. *Comparative Exercise Physiology* 15, 149–156.

Tanner, J.C., Rogers, C.W. and Firth, E.C. (2013) The association of 2-year-old training milestones with career length and racing success in a sample of Thoroughbred horses in New Zealand. *Equine Veterinary Journal* 45, 20–24.

Verhaar, N., Rogers, C.W., Gee, E., Bolwell, C. and Rosanowski, S.M. (2014). The feeding practices and estimated workload in a cohort of New Zealand competition horses. *Journal of Equine Veterinary Science* 34, 79–84.

7 Spatial Factors

Chris W. Rogers MAgrSc, PhD*

Massey University, Palmerston North, New Zealand

Introduction 96
Territoriality 96
Home range and core home range 96
Home range estimates 97
Domestic horses at pasture 97
Stabling and stall environment 98
Spatiality 99
Welfare and Spacing 101
Spatial needs – minimal standards or optimal environment? 101
Implications for management and sport 101
References 102

Introduction

The evolutionary path of the horse has greatly shaped its behaviour and its spatial interactions within its environment. We can obtain data on what is natural for a horse from observations of feral horses and herds. Conclusions drawn from these observations reinforce our understanding of the horse as a cursorial browser. Hence movement and flight responses significantly underpin all social and spatial behaviour patterns. As a cursorial browser, the availability and scarcity of resources (food and water) heavily influence the distances covered and the horse's home range. Under optimal conditions, horses will comfortably cover a range of about 7–15 km per day browsing. As resources become scarce, the distances travelled can increase to up to 55 km per day. Therefore, it is essential when reflecting on observations from feral herds to consider the effects that resource availability has on the data presented.

Somewhat surprisingly, we have relatively limited data on the spatial ecology of the horse, even under domestic management conditions. For feral horses, most of the published data are over 30 years old. Only recently are we starting to obtain some rich and robust data obtained via high-resolution global positioning satellite (GPS) tracking units and other approaches. These recent publications have contributed greatly to our understanding of how horses utilize their environment and their spatial ecology.

Territoriality

Home range and core home range

The 'home range' is a widely used term within the published literature, but its definition remains imprecise. In the broadest context, the home range represents 'an interplay between the environment and an animal's understanding of that environment; that is, its cognitive map' (Powell and Mitchell, 2012). Suppose this is used as our basis for defining the home range of a horse. In that case, it clearly demonstrates that the home range is plastic and varies dependently on available resources, the time of the year(s), and the evolutionary programmed innate behaviour of the animals within this environment. This may partially explain the quite different estimates within the literature for the home range for feral horses and equids in general, and the

*Corresponding author: c.w.rogers@massey.ac.nz

DOI: 10.1079/9781789242133.0007

difficulty in directly extrapolating or applying these to domestic horses managed at pasture or in a stall or loose box environment.

Using GPS data, we can apply greater precision in defining the spatial ecology of different species. It enables techniques such as utilization distributions to identify the home range and areas of concentrated use, described as the 'core range' or 'core home range' within the home range. In the context of horses, core home ranges may represent an area of concentrated grazing before the herd moves on to a new area for grazing.

Home range estimates

Irrespective of the equid studied, the home ranges of herds do not appear to be mutually exclusive and can overlap with those of other herds. These home ranges do not appear to be defended, but rather herds operate under conditions of mutual avoidance (King, 2002). Ranges can be actively shared, as at a water hole or when a herd passes through another. In winter, when bonds weaken, bands may split and then recombine as spring approaches (Ford and Keiper, 1979).

The reintroduction of Przewalski horses into their natural habitat in Mongolia has provided interesting insights into establishing home ranges and essential components of a home range (King, 2002). The key components, a water source, somewhere to rest (a wooded area or rocky outcrop), and pastures for grazing reflect the horse's basic needs and the plasticity of the home range size reported. This, in part, may reflect the lack of constraints on expansion and the vegetation source. During observation (visual recognition rather than GPS tracking), the Przewalski herds have been noted to have had home ranges of up to 1158 ha, with the development of the home range slowly expanding from the site of the original release. The pattern of expansion and evolution of the home range from the original release site for these equids reflects the observation that they use visual and olfactory cues to provide a 'cogitative map' of the space around them, preferring known routes and forgetting or ignoring those not utilized in a long time (Solstad *et al.*, 2008; Powell and Mitchell, 2012; Fischler *et al.*, 2019). Subsequent analysis of telemetry and GPS data has refined the estimates of home range and the mean distance travelled by the Przewalski horses. These estimates were of a daily (straight line) distance travelled of 3.5 km, and home ranges of 471 km^2 (range 152–826 km^2) that more closely agree with data from the United States of America and Australia on feral horse populations (Kaczensky *et al.*, 2008)

As indicated above, the distance covered per day by feral horses is highly influenced by the relative distance between their preferred pasture and water source. Feral horses in the Australian outback cover 15.9 km per day and, in extreme cases, up to 55 km per day, greater than the 9 km per day reported for feral horses in South Western Wyoming (USA). The core range of the Wyoming horses was 7.4 km^2 (standard error 1.3 km^2), and the summer home range was 40.4 km^2 (standard error 6.7 km^2), very similar to the kernel home range (48.2 km^2) reported for feral horses in Alberta, Canada (Henning *et al.*, 2018). In the Kaimanawa ranges of New Zealand, an area of high horse density, relatively abundant forage and a physically constrained area, have influenced the observation of many much smaller and overlapping home ranges from 0.96 to 17.7 km^2 (Linklater *et al.*, 2000).

Domestic horses at pasture

Extrapolation of feral horse data to horses in domestic or commercial management conditions is difficult. In part this is because conventional management by humans markedly alters the social structure of cohorts of horses. Horses used in equestrian or other sports may be more analogous to bachelor herds (single or small groups of geldings). Only broodmares on larger commercial farms are in social structures similar to that encountered with a feral herd (except for no resident stallion).

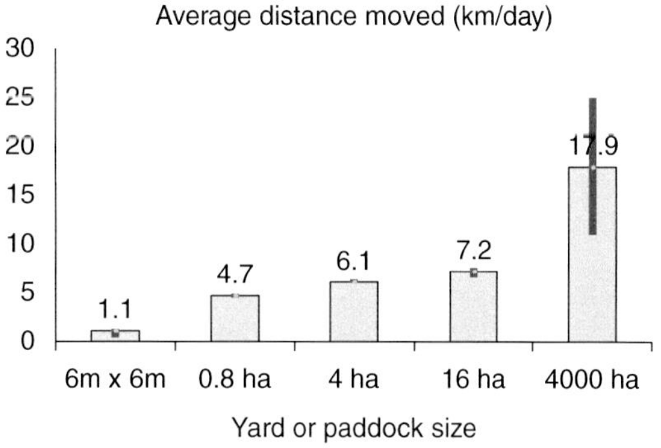

Fig. 7.1. Distances covered by horses within different sized yards and paddocks. Image modified from Hampson *et al.* (2010).

In herds of semi-feral Przewalski horses, daily bouts of herd movement range from 130 to 1600 m, with the vast majority of herd or cohort movement being short distances of <480 m (~83%) and at low speed (walking). In these herds, movement as a group accounts for 10% or more of the daily time budget, and the activity of grazing is consistently recorded before and after movement (Bourjade *et al.*, 2009). In the periods before movement, the stimuli for movement is initiated by several group members, thus qualifying the process as a 'partially shared consensus decision'. This observation contrasts with the traditional view of a single and consistent leader within the band.

For cohorts of domestic horses at pasture, the movement pattern appears similar to that reported for feral horses. The majority of activity consists of the hybrid activity of slow walk-grazing. Paddock size appears to provide a partial constraint to total daily distance moved by horses in conventional management systems. In a 6 × 6 m pen, daily distance travelled can be as little as 1.1 km per day. With increasing paddock size, there is an increase in total distance covered which appears to plateau at 6–7 km per day once the paddock size reaches 4 ha (Fig. 7.1) (Hampson *et al.*, 2010). This plateau in daily distance covered in a 4 ha paddock is very similar to the core home range reported for the feral horses in Wyoming and may indicate that this is the typical movement pattern for horses when feed is adequate but there is no limiting constraint in the grazing area. Hampson *et al.* (2010) proposed that at pasture the mean daily distance travelled could be estimated using the following equation: distance = 0.72 (standard error 0.029) × ln (paddock size in hectares) + 5.08 (standard error 0.094) (R^2 = 0.997). This formula may assist those in trying to estimate the spatial requirements for domestic horses.

In pasture-based systems, there has been an increased interest in the provision of lanes or 'racetracks' in various configurations (generally an area defined with temporary electric fence tape) within the paddock in an attempt to increase the activity of pasture-kept horses (generally those with 'thrifty phenotypes'). When pasture activity (distance travelled based on GPS) was compared between various configurations, it appeared that the more complex the paddock configuration (e.g. spiral design), the lower the activity of the horse. There is no difference in activity level between the open paddock and some of the simplest configurations (racetrack, etc.). However, establishing a novel feeding system that effectively forces horses to move to the other side of the paddock (yard) to obtain hay does result in a five-fold increase in activity (Hampson *et al.*, 2013). These data indicate that the innate drive to move within a pasture environment is constrained by paddock size. Additional increases in distance travelled can be stimulated via changing the feed access.

The establishment of areas of lawns (preferred grazing areas) and roughs (latrine areas) by horses kept at pasture implies, in a moderated form, the use of a cognitive map. Under conditions of adequate feed supply, an area of ~30% of effective pasture area remains as a latrine area (roughs). These roughs are spatially distributed across the pasture as a series of major areas (Fig. 7.2). The location of latrine areas is heavily conserved, and reintroduction of the herd, even after a period of cross grazing with ruminants, results in rapid re-establishment of these roughs. It is possible that the lawns under restricted pasture management represent the horses' core grazing area. During the day across the pasture, the pattern of movement is analogous to the pattern of movement observed in feral horses, albeit in a condensed format. The collection of the spatial ecology data via GPS of domestic horses at pasture could help refine this observation.

Stabling and stall environment

For many domestic horses (approximately 90% of horses in Europe) daily management involves an individual stable or loose box environment with some provision of turnout in small turnout yards or paddocks. While most national and state codes of welfare for horses suggest that horses should be provided with turnout time for free exercise, none appear to provide a suggested minimum time or area. Data from the literature indicate that given the opportunity with adequate feed and companionship, that activity alone is not a primary consideration. Most horses only seek approximately 15 min free turn out per day for a single turnout (turnout time increases to 45 min if it was with a companion or group of horses). Feed and companionship are consistently ranked in priority above forced exercise in preference tests (Lee *et al.*, 2011). These data imply that even considering the distance travelled during training and riding taken into account (e.g. typically 3–4 km per day for competition

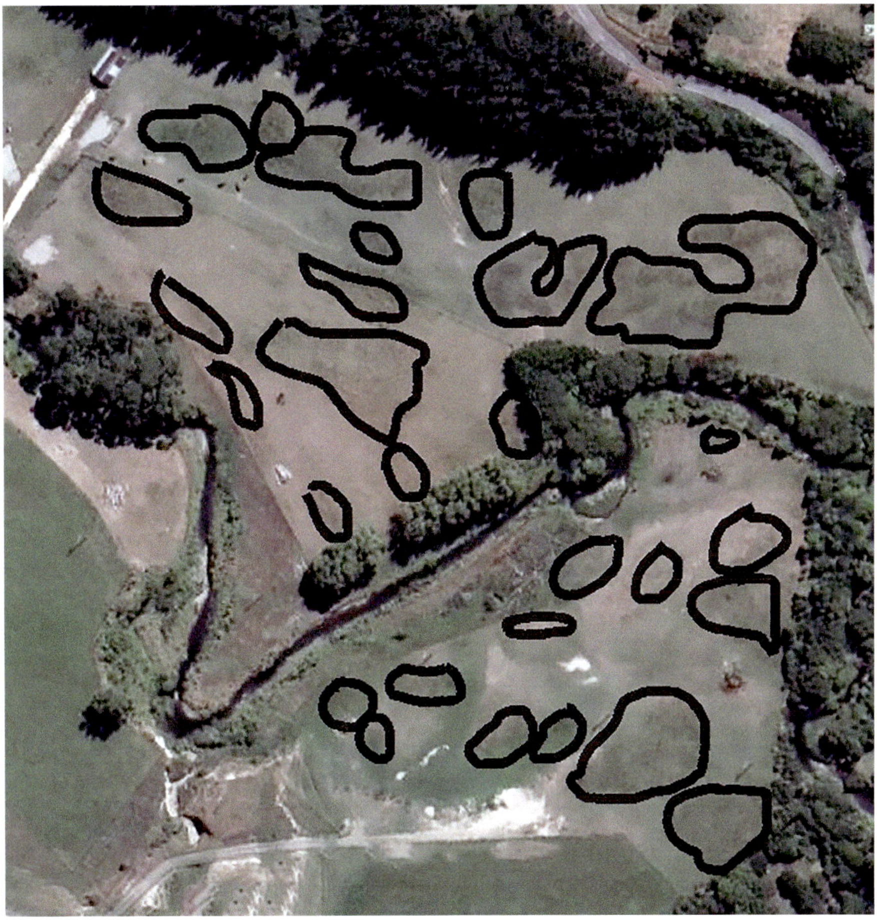

Fig. 7.2. Satellite monitoring of the persistence of the spatial distribution of latrine areas (roughs). Image represents one point in time from three paddocks with varying levels of grazing intensity. GPS data is overlaid to quantify both position and area (unpublished data, author).

jumpers), that provision of single-horse turnout may only just achieve the theoretical ideal of 6–7 km per day.

Spatiality

The keeping of most horses in Europe and many North American jurisdictions as singular animals in stables or loose boxes contrasts with the herd sizes and spatial distribution of feral horses. Feral horses are reported to have group sizes of up to 35 animals, but under 10 horses within a group is generally most common (Hartmann *et al.*, 2012). It is difficult to compare the spatial distribution of feral horses with those of domestic horses at pasture. However, it is generally accepted that an approximate distance of two horse lengths represents the space within which a horse can safely respond to agonistic behaviour without undue energy expenditure or risk of injury. There are limited reports accurately quantifying the consistency of spacing between individuals, either in a feral or a domesticated setting. It is currently proposed that spatially horses associate themselves with a nearest neighbour, often a conspecific of similar rank within the herd. The majority (60–70%) of these nearest neighbour observations have the two horses within 2 m of each other, and approximately 20% are separated by 3–10 m (Jørgensen *et al.*, 2009). When observing mobs or herds of horses, this often provides the appearance of a number of pairs of horses with closer spatial relationship or spacing than between the different pairs (Fig. 7.3).

Under domestic conditions, the number of agonistic interactions and injuries increases when horse density is increased (Roy *et al.* 2015). Most agonistic behaviours recorded relate to the inability of horses to maintain their individual space. Limited feed resources accentuate the number of agonistic behaviours.

To reduce stress and the frequency of agonistic behaviours, the density of horses at pasture should be sufficient to permit horses to maintain this individual space effortlessly. Under commercial breeding farm conditions broodmares and youngstock are often kept in cohorts of 4–10 horses within 2–10 ha (providing a density of 1.4–2.6 horses/ha), easily providing the opportunity for sufficient social spacing (Bengtsson *et al.*, 2018). Stocking density is generally driven by the need to provide sufficient pasture (kg DM pasture/ha) to meet daily nutrient requirements rather than directly because of social spacing. Sport horses at pasture are managed either singularly (50%) or as pairs (35%). Thus, the lower stocking density of 0.22 ha/horse is unlikely to provide difficulties with maintaining appropriate social spacing.

The flight distance reflects a horse's relative reactivity to novel stimuli or, in a herd environment, agonistic behaviour. There is a genetic component to flight distance and differences between breeds, and this needs to be considered when discussing differences in flight distances between horses. Flight distance reduces with greater investigative and exploratory behaviour, which are often used as proxy indicators of good welfare and management. Inconsistency of the individual composition of herds (frequent changes of group members) can lead to greater agonistic interactions. This can be observed as an increase in the horse's relative flight distance. Inconsistency in handling (incorrect or poor timing of signal and response) in sport horses has been associated with a reduced threshold for flight and increased flight distance. In young horses, the most consistent estimate of flight distance (in response to

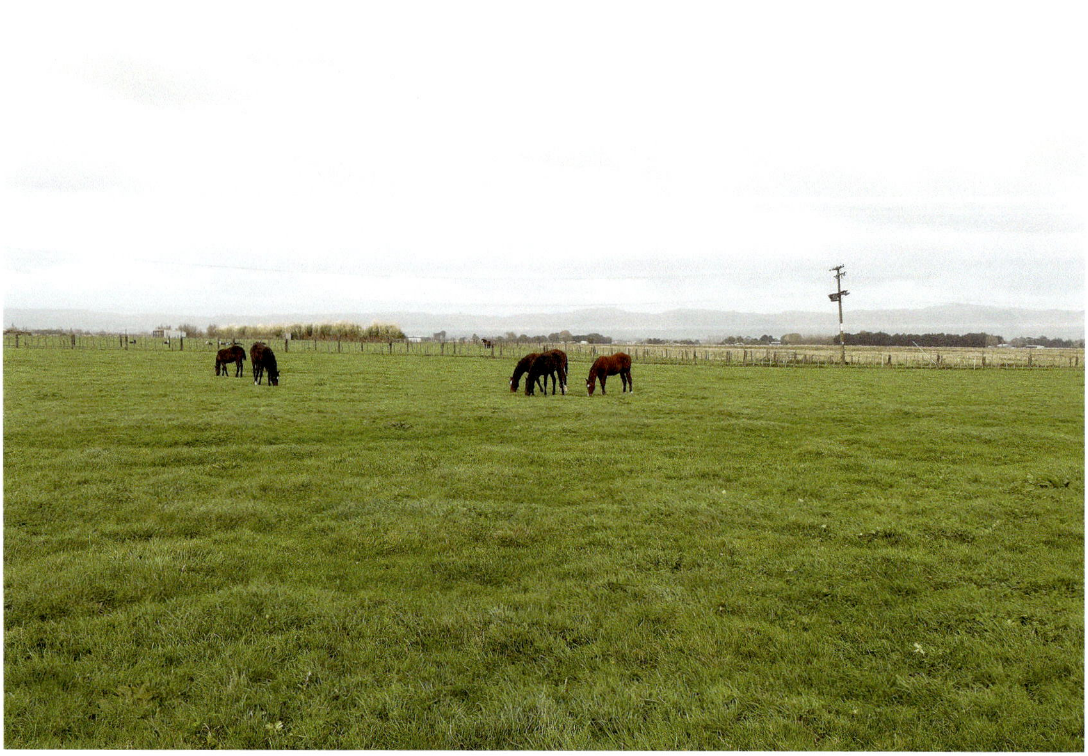

Fig. 7.3. Thoroughbred yearlings at pasture demonstrating typical spatial distribution with their nearest neighbours. Photo: author.

a novel umbrella stimulus) is 2.5 m. This provides a good reference point for the distance at which novel stimuli may provide management challenges when handling young horses. Appropriate (consistent) training of horses reduces the risk of injury to the handler or rider, as the strength of the association of signal and response should override the innate flight response. A dramatic observation of this mechanism occurs with the use of overshadowing (e.g. application of the park and step forward and back response) to prevent expression of the flight response to stimuli perceived as noxious (e.g. hair clippers).

Welfare and Spacing

Spatial needs – minimal standards or optimal environment?

Space requirements were historically viewed as those sufficient to contain the animal. Now it has been recognized that horses have a need for space, not only for containment but also to practise the social and maintenance patterns of innate behaviour. This change in welfare perspective can be seen in the adoption of the five domains perspective for animal welfare rather than minimum standards approach, which tended to be the reference point of the five freedoms approach (Mellor and Burns, 2020).

Implications for management and sport

The literature indicates that despite being a cursorial animal, provided with companionship and sufficient forage, horses can tolerate what initially may appear to be relatively restrictive management practices. However, if a five freedoms approach is taken, consideration must be given to provide management practices that provide a positive affective state and reflect what we interpret to be optimal management based on data from feral horses living in groups.

The major difficulty with applying the positive affective state approach has been the quantification of the metrics against which we can measure appropriate management. It is much easier to identify minimal management conditions below which there is a negative impact on the horse. This difficulty is highlighted by many of the codes of welfare and management identifying that horses housed singly in stables or loose boxes should be provided with turnout for free exercise but offer no prescription of what this should comprise. Because of this difficulty, there is often a requirement for a healthy degree of pragmatism in applying recommendations to horses and the respective management conditions (Fig 7.4).

In recognition of the spatial needs of the horse, the European Union recommends 330 m^2 per horse when placed out with other horses in a paddock for turnout purposes. Ideally, shelter should be provided for a horse during turnout. However, the nature and complexity of this are dependent on the local environment. What is perceived as the most suitable type of fencing for turnout appears to vary across countries, possibly reflecting the use of the horse, cultural preferences and cost. The primary

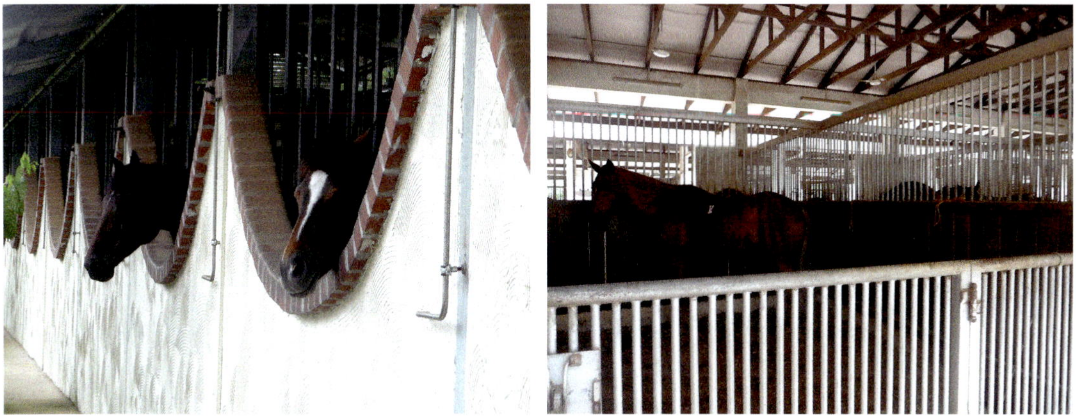

Fig. 7.4. Two examples of open and pragmatic stable design for a humid environment. Images of the Singapore Polo Club. Photo: Kylie Legg.

consideration is that the fencing is safe and robust enough to tolerate the impact of horses rubbing and pushing against structures or breaching them without injury.

The housing of horses should reflect the behavioural and physiological needs and the relative size of the horse. Loose boxes should be of sufficient size that a horse can lie down, rest in a natural position and get up unimpeded. Most loose boxes are now specified at 4 × 4 m (12 × 12 ft). A useful rough guide to check the sufficiency for horses of different sizes is that the internal linear dimensions should be 2.5 times the horse's height. A helpful metric to consider is 350 m^3 (800 ft^3) of cubic air space per horse to ensure sufficient airflow.

Adequate exercise and consistency of groups or cohorts permits a positive affective state and thus reduces the threshold for the flight response in the horses, improving welfare and reducing the risk of injury to the rider or handler. The ability of horses to form cognitive maps of their local environment should be considered when actively and thoughtfully introducing them to those that are new and unfamiliar. The use of a cognitive map may partially explain the success of arena familiarization with young sport horses, and why even seasoned sport horses often appear to recognize the orientation and layout of competition venues even if only visited annually.

References

Bengtsson, J., Rogers, C.W., Back, P.J., Emanuelson, U., Roca, J. *et al.* (2018) Characteristics of the grazing and farm management of broodmares on commercial Thoroughbred stud farms during spring. *New Zealand Journal of Animal Science and Production* 78, 88–91.

Bourjade, M., Thierry, B., Maumy, M. and Petit, O. (2009) Decision-making in Przewalski horses (*Equus ferus przewalskii*) is driven by the ecological contexts of collective movements. *Ethology* 115, 321–330.

Fischler, W.M., Joshi, N.R., Devi-Chou, V., Kitch, L.J., Schnitzer, M.J. *et al.* (2019) Olfactory landmarks and path integration converge to form a cognitive spatial map. *bioRxiv* 752360.

Ford, B. and Keiper, R.R. (1979) *The Island Ponies: An Environmental Study of Their Life on Assateague*. Morrow, New York.

Hampson, B.A., Morton, J.M., Mills, P.C., Trotter, M.G., Lamb, D.W. and Pollitt, C.C. (2010) Monitoring distances travelled by horses using GPS tracking collars. *Australian Veterinary Journal* 88, 176–181.

Hampson, B.A., De Laat, M.A., Monot, J., Bailliu, D. and Pollitt, C.C. (2013) Adaption of horses to a novel dynamic feeding system: Movement and behavioural responses. *Equine Veterinary Journal* 45, 481–484.

Hartmann, E., Søndergaard, E. and Keeling, L.J. (2012) Keeping horses in groups: A review. *Applied Animal Behaviour Science* 136, 77–87.

Henning, J.B., Beck, J.L. and Scasta, J.D. (2018) Spatial ecology observations from feral horses equipped with global positioning system transmitters. *Human-Wildlife Interactions* 12, 75–84.

Jørgensen, G.H.M., Borsheim, L., Mejdell, C.M., Søndergaard, E. and Bøe, K.E. (2009) Grouping horses according to gender - Effects on aggression, spacing and injuries. *Applied Animal Behaviour Science* 120, 94–98.

Kaczensky, P., Ganbaatar, O., Von Wehrden, H. and Walzer, C. (2008). Resource selection by sympatric wild equids in the Mongolian Gobi. *Journal of Applied Ecology* 6, 1762–1769.

King, S.R.B. (2002) Home range and habitat use of free-ranging Przewalski horses at Hustai National Park, Mongolia. *Applied Animal Behaviour Science* 78, 103–113.

Lee, J., Floyd, T., Erb, H. and Houpt, K. (2011). Preference and demand for exercise in stabled horses. *Applied Animal Behaviour Science*, 130, 91–100.

Linklater, W.L., Cameron, E.Z., Stafford, K.J. and Veltman, C.J. (2000) Social and spatial structure and range use by Kaimanawa wild horses (*Equus caballus: Equidae*). *New Zealand Journal of Ecology* 24, 139–152.

Mellor, D.J. and Burns, M. (2020) Using the Five Domains Model to develop welfare assessment guidelines for Thoroughbred horses in New Zealand. *New Zealand Veterinary Journal* 68, 150–156.

Powell, R.A. and Mitchell, M.S. (2012) What is a home range? *Journal of Mammalogy* 93, 948–958.

Roy, R.C., Cockram, M.S., Dohoo, I.R. and Ragnarsson, S. (2015).Transport of horses for slaughter in Iceland. *Animal Welfare* 24, 485–495.

Solstad, T., Boccara, C.N., Kroff, E., Moser, M.B. and Moser, E.I. (2008) Representation of geometric borders in the entorhinal cortex. *Science* 322, 1865–1868.

8 Equine Transport

Barbara Padalino DVM, PhD[1]* and Christopher B. Riley BVSc(Hons), PhD, Diplomate ACVS[2]

[1]*University of Bologna, Bologna, Italy;* [2]*Massey University, Palmerston North, New Zealand*

Introduction	104
Transport by Land	104
To slaughter	104
For racing	105
Non-commercial transport	106
Stressors During the Phases of Land Transport	107
Pre-loading	107
Loading	108
The loading ramp	108
In transit	109
Confinement and isolation	109
Space	109
Environment	109
Watering and feeding	110
Noise	110
Direction of travel	110
Duration of travel	111
Driver behaviour	112
After the journey	113
Physical Welfare	113
Traumatic injuries	113
Dehydration and weight loss	114
Laminitis, heatstroke and muscular problems	115
Gastrointestinal and respiratory problems	115
Behavioural Welfare Problems	116
Pre-loading	116
Loading	117
In transit	117
Unloading	117
Transport by Air	117
Transport by Water	118
References	120

*Corresponding author: barbara.padalino@unibo.it

 Fraser's the Behaviour and Welfare of the Horse (eds C.B. Riley, S.E. Cregier and A.F. Fraser)
DOI: 10.1079/9781789242133.0008

Introduction

Transport is among the most common management practices imposed upon the domestic horse. The earliest historical accounts describe the transport of horses in oar- or sail-powered ships, primarily for war and later for trade. Transport practices were developed by the Romans, improved upon by middle eastern nations in the early Middle Ages, and used in Europe from the 10th century onwards (Katić and Bajt, 2009). Land transport was first reported in the late 18th century, first by horse-drawn vehicles, then with steam engines by rail, and in motorized road vehicles for the first time shortly before World War I (Cregier, 1982). Currently, road transport is more common, movement by ship uncommon, and transport by air has steadily increased (Friend, 2001). Horses are perhaps the most frequently transported domesticated livestock species (Friend, 2001). The global transport of horses is a multibillion-dollar trade and a significant employer in the equine industry.

Despite the importance of horse transport, only recently have modern research approaches been applied to evaluate its consequences for equine welfare. An early review of the effects of road transport on horses found few objective research publications specific to the species (Cregier, 1982). Twenty years later, Friend (2001) found that equine transport welfare had become more strongly underpinned by objective research. Welfare issues identified included injury and physiological indicators of stress in commercially and non-commercially transported horses. During the past ten years, there has been a greater emphasis on understanding the welfare effects of land transport in smaller non-commercial vehicles. Emerging technologies and applying more complex approaches to data analyses now permit a more holistic understanding of the effects of transport on welfare and behaviour. This chapter reviews recent advances in our understanding of the behavioural, physical and physiological effects of transport on horses.

Transport by Land

In industrialized countries, horses kept primarily for pleasure or sport are frequently transported. The number of horse movements by road is too numerous to quantify globally. However, they fall into two main categories: commercial and non-commercial. Commercial transport must comply with codes of live animal transport that vary by country. In contrast, the non-commercial road transport of horses is almost completely unregulated. For this reason, evidence-based best practices must be identified, and guidelines developed and followed (Cregier, 2010). Generally, tame horses usually travel in single stalls, whereas unhandled horses are often transported in groups. Mares regularly travel loose with their foal within a box (Weeks *et al.*, 2012). The demographics of horse movements by road in New Zealand (Rosanowski *et al.*, 2013) and Great Britain (Robin *et al.*, 2011) inform disease control measures. Several surveys have documented the incidence of specific transport-related issues and injuries.

To slaughter

More than 6.6 million horses are transported to slaughterhouses annually (FAO, 2020). Many more movements are not documented. From a welfare perspective, slaughter horses are sometimes referred to as ‘the invisible horses’. Many travel to slaughterhouses in inappropriate conditions, and there is a clear need to improve their welfare (Messori *et al.*, 2016b). Horsemeat consumption became popular in Europe after World War II among those with low income. Nowadays, horsemeat is a highly priced delicacy in Europe, with over 530,000 transported to slaughter per year (Stull, 2001; FAO, 2020). In 2018, 47% of these horses were slaughtered in the Russian Federation, in the Ukraine 7.7%, in Spain 7.7%, in Romania 6.4%, in the United Kingdom 3.9%, and in Italy 3.8%, with smaller percentages in other European states (FAO, 2020). The trade is economically motivated throughout Europe, with meat from horses often originating from one country, transported to, slaughtered, and processed in others (Marlin *et al.*, 2011). This industry employs horse transport over long distances that warrant being more tightly regulated than is currently the case.

In the Americas, more than 1.3 million horses were transported to slaughter in 2018 (FAO, 2020). In the United States (USA), federal funding for the inspection of horse meat destined for human consumption was halted in 2007 following public pressure. This decision and the closure of USA slaughter plants has increased journey length for these horses as they are now diverted to slaughter plants in Canada and Mexico (Stull, 2012). Regional movements within the USA to the dispersal centres for international shipment are now less stringently monitored so that adverse consequences to their welfare are largely invisible (Roy and Cockram, 2015; Roy *et al.*,

2015a; Miranda-de la Lama *et al*., 2020). Horsemeat is still used in the USA for pet food, but there is little information on transport conditions for the 115,000 horses slaughtered domestically for this industry every year (FAO, 2020). In Canada, horses are also transported to slaughter over long distances, with a small number of the 127,000 killed annually consumed domestically; the rest are exported to Europe and Asia. In South America, horsemeat is popular, with approximately 400,000 transported to slaughter per year. However, few jurisdictions have appropriate legislation for protecting horses during transport with significant inadequacies in transport over long distances (Animal Welfare Foundation-Tiershutzbund Zürich, 2017).

Slaughter horses travel loose in trucks with variable loading densities (Fig. 8.1) (Weeks *et al*., 2012). In high-density compartments, horses can fall during shipment, resulting in injury or death; injuries due to kicking are less frequent (Whiting, 1999). Horses transported in mixed-age shipments have an increased risk of injury, especially foals (Roy *et al*., 2015a). In lower-density shipments, horses may have opportunities to escape aggressive situations, lowering their psychosocial stress (Collins *et al*., 2000). Aggressive behaviour during transport is influenced by individual horse temperament (Iacono *et al*., 2007).

The conduct of commercial shippers also affects transport welfare outcomes. For example, in a European study, 15% of the infringements during on-road inspections were issued to horse transporters (Padalino *et al*., 2020a). Fines were imposed for failure to identify the presence of live animals within the vehicle, missing or improper drinking systems, limited space allowance, the absence of ventilation systems, and lack of equipment to inspect animals. The Humane Society International (2012) has denounced the poor transport conditions of horses designated for slaughter and drawn attention to the trade in unbroken horses transported illegally over long distances. Further studies are needed to define optimal travel density and environment, particularly for unbroken horses, which constitute a significant percentage of horses transported to slaughter.

For racing

Despite the many horses specifically transported for racing, surprisingly little is known about its effects on performance. Available reports are somewhat

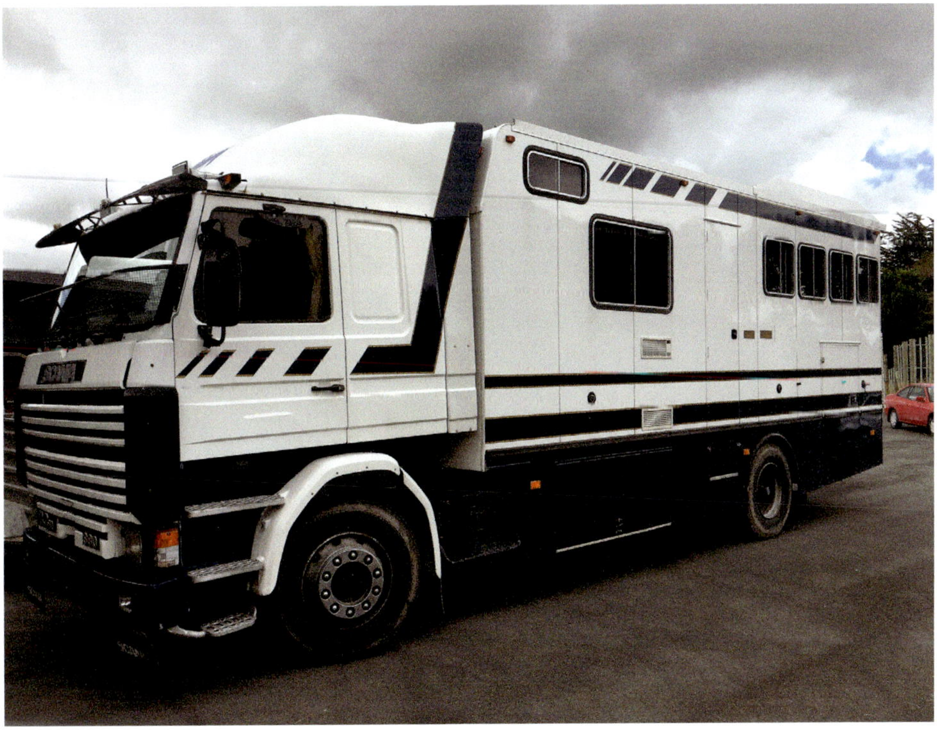

Fig. 8.1. Medium sized horse truck for transporting small groups of horses. Photo: C.B. Riley.

conflicting. For experienced horses, transport over short distances reportedly has little effect on performance (Beaunoyer and Chapman, 1987). However, journeys over longer distances may negatively affect the performance in closely contested races, particularly for horses transported forward facing displaying stress (Slade, 1987). Thoroughbreds are more likely to develop transport-related injuries and health issues than horses transported for recreation (Padalino, 2017). This is attributed to the combined stressors of transport and racing. Based on the increase in serum muscle enzymes caused by transport, a recovery period of 2 hours after 3 hours of travel is suggested for racehorses (Tateo *et al.*, 2012). Travel longer than 8 hours is discouraged before a competition, as it may compromise racing performance and requires several days for recovery (Linden *et al.*, 1991). Such journeys cause a drop in serum calcium and potassium and an increase in serum lactate and muscle enzymes (Padalino *et al.*, 2017a). Managing the transport of racehorses requires particular care, and the relationship between transport and racing needs more investigation.

Non-commercial transport

In contrast to most commercial operators, owners and drivers in the non-commercial sector frequently transport horses in individual compartments in smaller vehicles. These include one-to-three horse capacity trailers (floats) (Fig. 8.2) or trucks (horse boxes) (Fig. 8.3), often over shorter travel distances for recreational and competitive purposes (Weeks *et al.*, 2012). In many countries, non-commercial horse trailers do not require specific certification of their suitability for transporting animals (Cregier and Gimenez, 2015). Few amateur drivers are trained for conducting live animal transport, many have poor knowledge of regulations governing animal welfare during transport, some use improper vehicles, and often vehicle checks are not completed before departure. An Australian study of non-commercial horse transport found one in four participants had experienced an injury to a horse during transport, confirming that the non-commercial vehicular movement of horses poses a welfare hazard similar to that reported for commercial transport

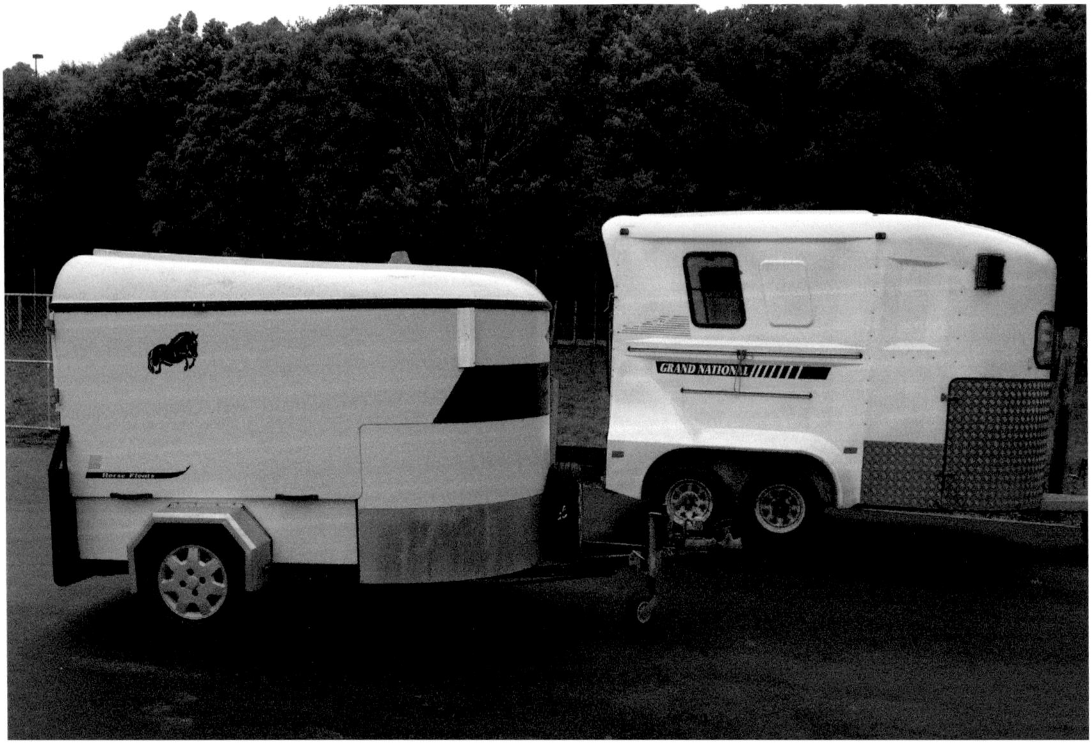

Fig. 8.2 Forward facing two-horse trailers (floats). Note, the float in the foreground has been built using a non-reinforced utility trailer chassis. This latter design is not recommended by the authors. Photo: C.B. Riley.

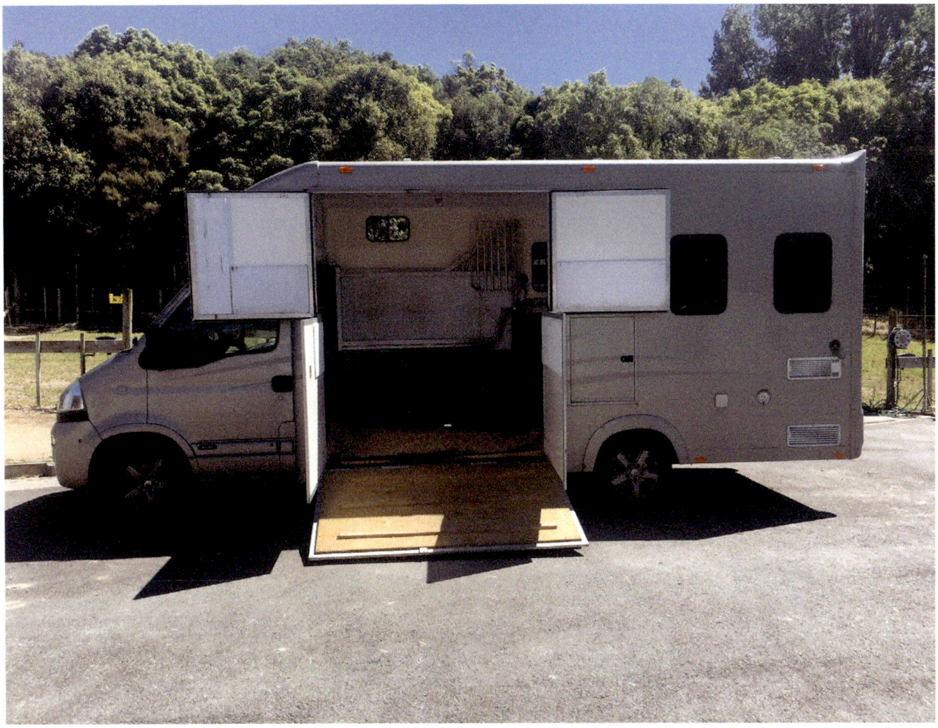

Fig. 8.3. Small horse truck (horse box) as commonly used for equine road transport in Europe. Photo: C.B. Riley.

(Riley *et al.*, 2016). In the United Kingdom, 97% of the respondents to a survey of incidents during road transport moved horses using non-commercial means (Hall *et al.*, 2020). Most (85%) had not completed driver training for livestock transport, and 16% reported a transport-related accident. Many horse owners and trainers responsible for the movement of horses by road do not comply with livestock transport policy because they are uninformed about recommended or required practices. Nevertheless, many indicate that they would like to have better knowledge of best practices. Thus, the main recommendation to safeguard the health and welfare of the horse during non-commercial transport is that all are educated on risk factors for injury and behavioural problems and how to reduce them through best practice, and compliance with animal transport codes encouraged.

Stressors During the Phases of Land Transport

Transport encompasses four phases: pre-loading, loading, transport (the journey) and unloading on arrival. Acclimatization with the new environment is considered a post-travel phase.

Pre-loading

Important stressors during pre-loading include human contact, handling, restraint, and leaving a familiar environment and conspecifics. Handling includes how animals are touched, moved and interacted with during husbandry procedures. Physical restraint is often part of the handling procedure, and it is important to know how horses are likely to react to us when moving and restraining them. Age, sex, and physiological condition influence the behaviour of horses during pre-loading. Foals and yearlings are usually not trained extensively and can be significantly more difficult and riskier than older animals. Although stallions are generally assumed to be more difficult to handle than geldings, this difference may also be age dependent. The response of animals to handling and transport is influenced by their sensory capabilities, the visual field and flight zone (see Chapter 2). Behavioural indicators of discomfort during pre-loading include vocalization, attempts to escape, kicking or struggling. Identifying and managing stressful situations by responding to key behaviours is essential (Siniscalchi *et al.*, 2014). The ability to recognize and react appropriately to stress behaviours in horses reduces the risk of injury to the horse and handler and has a significant effect on equine welfare (Padalino *et al.*, 2018a).

Loading

Loading is among the most stressful components of transport for horse and owner (Waran, 1993). Climbing a ramp is a frightening experience for a naïve horse (Fig. 8.4). Fears result from stimuli such as apprehension of entering an enclosed space, the height of the step leading onto the ramp, and the instability and incline of the ramp (Houpt and Leib, 1993). These factors can result in inexperienced horses exhibiting extreme evasive behaviour and a strong reluctance to step onto the ramp. Interestingly, the heart rate during loading is usually higher than that occurring during transport, regardless of experience. The energy expended in climbing the ramp and fear contributes to the elevation in heart rate (Waran, 1993). Therefore, although horses may become accustomed to loading, even experienced horses are aroused.

Evasive behaviour during loading is typical of young horses, and the time taken to load is influenced by age. Yearlings take more time to load (6 min) than 2-year-olds (30 s), 3-year-olds (22 s), and those over three years (5 s) (Waran and Cuddeford, 1995). Loading fear is innate in the horse, but some environmental stimuli exacerbate it. For example, loading a horse directly from a brightly lit arena into a dark trailer (Cross *et al.*, 2008). Many horses fight during loading as a fear response, thus increasing stress and risking injury to the horse and handler. Rearing, pulling back, head-tossing, pawing and turning sideways are commonly exhibited. These behaviours are negatively reinforced when loading is aborted by the handler.

The loading ramp

The ramp on which the horse gains access to the transport vehicle is a stressor to many horses,

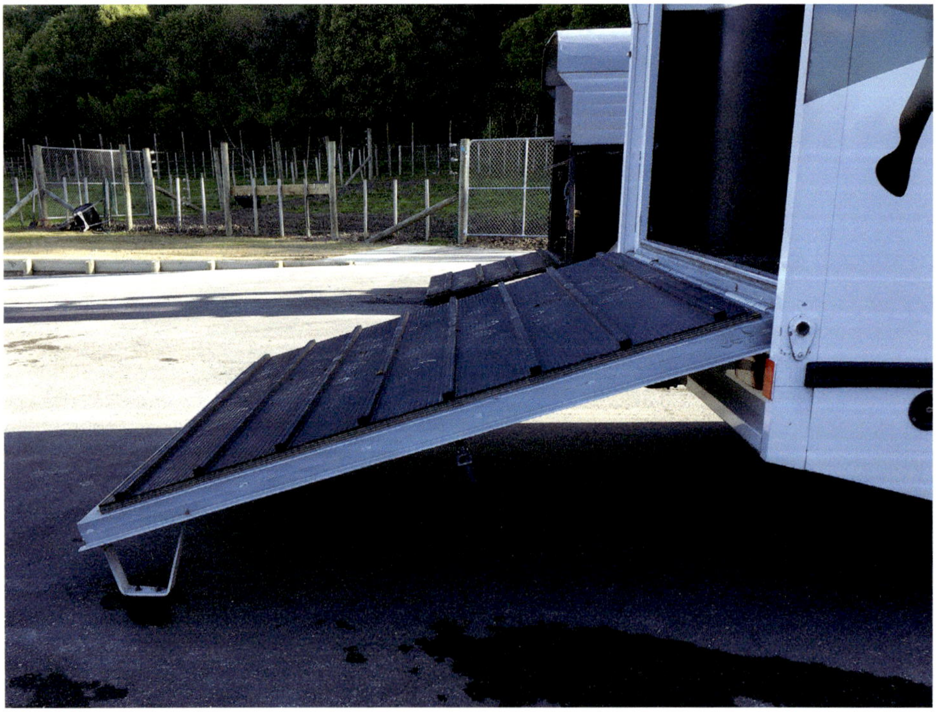

Fig. 8.4. Climbing a steep ramp can be a frightening experience for a horse. Photo: C.B. Riley.

particularly if it is very steep, moves, or makes a noise when the horse steps onto it. Quarter horses are stressed more during loading and stepping backwards off a 20 cm step than during unloading (Siniscalchi *et al.*, 2014). The stress associated with the ramp at unloading may result in some horses charging out of the trailer on arrival at the destination.

In transit

Vehicle movement stressors include confinement, isolation, density, unfamiliar neighbours, noise, vibration, position changes, keeping balance, driving skills, environmental challenges (i.e. temperature, humidity, ventilation, poor air quality) and fasting. Transport stress is a multi-factorial physical and emotional response, where the sympathetic nervous system shifts from alert to fear many times, and maximal effort expended in balance preservation. To maximize well-being during transport, the factors mentioned above should be considered and monitored. The magnitude of these stressors is strongly linked to the journey duration, vehicle design, road design and driver behaviour.

Confinement and isolation

Confinement and isolation are stressful and may suppress feeding behaviour during transport (Mal *et al.,* 1991). Once loaded, the horse is in a restricted space, either confined in an individual stall using partitions or experiencing pressure on individual space exerted by the other loose horses travelling in the same compartment. In both situations, confinement increases serum cortisol, a physiologic indicator of stress (Garey *et al.*, 2010). When travelling with a live companion, significantly less time is spent vocalizing, head-turning, head-tossing and pawing; eating behaviour increases. Heart rate and temperature are also significantly lower. Travelling with a mirror to provide surrogate companionship does not significantly affect physiological responses compared to travelling alone but reduces time spent turning the head, vocalizing and head-tossing; eating behaviour increases (Kay and Hall, 2009). Therefore, surrogate companionship in the form of an unbreakable mirror is preferable to travelling alone. However, where possible, a live companion is recommended. In the latter case, a compatible companion is preferable to reduce equine aggression-related injuries.

Space

Horses experiencing loss of balance, scrambling, abrupt braking and cornering are more agitated and anxious during the journey, possibly due to fear of falling inside the trailer (Riley, 2016). These responses are influenced by the amount of space provided during travel. Based on the risk of injury alone, the recommended loading density for loose horses in Canadian commercial transport vehicles is 1.2 m^2 per 500 kg horse (Whiting, 1999). This compares to a minimum allowance of 1.2 m^2 in Australia and 1.75 m^2 for long journeys in Europe (Eur-lex, 2005). However, many countries do not have regulations or operate under imprecise Office International des Epizooties (OIE)-based guidelines that don't address the horse's behavioural needs (Woods and Messori, 2014). The floor area alone may not account for a horse's needs. The European Union guidelines on the transport of slaughter horses recommend a minimum 10–20 cm space between partitions and animals (Messori, *et al.*, 2016a; Consortium of the Animal Transport Guides Project, 2017). Only recently have behavioural indicators and physiological measures of equine transport welfare been used to identify the space needs of horses on a commercial vehicle (Padalino and Raidal, 2020). For example, horses travelling in a wide bay of 1.9 m^2 show fewer balance-related movements, less leaning on the partitions, less frequent loss of balance and reduced vigilance. Our current evidence-based recommendation is that a minimum 1.9 m^2 be provided for the commercial transport of an average adult horse.

Environment

Poor ventilation in transport vehicles is linked to heat stress and pleuropneumonia (shipping fever), a severe bacterial infection of the airways and lungs. Smaller vehicles are often poorly ventilated, but there are no ventilation standards for non-commercial vehicles (Purswell *et al.*, 2006). In larger transport vehicles, the suitability of the trailer or truck's thermal environment has not been well determined for horses. The upper limit of the thermo-neutral zone in horses is not well defined, but at pasture they seek the comfort of shelter at 25 °C (Hartmann *et al.*, 2015). For Federation Equestre Internationale (FEI) competitions, these factors are used in the calculation of the wet bulb globe temperature index; values >28 require precautions to reduce thermal stress, and values >33 are not compatible with competition (Jeffcott, 1996; Marlin *et al.*, 2018). However, in transport vehicles, the limits set by the FEI are not valid and are often exceeded. In traditional trailers used during late summer–early autumn, inside-to-outside temperature differences range from 5.1 °C to 9.5 °C, decreasing with increased speed and open vents (Purswell *et al.*, 2010). Therefore, horses should not be transported during hot and humid days or when temperatures exceed 30 °C. This is often an impractical restriction in hot or arid countries. Therefore, increasing vent and window areas and adding fans have been suggested for transporting other species and should be used (Mitchell and Kettlewell, 2008). Wind speed in passively ventilated horse vehicles drops to zero when stationary. Air conditioners are recommended in transport conditions of high environmental temperature and humidity. If mechanical ventilation is unavailable, the vehicle should be parked in shaded areas with all windows and ramps open during rest stops (Waran *et al.*, 2007).

Animals produce CO_2 through respiration, ammonia in the urine and microorganisms in eliminations. Carbon monoxide may also contaminate the air. These gases compromise air quality within the confined space. Probes located at various positions within the trailer are used to measure temperature, humidity and air. Other probes in the vicinity of the horse's head measure concentrations of ammonia and other gases (Smith *et al.*, 1996). A commercial data logger can be used to collect data to inform improved transport practices in ways that neutralize environmental challenges and improve welfare.

The restrictive environment of the transport vehicle increases the risk of infectious disease spread during and after transport. When animals from different farms travel together, the pathogen transmission risk is significant. The loading of animals from different farms and of different ages should be avoided. Increasing the resting time and cleaning the interior during rest stops decreases transport stress and respiratory insults (Oikawa *et al.*, 2004). Since trailers and trucks are heavily contaminated with potentially harmful bacteria and spores after use, disinfection between shipments is recommended. An effective cleaning procedure requires cleaning with hot water and appropriate disinfectant concentrations, with scrubbing before and after the application of disinfectant to increase pathogen elimination (Böhm, 1998).

Watering and feeding

Racehorses are often offered hay in a net in transit because hay does not impair performance. In contrast, horses transported to slaughter are fasted to reduce the risk of faecal soiling and meat contamination. The quality of hay is important, and dry hay is a risk to horses prone to recurrent airway obstruction (RAO). Because horses develop signs of RAO after allergen (hay) exposure, it is better to use wet/dampened hay or pellets (Hotchkiss *et al.*, 2007). If hay is offered during the journey, soaking it and placing it on the floor lessens the dust risk. This also stimulates travelling horses to eat with a lowered head, reducing the development of respiratory diseases (Padalino *et al.*, 2018a). Horses are less willing to eat and drink in unfamiliar and stressful surroundings (Kay and Hall, 2009). Therefore, familiar water and food should be offered during planned rest periods. On long journeys, water should be offered while the engine is switched off, at least every 2–4 hours, especially when environmental temperatures are high (Houpt and Leib, 1993). It is deemed acceptable to remove all access to water and food for up to 24 hours during transport in many codes. This recommendation is a welfare concern, as 12 hours of fasting before or during travel increases the stomach pH and equine gastric ulcer syndrome (Padalino *et al.*, 2020b). The maximal journey duration without water should be amended in codes to reflect this finding.

Noise

Horses perceive high-frequency sounds and can be startled by sounds inaudible to humans (see Chapter 2). During loading, transport and unloading, noises arise from sources such as human voices, whips, animal vocalizations (e.g. barking dogs), noisy machinery, alarm bells/klaxon and compressed air brakes. Horses locate sounds with the ears rather than immediately looking at the origin of sounds. Therefore, they may react adversely during loading or unloading before our perception of the source of their distress. Intensive noise stimulation results in a central nervous system excitation, causing immune-system suppression, fatigue and cell death (Minka and Ayo, 2010).

Direction of travel

Most horse trailers and trucks accommodate transport with the horse facing to the front (i.e. the direction of travel) (Figs 8.5 and 8.6). However, horses transported facing forwards have increased licking behaviour, interactions with travel companions and stress behaviour compared to rear facing (Padalino and Raidal, 2020). In the forward-facing direction, horses have difficulty maintaining balance, experience increased anxiety-redirected behaviours and seek a social calming effect. Travelling in this direction causes arousal, with higher heart rates, heart rate variability and salivary cortisol, indicating greater stress on journeys of short-to-moderate duration (Schmidt *et al.*, 2010). Rear facing transport (i.e. facing away from the direction of travel) is associated with fewer impacts against the sides and ends of the trailers, less frequent loss of balance, and fewer directional adjusting movements (Fig. 8.7) (Smith *et al.*, 1994; Padalino and Raidal, 2020). Untethered horses prefer to travel rear-facing, and yearlings quickly learn that facing backwards is advantageous (Kusunose and Torikai, 1996). Individuals may have a travel preference based on previous experience. However, given the choice of travelling facing rearwards, horses are more likely to do so (Fig. 8.7).

Although the direction of travel is important for the ability of horses to keep their balance and minimize anxiety, it has not been clearly shown to affect their general health substantially. However, recent work by the authors suggests that behavioural problems and the risk of injury are affected by the direction of travel and vehicle type, with injury more likely to be associated with forward facing travel (Riley *et al.*, 2018).

Duration of travel

Journey duration is one of the most important risk factors for transport-related illness, and many transport codes include special requirements for longer journeys. Very long journeys (up to 4000 km) by commercial carriers for reasons other than slaughter carry a low risk of mortality (0.024%) and transport-related injuries or disease (2.8%) (Padalino *et al.*, 2015). These figures are much lower than those reported for owners transporting their horses (Riley *et al.*, 2016) and for horses transported to abattoirs (Grandin *et al.*, 1999; Marlin *et al.*, 2011; Roy *et al.*, 2015b; 2015c). Horses are more likely to die or become ill with colic or pleuropneumonia after 20 hours of transport. Even though horses are at greater risk of such illnesses, the maximal journey duration for horses allowed in many countries is still 24 hours. After 24 hours of transport, horses have a 6% loss in body weight on unloading, which persists at 3% loss at 24 hours after travel. These journeys are also associated with abnormalities in the white blood cell count and serum biochemistry, indicating significant stress and immune compromise (Maeda *et al.*, 2011; Padalino *et al.*, 2017a). Horses are more likely to develop a fever for journeys between 20 and 50 hours (1490–2920 km), although, on arrival, some of these horses initially return to normal rectal temperatures (Maeda and Oikawa, 2019).

Usually, horses used for equestrian activities and racing are transported over shorter distances (Padalino *et al.*, 2016b). Horses display more forward and backward movements during shorter (one hour) journeys than longer ones. Higher serum cortisol

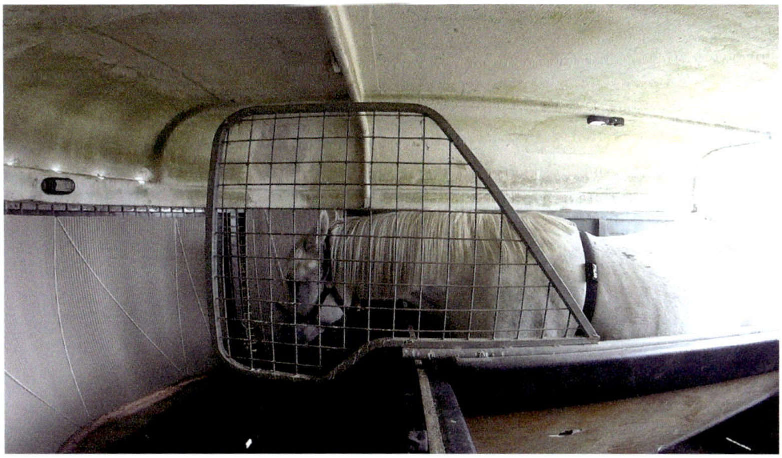

Fig. 8.5. Horse loaded for transport in a forward-facing trailer (float). Photo: C.B. Riley.

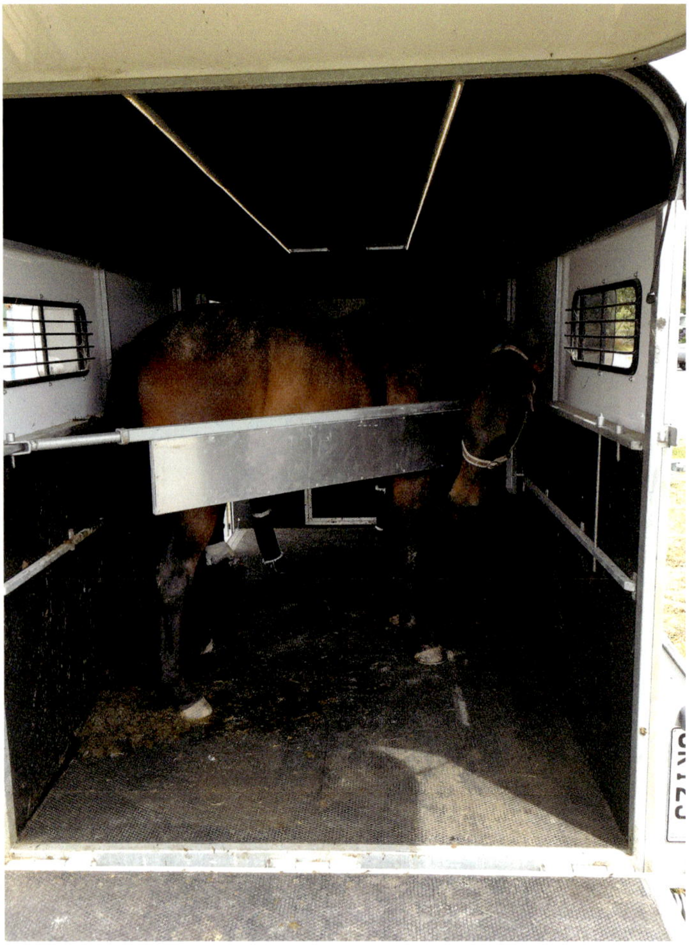

Fig. 8.6. Horse loaded in a forward angle float for the first time. Photo: C.B. Riley.

concentrations have been measured at unloading on short journeys, suggesting one hour is not sufficient time to adapt to travel (Tateo *et al.*, 2012). Indeed, the first hour of transport is the most critical, with horses more likely to display stress or become injured (Padalino *et al.*, 2018a). This means that short journeys require greater care to decrease these risks. Ultimately, both short and long trips are stressful for horses and require proper management. Longer trips have a greater effect on horse illness, whereas shorter trips pose a greater risk of injury.

Driver behaviour

Equine data are lacking, but driver experience is a recognized risk factor for heavy-vehicle accidents. Cattle are more likely to become injured when transported by less experienced drivers (Duke *et al.*, 2010). Driver skill, the ability to control the vehicle and style (i.e. how the vehicle is driven) greatly influence the horse's ability to balance, particularly during acceleration, deceleration, cornering and other difficult manoeuvres (West *et al.*, 1993). In horses, heart rate is correlated with muscular activity spent in balance preservation. Both are strongly affected by the driver's experience (Giovagnoli *et al.*, 2002). Road quality (motorway vs. minor road vs. city traffic) also affects the behaviour of transported animals (Schwartzkopf-Genswein *et al.*, 2012). European rules require the driver to demonstrate skill and ability in transporting animals. Nevertheless, driver distraction, such as mobile phone use while driving, is associated with a higher risk of equine injury (Fig. 8.8) (Riley *et al.*2016).

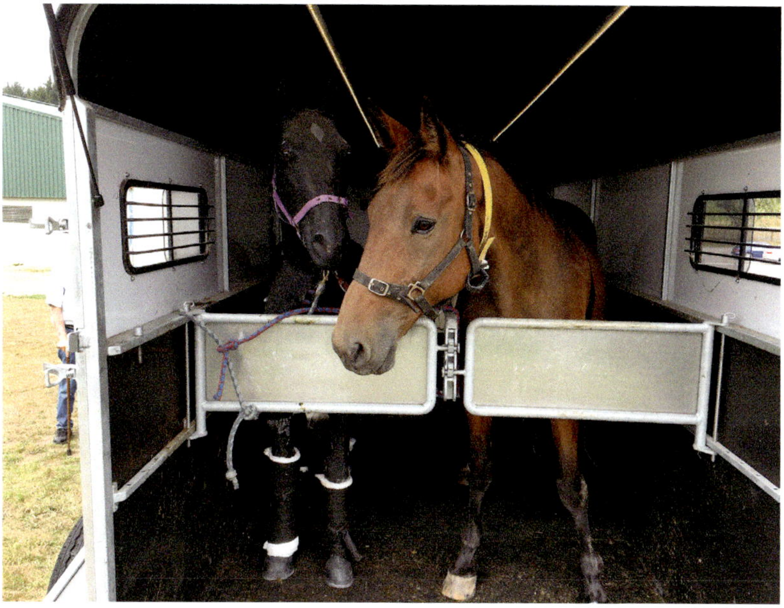

Fig. 8.7. Horse loaded in a rear-facing position with a mannequin companion to reduce social anxiety. Photo: C.B. Riley.

After the journey

Changes in housing, management and diet are well-known stressors. After a journey, horses show more interest in feeding than in other behaviours such as exploration and play, probably to recover from energy expenditure during road transport. To favour adaptation to its new environment, the horse is offered food and clean water on arrival, preferably the same food and water provided at the departure location. The transition to a new diet (if relevant) should be managed over 2–3 weeks (Padalino *et al.*, 2016a). Adaptation after a journey is more rapid when horses are kept with, or adjacent to, familiar stable companions on arrival at the destination. The recommended standard of care includes a period of quarantine to prevent disease spread and avoidance of intense exercise during long-distance transport recovery (Waran *et al.*, 2007).

Physical Welfare

Transport-related stressors most commonly result in stress-related physiological responses such as increases in heart and respiratory rates, heart rate variability and cortisol levels (Padalino, 2017). When a horse cannot cope, its immune system is affected, increasing the risk of severe health problems and death.

Traumatic injuries

The transport vehicle is the second most frequent source of trauma to horses after injuries in the paddock or yard (Darth, 2014). Limb injuries associated with the loading ramp are common. During the journey, halter rubbing at the poll or muzzle and tail rubbing are specific types of abrasion. Wither wounds can be caused through contact with the vehicle ceiling, while leg wounds most commonly occur due to loss of balance or footing after braking and cornering. Rapid and extreme braking can result in vertebral fracture and dislocation in forward-facing horses restrained with short tie-ropes (Mansmann and Woodie, 1995).

The incidence of transport-related horse injuries has been most extensively studied for horses moved by road using commercial companies and varies from 1.6% to 33% depending upon the population studied (Marlin *et al.*, 2011; Roy *et al.*, 2015a; Miranda-de la Lama *et al.*, 2020). Swedish horse owners report a 12% frequency of horse injury during loading, and 5% of these handlers are injured concurrently with the horse (Yngvesson *et al.*, 2016). In Australia, injuries associated with commercial and non-commercial equine transport averaged 22% annually over two years (Padalino *et al.*, 2016a). In another Australian study of non-commercial horse transport at equestrian events, 25% of the owners experienced a transport-related injury

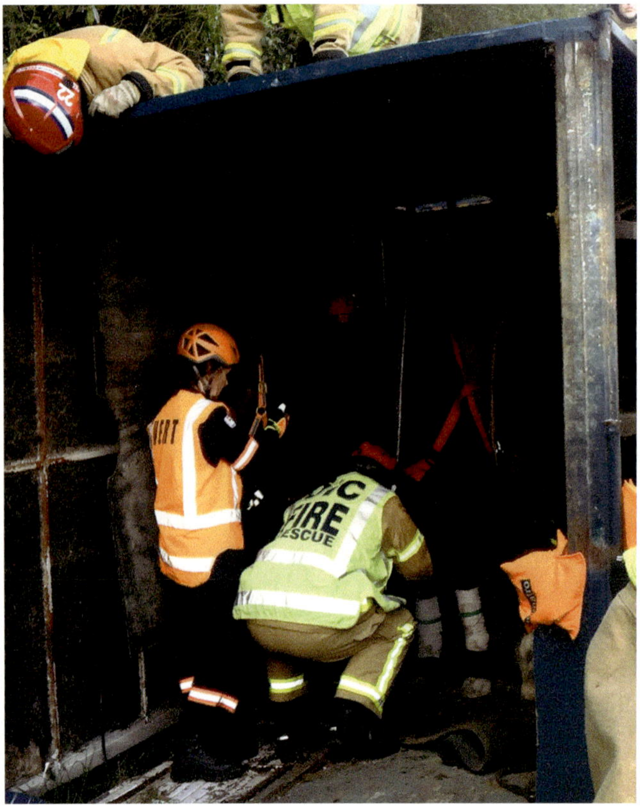

Fig. 8.8. Horses are rescued from a truck that has rolled onto its left side after trying to avoid collision with an oncoming vehicle that crossed the centre line. Photo: C.B. Riley.

within a 15-year period (Riley *et al.*, 2016). In New Zealand, 18% of participants report having a horse injured within the last year, with most occurring in transit (Padalino *et al.*, 2018c). Injuries range from shallow cuts to fractures. In the professional equine industry, breed, journey duration, failing to perform a mechanical check, behavioural problems and horse training for transport are strongly associated with the risk of injury. Other human factors related to the risk of horse injury during transport include the age of the driver (younger versus older), the choice to use protective equipment on the horse and the administration of sedation (Padalino *et al.*, 2016b). Injuries during transport can also be related to motor vehicle accidents (Hall *et al.*, 2020).

Dehydration and weight loss

During and after transport, mild to severe dehydration occurs, with the severity influenced by environmental and journey conditions. Even when water is available, horses tend to dehydrate during a journey, predisposing them to colic and other illnesses. Moderate to severe dehydration can lead to serious metabolic conditions such as heat stroke, laminitis, colon impaction, pneumonia and muscle problems. Dehydration also affects renal function, and this is particularly relevant for horses undergoing medical treatment. Early stages of dehydration are difficult to determine; horses may have up to 5% dehydration without showing outward signs. For the athletic horse, as little as 2–3% dehydration affects performance. Therefore, preventing dehydration is extremely important for any horse travelling to compete (Marlin, 2004). Capillary refill time (CRT), a simple non-invasive measure of hydration, is evaluated by gently pressing on the gum with a fingertip and timing how long it takes the blanched area to become pink again; normally <2 s (Dalla Costa *et al.*, 2014). Therefore, CRT should be monitored before, during and after the journey. When CRT is >3 s, water should be offered. If necessary, veterinary assisted rehydration techniques can be implemented. Monitoring body weight loss by girth tape following a journey is also recommended. After an 8-hour journey, bodyweight loss due to dehydration takes >24 hours to recover, so at least one day of rest post journey is recommended. Horses should not be exercised until they recover.

There are several techniques used to minimize the risk and extent of dehydration. Familiarizing horses with a water-normalizing substance, such as apple flavouring, can offset any difference in water taste during transport and at the destination (Mars *et al.*, 1992). Mineral oil or electrolyte-enriched water via nasogastric tube has been used successfully pre-transport to prevent gastrointestinal impaction. Veterinary administration of the oil recommended to prevent it from being passed into the lungs and causing fatal pneumonia. Mineral oil may affect the absorption of other nutrients. Electrolytes should not be given in a concentrated form (such as paste) close to a stressful event such as transport and should always be given as an iso-osmotic solution. Stopping during long-haul transport every 4–6 hours and overnighting horses at least every 12–16 hours reflects current best practice. During stops, horses suffering moderate or severe dehydration and related health problems should be examined by a veterinarian. Oral electrolytes and water can be given via a nasogastric tube to mild or moderately dehydrated horses or intravenously if dehydration is severe. The stomach of a 450–500 kg horse can accommodate 6–8 L of electrolyte-enriched water every 15 min for 1–2 hours (Mansmann and Woodie, 1995).

Laminitis, heatstroke and muscular problems

Laminitis, heatstroke, and muscular problems are common consequences of transport (Mansmann and Woodie, 1995; Marlin, 2004). Moderate dehydration can initiate abnormalities in blood flow to the hooves, thereby inducing laminitis. This problem may be accentuated by the hoof inflammation associated with removing shoes in normally shod horses. Other factors that increase the risk of laminitis include the duration of the journey relative to the horse's fitness, carbohydrate (concentrate) intake during the journey and potential endotoxic disorders initiated by travel. Preventive measures include not changing the horses' shoeing status, adding frog support to higher-risk horses and reducing carbohydrate intake before and during road transport (Mansmann and Woodie, 1995).

Heatstroke occurs when horses cannot regulate their body temperature in response to thermal stress and/or dehydration. This may be associated with high ambient temperatures, lack of vehicle ventilation and high humidity (Padalino *et al.*, 2018a). To reduce heatstroke risk, journeys should be planned after checking weather forecasts; temperature, humidity and airflow inside the vehicle monitored. In warm climates during spring and summer, the risk is highest during the daylight hours. Travel during these times should be minimized. Dehydration is a major contributor to the development of heatstroke, so horses should have access to water and feed *ad libitum* before journeys and watered at least every 4 hours en route (World Horse Welfare *et al.*, 2014). Horses within the thermal comfort zone can also develop heatstroke due to agitation (Weeks *et al.*, 2012). It is therefore vitally important to minimize transport stress. As previously mentioned, the first hour of the journey may be the most stressful. Therefore, horses can suffer from heatstroke during short journeys or at the beginning of a long journey in hot or humid conditions. Muscular problems are associated with the lack of assessment of fitness for travel, journeys of medium duration and non-commercial transport (Padalino *et al.*, 2017a).

Gastrointestinal and respiratory problems

The gastrointestinal and respiratory systems are more affected by protracted transport stress than short journeys (Leadon and Hodgson, 2014). The frequency of gastrointestinal problems reported in surveys ranges from 24% to 27% for long-distance journeys and for respiratory problems, 27% to 38% (Padalino, 2015; Padalino *et al.*, 2016b). Gastrointestinal motility is reduced during transport and may explain why horses tend to develop gastroenteric problems during and after the journey. Severe intestinal inflammation and diarrhoea (enterocolitis) have been linked to road transport (McClintock and Begg, 1990). Transport stress may affect the gastrointestinal microbiota in some horses, such that *Salmonella* and *Clostridium* species become predominant, causing enterocolitis

(Feary and Hassell, 2006). In some geographic regions, transport-related enterocolitis is a common condition and frequently fatal (Padalino *et al.*, 2016b). Other common gastrointestinal problems include diarrhoea without fever, colic and stomach ulcers. Diarrhoea without fever may be a sign of activation of the sympathetic system and is associated with stress and handler experience, highlighting the importance of professional management to reduce this risk. Gastric ulceration is associated with the fasting and transport of horses. The severity and rapid development (within 12 hours) of ulceration in some horses fasted before travel suggests that access to feed until departure, and potentially during transport, is important (Padalino *et al.*, 2020b).

Transport pneumonia (i.e. shipping fever or pleuropneumonia) is commonly associated with long-distance transport, with up to 10% of horses affected (Austin *et al.*, 1995; Padalino *et al.*, 2015; Maeda and Oikawa, 2019). Transport stress and lack of opportunity to lower the head allows the proliferation of the commensal bacteria within the airways and a change in the balance of the bacteria to species more likely to invade the lower respiratory tract. The combination of opportunistic bacterial proliferation (usually Pasteurellaceae or *Streptococcus equi* subspecies *zooepidemicus*) and immunocompromise associated with transport stress results in the infection of the airways, lungs and pleural cavity (Padalino *et al.*, 2017b). Thoroughbred racehorses are more likely to suffer from this problem. Journey duration and the head position are the most important risk factors, so tying the head up is discouraged (Raidal *et al.*, 1995; Stull and Rodiek, 2002). Monitoring the horse's behaviour en route (licking or chewing frequency, evasive behaviour frequency, duration of lowered head) may be useful in identifying those at risk of developing respiratory diseases (Padalino *et al.*, 2018a). To adopt the beneficial lower head position, horses need to experience low levels of stress before and during transport, travel in larger bays, long or no tying, travel in a quiet environment, motivated to lower their heads by offering food and by habituating them to transport by appropriate training methods (Padalino *et al.*, 2018). The assessment of the horse's fitness for travel is mandatory within some transport codes but does not include a specific respiratory system examination. For horses in preparation for long journeys, veterinary auscultation may be performed as part of their assessment for fitness. Post-travel management is also essential to reduce the risk of respiratory disease. However, codes of transport generally do not include any guidelines for the length of this period.

Behavioural Welfare Problems

Transport-related behavioural problems (TRBPs) are behaviours that impede the welfare or safety of the horse or handler during the transport process (Houpt, 1982). They increase the risk of physical injuries and fatalities in horses and humans, damage to property and vehicles, negative human–horse relationships, psychological damage to humans, and the wastage of horses with unresolved behavioural problems. They are categorized according to the phases of transport: pre-loading, loading, travelling and unloading. In Australia, almost 39% of people surveyed reported having one or more horses exhibiting TRBPs during pre-loading (28%), loading (51%), travelling (42%) and unloading (16%) (Padalino *et al.,* 2017a). In New Zealand, 22% of handlers reported TRBPs during pre-loading. Of these, 8% occurred during pre-loading, 31% during loading, 53% while travelling and 7% during unloading (Padalino *et al.,* 2018b). TRBPs are an indicator of compromised welfare and an associated risk of injury during transport. Horses showing TRBPs should not be forced to load or travel. They should be re-trained using equine learning theory principles, restarting from in-hand control before introducing the transport vehicle.

Pre-loading

Through associative learning, horses recognize features of the pre-loading routine (e.g., fitting of protective equipment and the presence of a transport vehicle) and associate them with past travel experiences (Weeks *et al.*, 2012) (see Chapter 1). Horses who have experienced problematic travel, such as falls, tend to exhibit increased TRBPs during pre-loading (Leadon *et al.*, 2008). Preloading TRBPs include signs of anxiety such as vocalization, pawing, heightened locomotion and shaking (Waran *et al.*, 2007; Padalino, 2015). Unsurprisingly, as pre-loading handling is typically when horses start to interact with people, the relationship between the horse and handler contributes to the horse's risk of displaying a TRBP (Padalino *et al.*, 2017a). It is important to apply an effective and humane handling routine underpinned by knowledge that recognizes and mitigates stress to prevent pre-loading TRBPs.

Loading

Loading TRBPs are frequently displayed as avoidance strategies such as rearing, pulling away sideways or backwards, or stress-related behaviours, including pawing, kicking out, bolting or head shaking (Lee *et al.*, 2001). Unpredictable or elevated avoidance behaviour combined with the horse's size and proximity to humans leads to a significant risk of injury to the horses and handlers. One survey estimated that as many as 12% of handlers are injured during loading, including 5% at the same time as the horse (Yngvesson *et al.*, 2016). Loading TRBPs can also result in the unintentional reinforcement of undesirable behaviour and rapidly lead to negative associations between the horse and handler (Ferguson and Rosalez-Ruiz, 2001). Common reasons for horse-related injuries linked to TRBPs include inadequate training and miscommunication, often due to insufficient knowledge of horse behaviour (Padalino *et al.*, 2018b). The properties of the trailer are a significant contributory factor to TRBPs; the dark interior, the hollow sound of the ramp, and the instability of both ramp and vehicle are likely to be fear-invoking stimuli for the horse (Houpt, 1986). Horses demonstrate less aversive behaviour when stepping directly into the trailer than walking up a ramp (Murphy and Hennessy, 2007).

Loading TRBPs can cause time disruptions and frustration, including cancellation of attendance at competitions due to the inability to load (Yngvesson *et al.*, 2016). Almost 9% of horses at an equine veterinary hospital experienced horse-loading events upon discharge associated with loading TRBPs. Although perhaps not a large percentage, 75% required staff assistance and 25% caused time delays of over 30 min. Owners are encouraged to address TRBPs early and before the need for emergency transport for veterinary treatment (Hancock and Pearson, 2014).

In transit

During transit, horses cope with many auditory and physical stressors. TRBPs are manifestations of a very high level of arousal generated by a multitude of stressors to which horses attempt to adapt. TRBPs during travel include vocalizing, head tossing, pawing, scrambling, head turning, kicking out at the vehicle, biting and kicking directed at travelling companions, and reduced feeding or drinking (York *et al*, 2017). These behaviours can lead to injuries from contact with vehicle components, by such actions as kicking the vehicle walls or dividers or by loss of balance, which may result in a fall (Padalino *et al.*, 2015). The heart rates of novice horses are consistently higher inside a standard stationary trailer compared with when outside.

Many studies relating to potential contributors to TRBPs have investigated the impacts of vehicle design, lighting, orientation, distance, isolation, driving skills, and road quality (York *et al.*, 2017; Riley *et al.*, 2018). However, results are often conflicting because these factors vary widely among studies. More evidence-based studies are needed to understand better how to minimize stress in transit and the incidence and consequences of TRBPs (Table 8.1). Since the inability to cope with transport stress is a risk factor for transport-related diseases (i.e. shipping fever, colic, heat stroke), the positive association between TRBPs (indicative of a failure to adapt to stress) and the development of transport-related diseases is clear.

Unloading

Unloading TRBPs include a reluctance to exit the vehicle after prolonged immobility and bolting at the first opportunity. The latter behaviour is a flight response. Unloading TRBPs may be exacerbated if the ramp is excessively steep or slippery, the horse is lame or anxious about the unloading environment, or in a vehicle that requires horses to be unloaded backwards, preventing them from seeing behind (Padalino *et al.*, 2017a). Like other behavioural problems, unloading TRBPs can result in injuries to horse and handler. Slaughter horses that exhibit unloading TRBPs risk being punished by handlers, resulting in additional injuries and poor horse welfare outcomes (Messori *et al.*, 2016b).

Transport by Air

The first reported transport of horses by aeroplane occurred during the early 1920s. Mass air transport was used to transfer and parachute horses and mules into theatres of war during World War II (Cregier, 2001). The first racehorses were flown across the Atlantic in 1946, and thereafter air travel

Table 8.1. Recommendations for the welfare-oriented road transport of horses.

The driver/handler should
Be educated on equine transport risk factors, best practices, codes and policies
Always conduct transport with the highest levels of professional competence
Have horse handling and driving skills
Before the journey
Plan and manage the journey carefully to minimize transport stress, considering: journey duration/journey route/rest stops/seasonal temperature and humidity/driver fatigue/food and water
Inspect the transport vehicle to ensure it is good repair: hitch/brakes/lights/suspension/structures (floor, sides, partitions)/tyres (wear and pressure)/mechanical (truck or tow vehicle)
Train horses for loading and travelling using habituation and self-loading approaches
Provide access to hay and water *ad libitum* before travelling
Carefully assess fitness for travel
Consider a veterinary examination of the respiratory tract for long journeys (>20 hours)
Do not transport injured or sick horses without consulting veterinarian
During the journey
Protective equipment such as boots and rugs should only be used where horses have been habituated, checked during the journey and used only for short journeys
Arousing stimuli during transport should be kept to a minimum
Environmental parameters should be monitored during transport
Horses should be allowed to lower their head to floor level during transport
Horses should have enough space to spread their legs for balance
Long fasting during transport should be avoided
Horse behaviour en route should be monitored via cameras (not by the driver)
After the journey
The horse should be carefully assessed for: injury/illness/dehydration/pain
After long journeys, visual inspection, monitoring temperature, gut and lung sounds are recommended at least once daily for five days to promptly monitor for disease
Closely monitor horses that spend most of their journey with the head elevated or perform stress-related behaviours (e.g. licking/chewing, pawing)
Allow the horse to rest for at least 24 hours following road journeys longer than 8 hours
Horses should be allowed to lower their heads for as long as possible after transport; therefore, keeping horses on pasture post-travel is recommended

for competitive purposes has increased (Judge, 1969; Küper and Schäffer, 2004). Air transport is an integral part of international competition and the breeding of high-performance horses (Hurley *et al.*, 2016). Nowadays, horses travel in partitioned air stables or jet stalls designed to accommodate a maximum of three horses, side by side, in wide-bodied jets (Leadon *et al.*, 2008). The jet stalls are loaded with horses on the ground and, once cleared by authorities, transferred into the aircraft's cargo bay. During the flight, access to the stalls is provided at the front for feeding and watering by specially trained grooms.

The most stressful phases of air transport are loading, unloading, departure and landing (Stewart *et al.*, 2003). Aggression, submission, heart rate and weight shifting to maintain balance increase during ascent and descent. During level flight, horses have normal resting heart rate values and engage in resting behaviours, indicating that they may settle better to air than road transport (Munsters *et al.*, 2013). There are injury and disease risks. Some horses resent prolonged confinement and suffer injury or death (Leadon *et al.*, 2008). Injured horses may require sedation, but this can be dangerous for the groom to administer. Despite being given water every 4–6 hours during their journey, horses may lose about 20 kg on a journey that lasts 24 hours. Quarantine regulations are generally applied after air travel to minimize biosecurity risks. However, restraint in the quarantine boxes can cause an increase in heart rate associated with environmental stress (Ohmura *et al.*, 2012). On arrival, pleuropneumonia occurs in as many as 11% of horses and 60% of flights when travelling from temperate to more humid climates (Hurley *et al.*, 2016). Most of these horses do not have a fever or show signs until 24–48 hours after the flight (Oertly *et al.*, 2017). Journey duration is a risk factor for disease, but this is difficult to control in the face of flight delays and quarantine requirements. On arrival, horses need sufficient time to acclimatize to the new environmental conditions and local feedstuffs (Marlin *et al.*, 2001).

Transport by Water

The transport of horses and mules by sea played an important part in the European colonization of the Americas and Oceania, and during the first half of the last century, in theatres of war (Leadon *et al.*, 2008; Katic and Bajt, 2009). Sea transport is still used because it is the least costly approach for large numbers of slaughter horses travelling from South America to Europe (Giovagnoli, 2008). Feral horses have been shipped in this way from Argentina for recreational and breeding uses in Italy (Cavallone *et al.*, 2002). In modern cargo ships, horses travel in boxes that range in dimension from 4.5×4.5 m^2 to 6.0×4.5 m^2 and have access to a sand yard to exercise during the voyage (Waran *et al.*, 2007). The key disadvantages of sea transport include the lengthy duration and risk of injury. Horses well accept long transfers by ship. However, horses can develop medical problems associated with changes in management and conditions or hierarchical conflicts associated with adapting to the new stalls and social groupings during and after the journey (Cavallone *et al.*, 2002).

Horses may be transported on coastal waterways, rivers, and lakes on ferries also called 'roll on/roll off' (RORO) transport. Smaller boats are also used (Fig. 8.9). In the ferry, horses travel in their trailer or truck; by law, this is considered a rest period. However, horses are still confined and often fasted. A major concern of ferry transport is the limited airflow and ventilation within the cargo hold because of the risk of intoxication by carbon monoxide and heat stroke. In 2018, 13 polo horses transported in the hold of a ferry from Tasmania to mainland Australia died of suspected asphyxiation despite many previous uneventful shipments on the same ferry. In many jurisdictions, live animals may only be loaded in the decks of the ship (i.e. not the hold) to provide better air circulation. Ferries must be equipped with fans to ensure the best airflow possible. However, horses that travel inside their vehicle on the boat are often not provided with forced ventilation. When combined with small windows and positional readjustment movements, the temperature inside their vehicle is at least 3–4 °C higher than the environmental temperature (Padalino, 2015). Therefore, particular attention should be given to the weather forecast when planning to move horses by ferries over long distances (>8 hours), avoiding transporting horses in a RORO ferry when the environmental temperature exceeds 27 °C, or the humidity exceeds 80%. Although there are many media reports of horses found dead after ferry transport, there are no data on the incidence of these and other transport-related health problems.

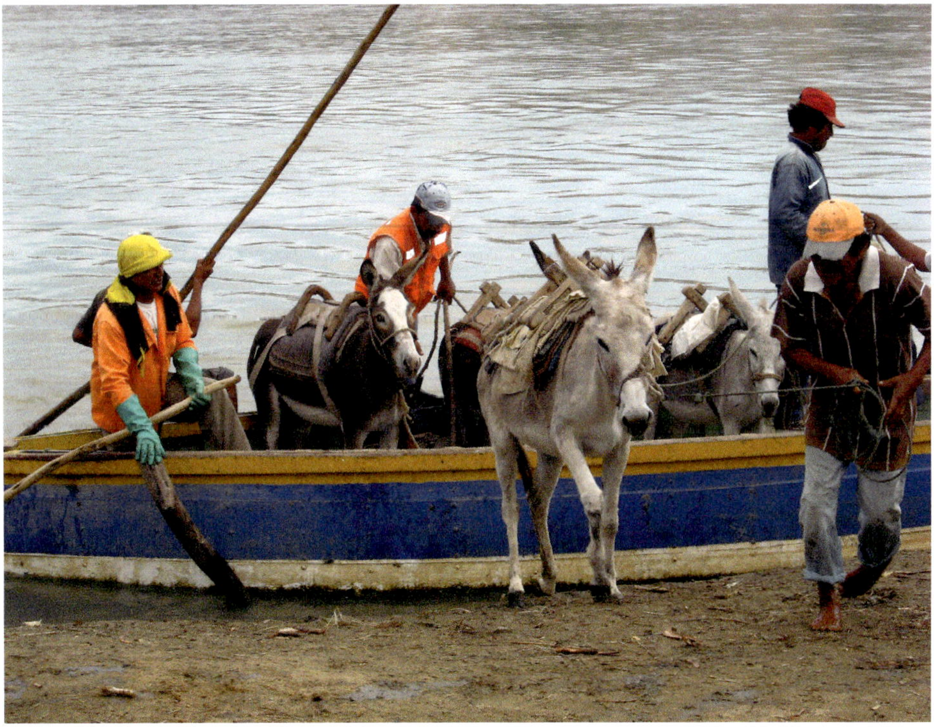

Fig. 8.9. Donkeys exit an open boat with human passengers after a river crossing in Northern Peru. Photo: C. B. Riley.

References

Animal Welfare Foundation-Tiershutzbund Zürich (2017) Production of Horsemeat in Argentina and Uruguay. Available at: https://www.animal-welfare-foundation.org/en/blog/uruguay-argentina-horsemeat-production-2 (accessed 23 January 2022).

Austin, S.M., Foreman, J.H. and Hungerford, L.L. (1995) Case-control study of risk factors for development of pleuropneumonia in horses. *Journal of the American Veterinary Medical Association* 207, 325–328.

Beaunoyer, D. and Chapman, J. (1987) Trailering stress on subsequent submaximal exercise performance. *Proceedings of 11th Equine Nutrition and Physiology Symposium*. Oklahoma State University, Stillwater, OK, pp. 379–384.

Böhm, R. (1998) Disinfection and hygiene in the veterinary field and disinfection of animal houses and transport vehicles. *International Biodeterioration & Biodegradation* 41, 217–224.

Cavallone, E., Di Giancamillo, M., Secchiero, B., Beloli, A., Pravettoni, D. and Rimoldi, E.M. (2002) Variations of serum cortisol in Argentine horses subjected to ship transport and adaptation stress. *Journal of Equine Veterinary Science* 22, 541–545.

Collins, M.N., Friend, T.H., Jousan, F.D. and Chen, S.C. (2000) Effects of density on displacement, falls, injuries, and orientation during horse transportation. *Applied Animal Behaviour Science* 67, 169–179.

Consortium of the Animal Transport Guides Project (2017) *Guide to Good Practices for the Transport of Horses Destinated for Slaughter*. Wageningen Livestock Research, Wagenigen, Netherlands. Available at: www.animaltransportguides.eu/wp-content/uploads/2016/05/Animal-Transport-Guides-Horses-2017.pdf (accessed 23 January 2022).

Cregier, S.E. (1982) Reducing equine hauling stress: A review. *Journal of Equine Veterinary Science* 2, 186–198.

Cregier, S.E. (2001) Burma's long-eared paratroops. *Journal of Equine Veterinary Science* 21, 519–523.

Cregier, S.E. (2010) Best practices: surface transport of the horse. *Proceedings of Animal Transportation Association*, AATA Education Committee, Canada, p. 1e29.

Cregier, S.E. and Gimenez, R. (eds) (2015) *Non-commercial Horse Transport: New Standards for Trailers in Canada*. Cregier S., Montague, Canada.

Cross, N., van Doorn, F., Versnel, C., Cawdell-Smith, J. and Phillips, C. (2008) Effects of lighting conditions on the welfare of horses being loaded for transportation. *Journal of Veterinary Behavior: Clinical Applications and Research* 3, 20–24.

Dalla Costa, E., Murray, L., Dai, F., Canali, E. and Minero, M. (2014) Equine on-farm welfare assessment: A review of animal-based indicators. *Animal Welfare* 23, 323–341.

Darth, A.C. (2014) Identifying causes and preventing injuries to horses. Swedish University of Agricultural Sciences, Uppsala, Sweden. Available at: https://stud.epsilon.slu.se/7223/ (accessed 28 January 2022).

Duke, J., Guest, M. and Boggess, M. (2010) Age-related safety in professional heavy vehicle drivers: A literature review. *Accident Analysis and Prevention* 42, 364–371

Eur-lex (2005) Animal welfare during transport – EU rules. Available at: www.eur-lex.europa.eu/legal-content/EN/TXT/?uri=uriserv:f83007 (accessed 1 October 2015).

FAO (Food and Agricultural Organisation of the United Nations) (2020) FAOSTAT. Available at: www.fao.org/faostat/en/#data/QL (accessed 18 June 2020).

Feary, D.J. and Hassel, D.M. (2006) Enteritis and colitis in horses. *Veterinary Clinics of North America: Equine Practice* 22, 437–479.

Ferguson, D.L. and Rosales-Ruiz, J. (2001) Loading the problem loader: the effect of target training and shaping on trailer-loading behavior of horses. *Journal of Applied Behavior Analysis* 34, 409–423.

Friend, T. (2001) A review of recent research on the transportation of horses. *Journal of Animal Science* 79(E-Suppl), E32–E40.

Garey, S.M., Friend, T.H., Sigler, D.H. and Berghman, L.R. (2010) The effects of loose group versus individual stall transport on glucocorticosteriods and dehydroepiandrosterone in yearling horses. *Journal of Equine Veterinary Science* 30, 696–700.

Giovagnoli, G. (2008) *Manuale teorico-pratico sul trasporto del cavallo*. Mursia Editore, Milano, Italy, p. 1.

Giovagnoli, G., Trabalza Marinucci, M., Bolla, A. and Borghese, A. (2002) Transport stress in horses: An electromyographic study on balance preservation. *Livestock Production Science* 73, 247–254.

Grandin, T., McGee, K. and Lanier, J. L. (1999) Prevalence of severe welfare problems in horses that arrive at slaughter plants. *Journal of the American Veterinary Medical Association* 214, 1531–1533.

Hall, C., Kay, R. and Green, J. (2020) A retrospective survey of factors affecting the risk of incidents and equine injury during non-commercial transportation by road in the United Kingdom. *Animals* 10, 288.

Hancock, E. and Pearson, G. (2014) A pilot study investigating the prevalence of loading problems at an equine referral hospital. *Conference Proceedings 10th International Equitation Science Conference*. 6–9th August 2014, Bredsten, Denmark, pp. 76.

Hartmann, E., Hopkins, R.J., Blomgren, E., Ventorp, M., von Brömssen, C. *et al.* (2015) Daytime shelter use of individually kept horses during Swedish summer. *Journal of Animal Science* 93, 802–810.

Hotchkiss, J., Reid, S. and Christley, R. (2007) A survey of horse owners in Great Britain regarding horses in their care. Part 2: Risk factors for recurrent airway obstruction. *Equine Veterinary Journal* 39, 301–308.

Houpt, K. (1982) Misbehavior of horses: Trailer problems. *Equine Practice* 4,12–16.

Houpt, K.A. (1986) Stable vices and trailer problems. *The Veterinary clinics of North America. Equine Practice* 2, 623–633.
Houpt, K. and Lieb, S. (1993) Horse handling and transport. Grandin, T. (ed.) *Livestock Handling and Transport CAB International*, Wallingford, UK, pp. 233–252.
Hurley, M., Riggs, C., Cogger, N. and Rosanowski, S. (2016) The incidence and risk factors for shipping fever in horses transported by air to Hong Kong: Results from a 2-year prospective study. *The Veterinary Journal* 214, 34–39.
Iacono, C., Friend, T., Keen, H., Martin, T. and Krawczel, P. (2007) Effects of density and water availability on the behavior, physiology, and weight loss of slaughter horses during transport. *Journal of Equine Veterinary Science* 27, 355–361.
Jeffcott, L.B. (1996) Use of the wet bulb globe temperature (WBGT) index to quantify environmental heat loads during three-day event competitions. *Equine Veterinary Journal Supplement* 22, 3–6.
Judge, N. (1969) Transport of horses. *Australian Veterinary Journal* 45, 465–469.
Katić, I. and Bajt, V.V. (2009) On the water transport of animals with special reference to Denmark. *Acta Medico-Historica Adriatica* 7, 39–48.
Kay, R. and Hall, C. (2009) The use of a mirror reduces isolation stress in horses being transported by trailer. *Applied Animal Behaviour Science* 116, 237–243.
Küper, S. and Schäffer, J. (2004) Pegasos braucht keine Flügel mehr: Der Flugtransport von Pferden 1924–2000. *Pferdheilkunde*, 20, 159–172.
Kusunose, R. and Torikai, K. (1996) Behavior of untethered horses during vehicle transport. *Journal of Equine Science*, 7, 21–26.
Leadon, D.P. and Hodgson, D.R. (2014) Transport of horses. In: *The Athletic Horse: Principles and Practice of Equine Sports Medicine*, 2nd edn. Elsevier-Saunders, St. Louis, Missouri, pp. 155–161.
Leadon, D., Waran, N., Herholz, C. and Klay, M. (2008) Veterinary management of horse transport. *Veterinaria Italiana,* 44, 149–163.
Lee, J., Houpt, K. and Doherty, O. (2001) A survey of trailering problems in horses. *Journal of Equine Veterinary Science* 21, 235–238.
Linden, A., Art, T., Amory, H., Desmecht, D. and Lekeux, P. (1991) Effect of 5 different types of exercise, transportation and ACTH administration on plasma cortisol concentration in sport horses. *Equine Exercise Physiology* 3, 391–396.
Maeda, Y. and Oikawa, M. (2019) Patterns of rectal temperature and shipping fever incidence in horses transported over long distance. *Frontiers in Veterinary Science* 6, 27.
Maeda, Y., Tomioka, M., Hanada, M. and Oikawa, M. (2011) Changes in peripheral blood lymphocyte and neutrophil counts and function following long-term road transport in Thoroughbred horses. *International Journal of Applied Research in Veterinary Medicine* 9, 284–289.
Mal, M., Friend, T., Lay, D., Vogelsang, S. and Jenkins, O. (1991) Physiological responses of mares to short term confinement and social isolation. *Journal of Equine Veterinary Science* 11, 96–102.
Mansmann, R.A. and Woodie, B. (1995) Equine transportation problems and some preventives: A review. *Journal of Equine Veterinary Science* 15, 141–144.
Marlin, D.J. (2004) Transport of horses. In: *Equine Sports Medicine and Surgery*. Elsevier-Saunders, St. Louis, Missouri, pp. 1239–1250.
Marlin, D.J., Schroter, R.C., White, L., Maykuth, P., Matthesen, G. *et al.* (2001) Recovery from transport and acclimatisation of competition horses in a hot humid environment. *Equine Veterinary Journal* 33, 371–379.
Marlin, D., Kettlewell P., Parkin, T., Kennedy, M., Broom, D. *et al.* (2011) Welfare and health of horses transported for slaughter within the European Union Part 1: Methodology and descriptive data. *Equine Veterinary Journal* 43, 78–87.
Marlin, D., Misheff, M. and Whitehead, P. (2018) Optimising performance in a challenging climate. *Proceedings FEI Sports Forum*, Lausanne, Switzerland, pp. 26.
Mars, L.A., Kiesling, H., Ross, T., Armstrong, J. and Murray, L. (1992) Water acceptance and intake in horses under shipping stress. *Journal of Equine Veterinary Science* 12, 17–20.
McClintock, S.A. and Begg, A.P. (1990) Suspected salmonellosis in seven broodmares after transportation. *Australian Veterinary Journal* 67, 265–267.
Messori, S., Ouweltjes, W., Visser, K., Dalla Villa, P., Spoolder, H. *et al.* (2016a) Improving horse welfare at transport: definition of good practices through a Delphi procedure. *Book of Abstracts of the 67th Annual Meeting of the European Federation of Animal Science*. 26th August to 2 September 2016, Belfast, Ireland, pp. 404
Messori, S., Visser, E.K., Buonanno, M., Ferrari, P., Barnard, S. *et al.* (2016b) A tool for the evaluation of slaughter horse welfare during unloading. *Animal Welfare* 25, 101–113.
Minka, N. and Ayo, J. (2010) Physiological responses of food animals to road transportation stress. *African Journal of Biotechnology* 9, 40.
Miranda-de la Lama, G.C., Gonzales-Castro, C.A., Gutierrez-Piña, F.J., Villarroel, M., Maria, G.A. *et al.* (2020) Welfare of horses from Mexico and the United States of America transported for slaughter in Mexico: Fitness profiles for transport and pre-slaughter logistics. *Preventive Medicine* 180, 105033.
Mitchell, M.A. and Kettlewell, P.J. (2008) Engineering and design of vehicles for long distance road transport of livestock (ruminants, pigs and poultry). *Veterinaria Italiana* 44, 201–213.

Munsters, C., de Gooijer, J.W., van den Broek, J. and van Oldruitenborgh-Oosterbaan, M.S. (2013) Heart rate, heart rate variability and behaviour of horses during air transport. *Veterinary Record* 172, 15.

Murphy, J. and Hennessy, K. (2007) Trailer for horses: some transport systems may be less problematic for the naive horse during loading. *3rd International Equitation Science Conference*. East Lansing, Michigan.

Oertly, M., Gerber, V., Anhold, H. and Pusterla, N. (2017) The accuracy of serum amyloid a in determining early inflammation in horses following long-distance transportation by air. *Proceedings of the 63rd Convention of the American Association of Equine Veterinary Practitioners* 63, 460–461.

Ohmura, H., Hobo, S., Hiraga, A. and Jones, J.H. (2012) Changes in heart rate and heart rate variability during transportation of horses by road and air. *American Journal of Veterinary Research* 73, 515–521.

Oikawa, M.A., Takagi, S. and Yashiki, K. (2004) Some aspects of the stress responses to road transport in Thoroughbred horses with special reference to shipping fever. *Journal of Equine Science* 15, 99–102.

Padalino, B. (2015) Effects of the different transport phases on equine health status, behavior, and welfare: A review. *Journal of Veterinary Behavior: Clinical Applications and Research* 10, 272–282.

Padalino, B. (2017) Transportation of horses and the implications for health and welfare. PhD Thesis. The University of Sydney.

Padalino, B. and Raidal, S.L. (2020) Effects of transport conditions on behavioural and physiological responses of horses. *Animals* 10, 160.

Padalino, B., Barrasso, R., Tullio, D., Zappaterra, M., Costa, L.N. *et al.* (2020a) Protection of animals during transport: Analysis of the infringements reported from 2009 to 2013 during on-road Inspections in Italy. *Animals* 10, 356.

Padalino, B., Davis, G.L. and Raidal, S.L. (2020b) Effects of transportation on gastric pH and gastric ulceration in mares. *Journal of Veterinary Internal Medicine*, 34, 922–932.

Padalino, B., Hall, E., Raidal, S., Celi, P., Knight, P. *et al.*, (2015) Health problems and risk factors associated with long haul transport of horses in Australia. *Animals*, 5, 1296–1310.

Padalino, B., Raidal, S.L., Hall, E., Knight, P., Celi, P. *et al.* (2016a) A survey on transport management practices associated with injuries and health problems in horses. *PloS ONE* 11(9), e0162371.

Padalino, B., Raidal, S., Hall, E., Knight, P., Celi, P. *et al.* (2016b) Survey of horse transportation in Australia: issues and practices. *Australian Veterinary Journal* 94, 349–357.

Padalino, B., Henshall, C., Raidal, S.L., Knight, P., Celi, P. *et al.* (2017b) Investigations into equine transport-related problem behaviors: survey results. *Journal of Equine Veterinary Science* 48, 166–173.e162.

Padalino, B., Raidal, S.L., Carter, N., Celi, P., Muscatello, G. *et al.* (2017a) Immunological, clinical, haematological and oxidative responses to long distance transportation in horses. *Research in Veterinary Science* 115, 78–87.

Padalino, B., Raidal, S.L., Knight, P., Celi, P., Jeffcott, L. *et al.* (2018a) Behaviour during transportation predicts stress response and lower airway contamination in horses. *PloS ONE* 13(3), e0194272.

Padalino, B., Rogers, C.W., Guiver, D., Bridges, J. and Riley, C.B. (2018b) Risk factors for transport-related problem behaviors in horses: a New Zealand survey. *Animals* 8, 134.

Padalino, B., Rogers, C.W., Guiver, D., Thompson, K.R. and Riley C.B. (2018c) A survey-based investigation of human factors associated with transport related injuries in horses. *Frontiers in Veterinary Science* 5, 294.

Purswell, J.L., Gates, R.S., Lawrence, L.M., Jacob, J.D., Stombaugh, T.S. *et al.* (2006) Air exchange rate in a horse trailer during road transport. *Transactions of the ASABE* 49, 193–201.

Purswell, J.L., Gates, R.S., Lawrence, L.M. and Davis, J.D. (2010) Thermal environment in a four-horse slant-load trailer. *Transactions of the American Society of Agricultural and Biological Engineers* 53, 1885–1894.

Raidal, S.L., Love, D.N. and Bailey. G.D. (1995) Inflammation and increased numbers of bacteria in the lower respiratory tract of horses within 6 to 12 hours of confinement with the head elevated. *Australian Veterinary Journal* 72, 45–50.

Riley, C.B. (2016) Mechanical and behavioral responses of horses during non-commercial trailer transport – a pilot study. *42nd Animal Transport Association Conference*, Lisbon.

Riley, C.B., Noble, B.R., Bridges, J., Hazel, S.J. and Thompson, K. (2016) Horse injury during non-commercial transport: Findings from researcher-assisted intercept surveys at Southeastern Australian equestrian events. *Animals* 6, 65.

Riley, C.B., Rogers, C.W. and Padalino, B. (2018) Effects of vehicle type, driver experience and transport management during loading and in-transit on the welfare of road transported horses in New Zealand. *New Zealand Journal of Animal Science and Production* 78, 92–95.

Robin, C.A., Wylie, C.E., Wood, J.L.N. and Newton, J.R. (2011) Making use of equine population demography for disease control purposes: Preliminary observations on the difficulties of counting and locating horses in Great Britain. *Equine Veterinary Journal*, 43, 372–375.

Rosanowski, S.M., Cogger, N., Rogers, C.W., Bolwell, C.F., Benschop, J. *et al.* (2013) Analysis of horse movements from non-commercial horse properties in New Zealand. *New Zealand Veterinary Journal* 61, 245–253.

Roy, R.C. and Cockram, M.S. (2015) Patterns and durations of journeys by horses transported from the USA to Canada for slaughter. *Canadian Veterinary Journal* 56, 581–586.

Roy, R.C., Cockram, M.S. and Dohoo, I.R. (2015a) Welfare of horses transported to slaughter in Canada: Assessment of welfare and journey risk factors affecting the welfare. *Canadian Journal of Animal Science* 95, 509–522.

Roy, R.C., Cockram, M.S., Dohoo, I.R. and Ragnarsson, S. (2015b) Transport of horses for slaughter in Iceland. *Animal Welfare*, 24, 485–495.

Roy, R.C., Cockram, M.S., Dohoo, I.R. and Riley, C.B. (2015c) Injuries in horses transported to slaughter in Canada. *Canadian Journal of Animal Science* 95, 523–531.

Schmidt, A., Möstl, E., Wehnert, C., Aurich, J., Müller, J. *et al.* (2010) Cortisol release and heart rate variability in horses during road transport. *Hormones and Behavior* 57, 209–215.

Schwartzkopf-Genswein, K.S., Faucitano, L., Dadgar, S., Shand, P., González, L.A. *et al.* (2012) Road transport of cattle, swine and poultry in North America and its impact on animal welfare, carcass and meat quality: A review. *Meat Science* 92, 227–243,

Siniscalchi, M., Padalino, B., Lusito, R. and Quaranta, A. (2014) Is the left forelimb preference indicative of a stressful situation in horses? *Behavioural Processes* 107, 61–67.

Slade, L.M.J. (1987) Trailer transportation and racing performance. *10th Equine Nutrition and Physiology Symposium*, Fort Collins, Colorado.

Smith, B.L., Jones, J.H., Carlson, G.P. and Pascoe, J.R. (1994) Body position and direction preferences in horses during road transport. *Equine Veterinary Journal* 26, 374–377.

Smith, B.L., Jones, J.H., Hornof, W., Miles, J., Longworth, K.E. *et al.* (1996) Effects of road transport on indices of stress in horses. *Equine Veterinary Journal* 28, 446–454.

Stewart, M., Foster, T.M. and Waas, J.R. (2003) The effects of air transport on the behaviour and heart rate of horses. *Applied Animal Behaviour Science* 80, 143–160.

Stull, C.L. (2001) Evolution of the proposed federal slaughter horse transport regulations. *Journal of Animal Science* 79(E-Suppl), E12–E15.

Stull, C.L. (2012) The journey to slaughter for North American Horses. *Animal Frontiers* 2, 68–71.

Stull, C.L. and Rodiek, A.V. (2002) Effects of cross-tying horses during 24 h of road transport. *Equine Veterinary Journal* 34, 550–555.

Tateo, A., Padalino, B., Boccaccio, M., Maggiolino, A. and Centoducati, P. (2012) Transport stress in horses: Effects of two different distances. *Journal of Veterinary Behavior: Clinical Applications and Research* 7, 33–42.

The Humane Society International (2012) Long distance horse transports in the European Union. Available at: https://www.hsi.org/wp-content/uploads/assets/pdfs/horses_EU_long-distance_horse_transports_in_EU.pdf (accessed 23 January 2022).

Waran, N.K. (1993) The behaviour of horses during and after transport by road. *Equine Veterinary Education* 5, 129–132.

Waran, N.K. and Cuddeford, D. (1995) Effects of loading and transport on the heart rate and behaviour of horses. *Applied Animal Behaviour Science* 43, 71–81.

Waran, N., Leadon, D. and Friend, T. (2007) The effects of transportation on the welfare of horses. Waren, N. (ed.) *The Welfare of Horses*. Springer, Houten, Netherlands, pp. 125–150.

Weeks, C.A., McGreevy, P. and Waran, N.K. (2012) Welfare issues related to transport and handling of both trained and unhandled horses and ponies. *Equine Veterinary Education* 24, 43–430.

West, R., French, D., Kemp, R. and Elander, J. (1993) Direct observation of driving, self reports of driver behaviour, and accident involvement. *Ergonomics* 36, 557–567.

Whiting, T. (1999) Maximum loading density of loose horses. *Canadian Journal of Animal Science* 79, 115–118.

Woods, J. and Messori, S. (2014) Animal transport legislation and conditions of long distance transport. *CP2 Final Conference,* Kurhaus, Scheveningen, The Hague, 7 May 2014.

World Horse Welfare, FVE, FEEVA, Animal Transportation Association, Animals' Angels and The Donkey Sanctuary (2014) *Practical Guidelines on the Watering of Equine Animals Transported by Road*. Available at: www.animaltransportguides.eu/wp-content/uploads/2017/03/EQUINE-Watering-Guidelines-ENG-5.pdf (accessed 23 January 2022).

Yngvesson, J., de Boussard, E., Larsson, M. and Lundberg, A. (2016) Loading horses (*Equus caballus*) onto trailers—Behaviour of horses and horse owners during loading and habituating. *Applied Animal Behaviour Science* 184, 59–65.

York, A., Matusiewicz, J. and Padalino, B. (2017) How to minimise the incidence of transport-related problem behaviours in horses: a review. *Journal of Equine Science* 28, 67–75.

9 Reproduction and Breeding

Erica K. Gee BVSc, PhD, Diplomate ACT*

Massey University, Palmerston North, New Zealand

Introduction	124
General Overview of Reproduction in the Horse	125
Breeding Behaviour in Free-ranging Herds	125
Breeding Management Under Human Control	128
Paddock breeding	128
In-hand breeding	129
Breeding older horses	131
Commercial Thoroughbred Breeding	131
Stallion Semen Collection and Artificial Insemination of Mares	133
Other Assisted Reproductive Technologies	134
Embryo transfer	134
Oocyte retrieval and intracytoplasmic sperm injection	134
Cloning	134
Abnormalities and Irregularities of Mare Reproductive Behaviour	134
Non-oestrus mares displaying oestrus-like behaviour	134
Prolonged oestrus behaviour	134
Aggression and stallion-like behaviour in mares	135
Mares not showing signs of oestrus during the normal breeding season	135
Abnormalities and Misunderstood Stallion Reproductive Behaviour	135
Masturbation	135
Low libido	135
Unruly stallions	135
Self-mutilation	135
Stallion-like behaviour in non-breeding horses	135
After castration	135
Colt foals	136
Summary	136
References	136

Introduction

Breeding can take place without human aid (for example, in feral herds and paddock breeding). However, with human involvement, breeding can be managed efficiently to maximize reproductive outcomes. Reproductive management under human control can have negative welfare implications for mares and stallions, often relating to failure to allow animals to display normal social and reproductive behaviours. In the breeding shed, interactions between the mare and stallion are very limited prior to mating, and restraint is used to reduce animal movement. Therefore, they have a reduced ability, or limited display, of normal reproductive behaviours.

*Corresponding author: e.k.gee@massey.ac.nz

DOI: 10.1079/9781789242133.0009

Outside of the breeding shed, management issues include extreme social isolation of the stallion and widespread misunderstanding of the normality of masturbation and erection in non-breeding situations (including in geldings). To minimize aberrant behaviours and optimize welfare states for breeding horses, knowledge of equine reproductive behaviour and reproductive management is essential for anyone actively involved in these practices.

General Overview of Reproduction in the Horse

The mare is a long-day, seasonal breeder, meaning that she is typically reproductively active during late spring, summer and autumn. In winter, reproductive activity ceases for most mares, especially those that have raised a foal in the previous breeding season. This period of reproductive inactivity is known as winter anoestrus, a prolonged period when the mare does not cycle (release an egg or ovum) and is incapable of becoming pregnant. The duration of anoestrus is influenced by daylight length, latitude, nutrition and environmental temperature. Around 20–25% of mares, especially those who are well-conditioned and did not have a foal at foot in the previous breeding season, continue cycling during winter.

Mares move from anoestrus into a transitional period (spring transition) in response to increasing daylight length. The transition is characterized by erratic periods of oestrus behaviour for 2–3 months, while follicles, structures that contain the developing ovum (egg), grow and regress on the ovaries without ovulation (release of the egg). Ovulation does not occur during the spring transition period; so, mares cannot become pregnant during this time, even though they may show strong interest in a stallion. Mares can only ovulate at the very end of the spring transition period and become pregnant if inseminated at this time.

Stallions are also long-day seasonal breeders but to a lesser extent than mares. In winter, the testicular size and spermatozoa numbers show some reduction. However, stallions are capable of breeding and achieving pregnancies all year round.

Once the mare has ovulated at the end of the spring transition period, she enters the breeding season, having regular cycles unless she becomes pregnant. The oestrous cycle is typically 21 days long and is divided into oestrus (in heat) and dioestrus (not in heat). During oestrus, which usually lasts 5–7 days, the mare responds to a stallion with increasingly positive teasing behaviour to the point that she will stand to be mated, often over several days. During dioestrus, the mare responds negatively to a stallion's responses. The teasing behaviours that are seen commonly in oestrus and dioestrus mares are summarized in Table 9.1.

Breeding Behaviour in Free-ranging Herds

The social organization and behaviour of feral horses are very similar worldwide (Linklater, 2000). Bands are stable groups of mature mares and their pre-dispersal offspring, with one or more stallions (Fig. 9.1). These stable groups have very strong social and reproductive bonds. Colts and fillies usually leave the herd around puberty (1–2 years of age) or after weaning (Linklater, 2000). On leaving, colts will usually join an unstable bachelor band, and fillies may join other groups of mares or pair up with a bachelor male.

The stallion actively guards and maintains or tends the mature mares within his herd, having many interactions to assess their receptiveness. The stallion also protects younger fillies but may allow them to stray during oestrus. Stallions may herd straying young foals back to the band and play with older foals. Stallions and bachelor males mark faecal piles of other horses with their own urine and faeces, leading to large piles of faeces (Fig. 9.2).

Breeding occurs mostly during the summer months, meaning that most foals are born the following summer (gestation length is around 340 days) when

Table 9.1. Percentage of behaviours shown in oestrus and dioestrus mares in the presence of a stallion. Fraser, 2010.

Behaviour shown	Percentage in oestrus	Percentage in dioestrus
Remained calm and stationary	>80	1–20
Raised tail away from the perineum	>80	1–20
Clitoral winking	>80	1–20
Posturing hind end towards stallion with a hind out foot	>80	1–20
Urinated promptly	41–60	1–20
Moved position reactively	21–40	>80
Held ears back stiffly	1–20	>80
Swished tail vigorously	1–20	>80

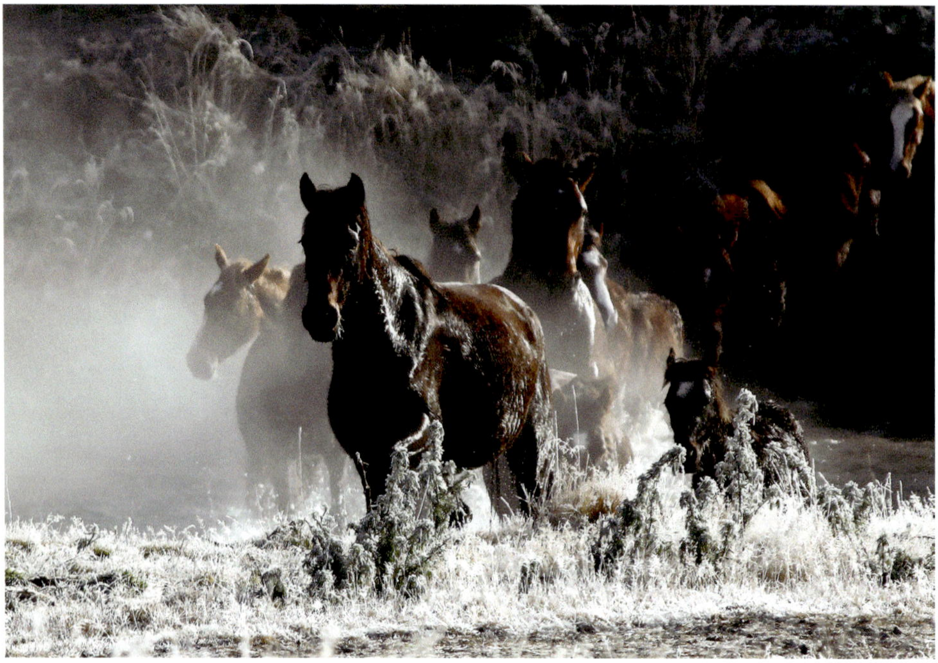

Fig. 9.1. A band of Kaimanawa of horses, the feral horses of New Zealand, cross a stream early in the morning. Photo: Margaret Leyland.

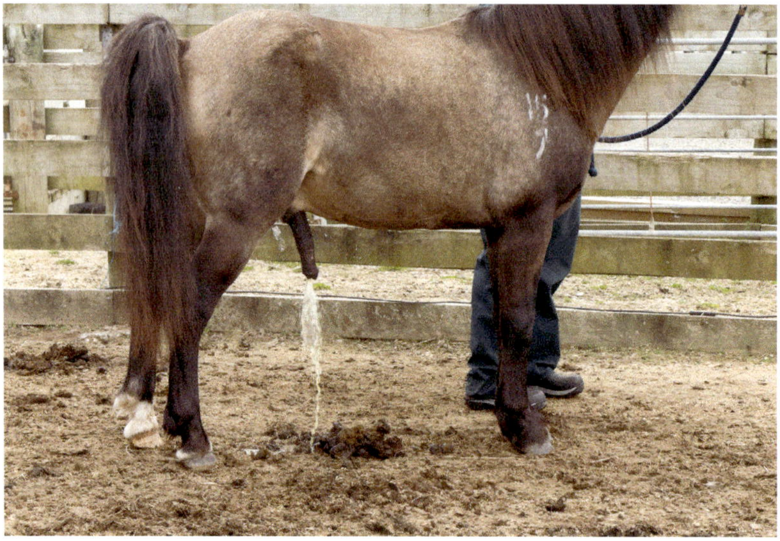

Fig. 9.2. A stallion urinating on a faecal pile. Photo: Avedon Photography.

food resources are likely to be most abundant. The stallion spends much of his time tending to individual band members, checking the oestrus status of each mare using a combination of visual, olfactory and auditory cues. The stallion will closely follow the oestrus mare and investigates any urine and faeces from her, often urinating over them (McDonnell, 2016). Only an approaching threat, such as another stallion that needs to be chased away, will interrupt the stallion (McDonnell, 2016). The initial interactions between the oestrus mare and stallion are nose to nose and often initiated by the mare in oestrus.

Over several days and many mare–stallion interactions, the mare in oestrus may become more attractive to the stallion and more receptive to his advances (McDonnell, 2000). Oestrus mares show a general increase in movement and may have relaxed facial expressions, with the ears turned to the side and the head slightly lowered (Crowell-Davis, 2007). When the mare is ready for breeding, she invites the stallion to investigate her hindquarters, often looking back at him with her head bent towards her flank (McDonnell, 2016). The oestrus mare will present the stallion with her hindquarters, allowing him to lick and nibble her coat over the withers, flanks, hindlimbs and buttocks (Fig. 9.3). The mare will elevate her tail or move it to the side and pass small amounts of urine followed by clitoral winking (Fig. 9.4). Many stallions will display flehmen in response (Fig. 9.5), perhaps to improve the olfactory signals of oestrus.

When receptive to breeding, mares adopt a stable standing position, with the hindlegs placed widely apart, for the stallion to mount. The stallion usually nuzzles or nips the flank and hocks of the mare, and she may turn her head back to allow muzzle to muzzle contact before he mounts (McDonnell, 2016). It is usual for both experienced and inexperienced stallions to first mount without an erection. When the stallion is assured that the mare will stand for breeding, he will mount with an erection, placing his front limbs in front of the mare's hips (Fig. 9.6). He may grasp the mare's mane (and sometimes neck) with his teeth. During breeding, the mare moves and postures to allow the stallion to penetrate and thrust. Pelvic thrusts enable quick intromission, and further pelvic thrusts quickly lead to ejaculation and tail flagging (the up and down movement of the stallion's tail). The stallion then typically rests on the mare after ejaculation, before the mare walks forward, ending the coupling. The stallion then investigates any urine or semen on the ground and continues to tend to the mare. Stallions may have a short refractory period after breeding and may be ready to breed again in 30 minutes. Mares may be bred multiple times in a day, over multiple days, for as long as she is in standing heat.

A stallion's interactions with dioestrus mares are much shorter than those with oestrus mares. Dioestrus mares show strong agonistic behaviours that may include squealing, kicking, laying ears back, baring the teeth and trying to move away. Experienced stallions usually

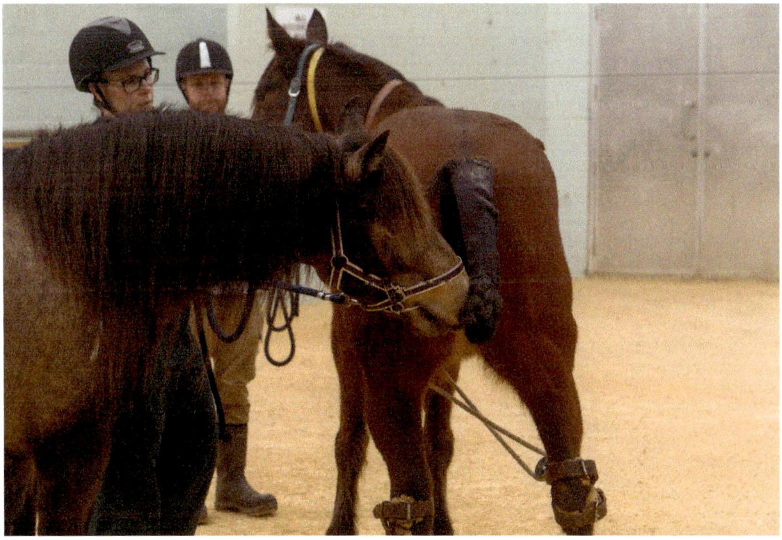

Fig. 9.3. Stallion investigating oestrus mare. Note the use of breeding hobbles to reduce the risk of the mare kicking the stallion. Photo: Avedon Photography.

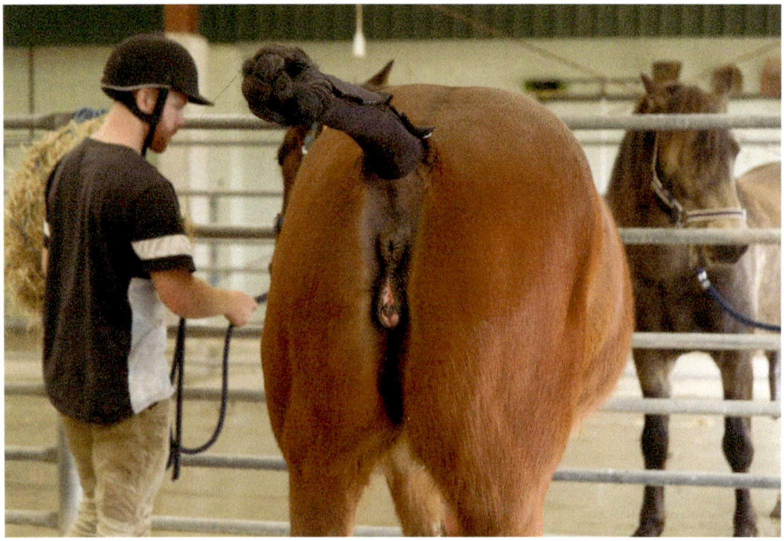

Fig. 9.4. Clitoral winking of oestrus mare in the presence of a stallion. Photo: Avedon Photography.

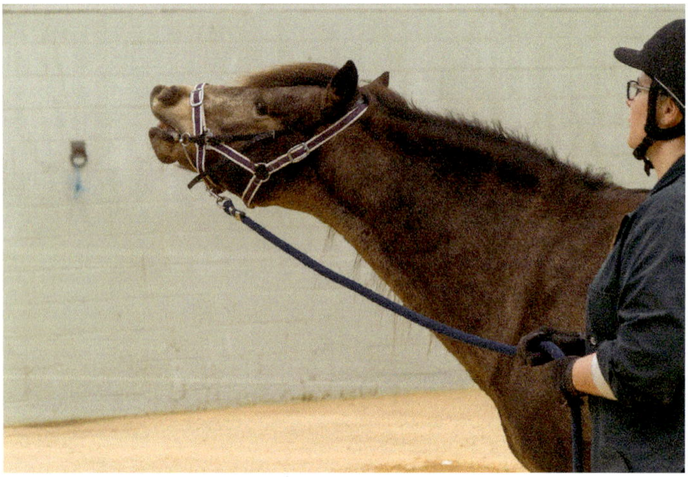

Fig. 9.5. Flehmen exhibited by a stallion. Photo: Avedon Photography.

move on from dioestrus mares to investigate other mares in the herd.

Breeding Management Under Human Control

Paddock breeding

With paddock breeding, a stallion is kept with mares within the confines of a paddock. If all mares are brought in together at the start of the breeding season, the artificially constituted herd can be stable and develop strong social and reproductive bonds, as in the free-ranging situation. In contrast, adding mares throughout the breeding season negatively affects herd stability, with more displays of agonistic behaviour increasing the risk of individual horse injury. Stallions used for paddock breeding may be of relatively low economic value.

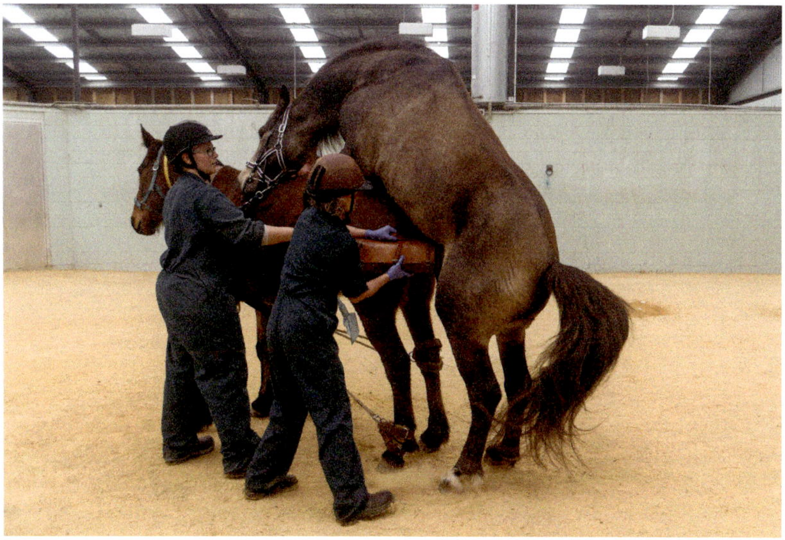

Fig. 9.6. A stallion is mounting an oestrus mare for collection via an artificial vagina. Photo: Avedon Photography.

In-hand breeding

In-hand breeding (live cover) requires human control of a mare and stallion that are only brought together for breeding. This may reduce the potential risk of injury to the stallion and mare during breeding but poses safety risks for their handlers and reduces opportunities for normal sexual behaviour between the mare and stallion.

Under human control, broodmares are usually kept in small herds of around 14 individuals at pasture in Australasia (Rogers *et al.*, 2007). In contrast, Iceland horse herds average 23 mares, whereas in the USA, 30% of establishments have more than 20 horses, 30% between 10 and 19, and 40% with 5 to 9 horses (USDA, 2016; Sigurjónsdóttir and Haraldsson, 2019). Mares in stable herds can develop strong social bonds and exhibit normal social behaviours. When herds are mixed, as frequently happens when groups are formed based on reproductive status, strong social bonds are difficult to form, and agonistic behaviour is more common, which can lead to a negative welfare state. Young, inexperienced mares face many social challenges when introduced to a herd and may lose weight, leading to an increased risk of early pregnancy losses.

Domesticated stallions are rarely kept in close physical distance to mares and do not have opportunities to show normal social behaviours. Stallion barns are common on commercial studs, where they are kept in individual boxes, but can hear, smell and sometimes see other stallions. This housing situation can lead to a bachelor herd effect for some stallions, with reduced testosterone concentrations, reduced libido and poorer conception rates. This state can often be alleviated by keeping the stallion in a location away from other stallions but where he can see mares or fillies nearby (McDonnell, 2016).

With commercial studs, the oestrus teasing behaviour of mares is often assessed using a less valuable stallion, such as a pony, rather than the breeding stallion to reduce the risk of injury to the sire. The 'teaser stallion' is used to elicit signs of oestrus or dioestrus behaviour in mares, often with solid separation between the mare and teaser stallion, such as a teasing wall. Both oestrus mares and stallions can show agonistic behaviour such as squealing and threatening to strike, especially when first introduced, posing a safety risk for handlers. Assessment of teasing behaviour is a skill that requires a good knowledge of normal mare and stallion behaviour, patience and persistence.

Typically, the teaser stallion and oestrus mare are first allowed head to head contact. Then, if the mare shows any positive teasing signs, the stallion is encouraged to investigate the back end of the mare, often over the teasing wall. Mares and stallions often vocalize during teasing, and more vocal stallions elicit oestrus signals more quickly than quiet stallions (Pickerel *et al.*, 1993). Initially, mares in oestrus may show mixed messages in response to the stallion, but oestrus behaviours become more positive with more interaction. Maiden mares and maiden mares with foals at foot often require more prolonged interaction with the teaser stallion before showing teasing signs. Foals are usually put in an adjacent enclosure during teasing to reduce the risk of injury to the foal while maintaining its visibility to the mare. Handling of pre-weaned foals by experienced handlers may result in transient signs of stress in the foal, but do not have long-term negative effects on the human–horse relationship (Górecka-Bruzda *et al.*, 2017).

The welfare of the teaser stallion is seldom considered. While he is encouraged to initiate courtship behaviour with multiple mares, he is not permitted to breed them. Poor understanding of oestrus teasing behaviour may mean that the teaser stallion is forced to interact with dioestrus mares, increasing the risk of injury to the teaser. Like breeding stallions, teasers are kept isolated from other horses, except while working. They are unable to partake in normal social behaviours.

In-hand breeding typically takes place in a breeding shed or barn, with some protection from the elements and good footing to reduce the risk of the stallion slipping when mounting and breeding. After confirming the mare is in strong standing heat by the teaser stallion, the mare is prepared for breeding. Her perineum is washed and dried, and the tail may be bandaged. Precautions are taken to reduce the risk of injury to both horses, especially the stallion, during breeding. Boots may be applied to the rear hooves of the mare to reduce the impact if she kicks the stallion. The mare is restrained with a halter and lead, with or without a chain over the nose or in the mouth or a twitch applied to her upper lip to reduce movement. Sometimes, a front leg is held by an attendant as the stallion mounts or a leg strap is used to hold the front leg up. A neck cape may cover the neck of a mare being bred to a stallion known to bite and break the skin. Some breeding capes have projections that the stallion can bite to help balance himself. A breeding roll can be placed across the rear thigh region of the mare to prevent the stallion from penetrating her reproductive tract too deeply. Well behaved stallions can be managed with a simple halter and lead rope. More commonly, after placing the halter and lead rope, a chain is placed through the mouth or over the nose for restraint during breeding. Alternatively, bits and bridles are used for restraint. Stallions that are known to bite or savage mares may also wear a muzzle to protect the mare and handlers.

Personnel used in the breeding shed may be required to wear personal protective equipment as a safety measure. Equipment ranges from leather boots and helmets to body protectors, depending on the stallion's temperament and behaviour. Normally, only a few experienced people are allowed in the breeding shed during breeding, including the mare handler, stallion handler, and sometimes an assistant to hold the mare's tail. Experienced stallion handlers usually have a good working relationship with the stallion in a non-breeding situation and in the breeding shed and use an appropriate level of restraint for the stallion. All personnel should understand that the vocalization and prancing by the stallion are normal breeding behaviours. The breeding shed should be relatively quiet with few distractions. A pen for restraint of the dam's foal is situated where the mare can easily see her foal while being bred.

After the mare is restrained, the stallion is brought to the breeding shed, where he is expected to gain an erection rapidly, mount once and breed the mare in a short space of time. The stallion's penis may be washed with warm water before and/or after breeding. The opportunity for the stallion to interact with the head and body of the mare is limited, with handlers often guiding the approach of the stallion directly to the mare's back end. The mare's restraints mean she cannot move forward when the stallion advances or when he mounts. False mounts (mounting without an erection) are discouraged by only allowing the stallion to mount when he has an erection. After the stallion has ejaculated, he is encouraged to dismount the mare rather than the mare walking forward as would happen without human intervention. The total breeding time may be only several minutes (McDonnell 2009). Repeat in-hand breeding every two days for as long as the mare shows signs of standing oestrus is normal practice if veterinary ultrasound scanning and drugs are not used routinely in broodmare management. Thus, the inclusion of a veterinarian in the breeding team may improve the welfare of the mare.

The welfare of the mare can be compromised in the breeding shed with the use of excessive restraint, the lack of opportunity to engage in normal courtship behaviours, and the greatly reduced ability to halt stallion advances. Mare restraints may provoke fear and resistance by the mare, further exacerbated by the inability to interact or react to the stallion, often seen as resistance to the stallion mounting (McDonnell, 2000). The welfare of the stallion may be compromised in the breeding shed, with little ability to display full courtship behaviour, and with poor handling resulting in inappropriate or excessive restraint and use of punishment for displaying normal breeding behaviours. Overuse of the stallion may result in a loss of libido.

Breeding older horses

Mare fertility starts to steadily decline by 13 years of age for light horse breeds, and relatively few mares over 18 years have live foals (Hanlon *et al.*, 2012; Scoggin, 2015). Older mares are more likely to have problems with excessive fluid in their uterus after breeding and are more prone to infections than young mares, sometimes requiring intensive veterinary management to improve pregnancy rates. Older mares have a higher pregnancy loss rate than younger mares (Hanlon *et al.*, 2012).

Commercial Thoroughbred Breeding

The Thoroughbred industry requires that all pregnancies result from live cover for offspring to be eligible for registration for racing. Breeding relies almost exclusively on in-hand breeding, where handlers manage the mare and stallion. Artificial breeding techniques are prohibited.

The Thoroughbred industry has an imposed breeding season that does not match the physiologic summer breeding season. For example, in New Zealand and Australia, the Thoroughbred breeding season starts on 1 September and ends by mid-December for most commercial stallions, with a length of 105 days. This compares to 150 days in the Northern Hemisphere (Hanlon *et al.*, 2012), with a trend to 120 days in the United Kingdom (Allen and Wilsher, 2012). The operational breeding season in the northern hemisphere runs from 15 February to the first week of July. Horse breeders try to get mares in foal as early as possible, so yearlings are older and larger at major sales, held in January and February in the Southern Hemisphere and in September and October in the Northern Hemisphere. This industry-imposed, short- and early-breeding season affects the management of mares and stallions.

In autumn (September), the start of the Thoroughbred breeding season in the Southern Hemisphere, around 80% of mares are not cycling (they are in winter anoestrus or the spring transition period) (Osborne, 1966). Breeders can advance the onset of spring transition using artificial lighting to mimic increasing day length, so non-pregnant mares are ready for breeding at the start of the imposed breeding season. Lights can be provided indoors in boxes (common in the northern hemisphere, where 100% of non-pregnant mares are put under lights) or outdoors in large yards by overhead lights. Outdoor lighting is used for about 35% of these mares in New Zealand (Hanlon *et al.*, 2012). Artificial lights are used to extend daylight hours at the end of the day, giving around 14–16 hours of light and 8–10 hours of darkness. In the Southern Hemisphere, mares are put under lights from 1 July to be ready for breeding from 1 September. In Europe and North America, mares are placed under lights by early December for 60–90 days until the mares start to cycle normally. An alternative to overhead lights are masks that emit blue light in one eye. Therefore, they can be worn in the paddock, giving similar results to artificial lights in advancing the breeding season (Murphy *et al.*, 2014). One potentially negative outcome of putting mares under lights is the early shedding of winter coats. For mares housed indoors, this is not an issue, provided the barn or stable is kept warm, but mares kept at pasture may need extra protection with rugs and shelter from inclement weather.

With commercial studs, the timing of breeding for an individual mare is usually decided by a combination of teasing results and findings from multiple veterinary transrectal reproductive ultrasound exams (scans). Teasing mares may be scanned every day or two during oestrus to monitor follicle growth and to check for fluid in the uterus. Mares are typically restrained in stocks for this scanning, and often a handler is present at the head, holding a lead rope attached to the mare's halter. Many mares do not require any additional restraint while in stocks (Ille *et al.*, 2016). A veterinarian's transrectal palpation and scanning are not considered a major stressor, with only small changes in stress indicators such as heart rate, heart rate variability, and salivary cortisol concentrations in non-pregnant mares (Ille *et al.*, 2016). However, with palpation and scanning, there is a potential risk of rectal tears that can result in bleeding, abdominal infection and death. To reduce the risk of rectal tears, mares that show aversive signs to rectal palpation and scanning may be sedated, a nose twitch applied, or drugs administered to sedate the mare or to relax the rectum.

In concert with a veterinary examination, drugs like human chorionic gonadotrophin (hCG) and deslorelin are used to induce ovulation in oestrus mares, ensuring that each is bred only once per cycle. Regular scanning in breeding mares only once per cycle with drugs to induce ovulation has several benefits. There is less contamination of the uterus with only one breeding, and uterine inflammation associated with breeding can easily be identified, treated and monitored by ultrasound. The length of dioestrus is shortened with the use of prostaglandin $PGF_{2\alpha}$ (known as short cycling a mare with PG).

Most mares ovulate one follicle containing an ovum each 21-day cycle. However, around 28% of Thoroughbred mares ovulate two ova each cycle (Davies Morel and Newcombe, 2008), increasing the likelihood of pregnancy each cycle and the risk of twin pregnancies. Standard doses of hCG used to induce ovulation may increase the number of ovulations in each cycle (Perkins and Grimmett, 2001). However, placentation in the mare has not evolved to carry twin pregnancies successfully; often, the mare aborts twin foetuses in late gestation. If she does give birth to one or two live foals, the survival rates of the offspring are poor, and the mare may need assistance during foaling. Due to the negative impacts of twin pregnancies, Thoroughbred mares routinely have multiple early pregnancy checks via transrectal ultrasound. This is to establish if twins are present, and if so, then reduce twins to singletons. If twin reductions are carried out early (14–16 days post-breeding or post-ovulation), the prognosis for the remaining twin is very good, with a similar rate of embryonic loss to a singleton pregnancy (Hodder *et al.*, 2008; Hanlon *et al.*, 2012). Before the widespread use of reproductive ultrasound examinations in mares, twins were the single major cause of abortions (Whitwell, 1980).

Thoroughbred mares are prone to poor vulval conformation as they age (Scoggin, 2015), allowing air and debris into the vagina, resulting in inflammation in the vagina and potentially the uterus, and reduced fertility. Vulval conformation is improved with a minor surgical procedure, commonly known as a Caslick, that sutures together the upper part of the vulval lips. The procedure is commonly performed with the mare restrained in stocks. Local anaesthetic is infused in the surgical area, with or without sedation or other forms of restraint, depending on the mare's behaviour. Based on personal communication, Hemberg *et al.* (2005) estimate that 70–80% of Thoroughbred mares have Caslick procedures. These are performed multiple times during a broodmare's life and must be reversed before foaling. Widespread poor vulval conformation may be due to the selection of mares and stallions for performance and pedigree rather than for their reproductive characteristics (Hemberg *et al.*, 2005).

Mares have their first postpartum oestrus, known as foal heat, starting 5–12 days after foaling. In New Zealand, around 32% of Thoroughbred mares are bred on foal heat. When specific selection criteria are adhered to (i.e. ovulation at day ten or later, less than 1 cm fluid in the uterus, no history of dystocia or retained foetal membranes), pregnancy rates are not different to those in mares bred on the subsequent cycle, with an overall first cycle pregnancy rate of 54% (Hanlon *et al.*, 2012). When the specific selection criteria are not applied, the conception rates for foal heat breeding may be as low as 20% (Blanchard *et al.*, 2012). The large number of mares bred on foal heat is driven by the short breeding season and the efforts to get mares pregnant as early as possible to maintain a yearly foaling pattern.

For stallions, veterinary management of mares allows popular stallions to have large books of mares, with each mare being served only once per cycle. While 40 mares were historically considered a suitable number for a stallion to breed in hand, veterinary management of mares means that popular Thoroughbred stallions have books of more than 100 mares in a season. In the short Thoroughbred breeding season, stallions commonly breed at least four times a day (Hanlon *et al.*, 2012). Large book sizes are associated with significantly lower first-cycle pregnancy rates compared to stallions with books of fewer than 100 mares (Hanlon *et al.*, 2012). Libido (the desire to breed) and fertility diminish for most stallions that are bred in hand more than once or twice a day (McDonnell, 2000). The Thoroughbred industry further increases stallion use by shuttling stallions via air transport, so they stand at stud for breeding in the Northern and Southern Hemisphere breeding seasons. Shuttling is reported to have no detrimental effect on first-cycle pregnancy rates (Lane *et al.*, 2016), indicating that shuttling stallions maintain their fertility despite the associated stress of long-distance transport.

Stallion Semen Collection and Artificial Insemination of Mares

Many breed registries, including those for Standardbreds and most sport horses, have widely adopted artificial insemination (AI) as the primary method of breeding mares. Stallion semen collection and AI of the mare enable the mare and stallion to be geographically isolated, thereby reducing transport stress. Semen life can be extended using products that increase the longevity of the spermatozoa, and extended semen can be used fresh or cooled to 4 °C for overnight transportation. Furthermore, semen from some stallions can be frozen and stored indefinitely in liquid nitrogen, meaning that a stallion's genetics can be used even after castration or death.

In this setting, most stallions are trained to jump a dummy mount (phantom), and semen is collected using an artificial vagina (Fig. 9.7). This approach reduces the risk of horse and personnel injuries in the breeding shed. Some stallions require no training to mount a dummy, while others need some training, usually in the presence of a mare in oestrus. The dummy mount is often permanently fixed in the breeding shed or barn, with enough room at the front and sides for the stallion to move around safely. The dummy mount may be adjustable in height and angle to best suit individual stallions. An oestrus mare may be restrained in stocks in the breeding shed. The flooring is usually non-slip and easily cleaned.

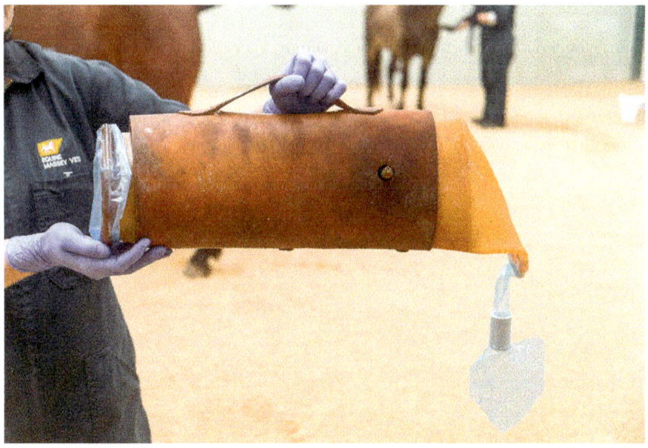

Fig. 9.7. Missouri-type artificial vagina for semen collection. It can be used with warm water and air to give a core temperature of around 48 °C. Photo: Avedon Photography.

The trained stallion usually quickly develops an erection when he enters the breeding shed and may not need the presence of a mare in oestrus. The stallion is trained to stand still while his penis is washed with warm water. He is then led to the phantom and encouraged to mount. On mounting, the stallion's penis is deflected into an artificial vagina, and the stallion thrusts and ejaculates quickly. Different types of artificial vaginas are used for semen collection; all provide the warmth and pressure that a stallion requires for ejaculation. After ejaculation, the stallion jumps off the phantom and is led from the breeding shed. Most popular stallions have semen collected every second day during the breeding season.

The collected ejaculate is taken into a laboratory close to the breeding shed. The semen is evaluated (volume, concentration and motility of spermatozoa) and extended to promote the longevity of the spermatozoa. Each extended ejaculate can be divided into multiple mare doses and sent to other sites or processed and frozen for future use.

The management of mares for breeding by AI relies on veterinary management with regular transrectal ultrasound examinations (often daily during oestrus) and the use of drugs to induce ovulation so that mares are bred just once per cycle. Many breeding centres do not use teaser stallions, so mares may never interact with a mature male horse. Insemination is carried out with the mare restrained in stocks and, depending on the country's regulations, may be carried out by veterinarians or trained laypeople. The tail is wrapped, and the perineal region washed, often with warm water and soap, then dried with paper towels. The inseminator wears a sterile full-length sleeve, and the semen is drawn into a syringe with an insemination pipette. The pipette is then introduced in the gloved and lubricated hand through the vulval lips, advanced to the vagina, and then passed through the cervix. The extended semen is placed in the uterus of the mare. Most mares do not require additional restraint for AI and appear to tolerate the procedure well. AI is considered as likely to be minimally painful or stressful for the mare (Campbell and Sandøe, 2015).

The welfare of stallions in semen collection programmes may be improved by reduced injury risk using a dummy mount and breeding only once every second day. However, they face negative welfare effects from little to no interactions with oestrus mares and opportunities to display courtship and tending behaviours. The welfare of mares (and their foals) in IA programmes may be improved because of the reduced risk of injury with no stallion interaction and a reduced need for transport. However, there are few to no opportunities for mares to display normal breeding behaviours.

Other Assisted Reproductive Technologies

Embryo transfer

Embryo transfer (ET) technologies mean that mares who cannot carry their own pregnancies to term (either due to competition commitments or reproductive pathology) can still contribute their genetics. Frozen stallion spermatozoa can be used for breeding many years after a stallion has died or even after he has been castrated. Embryos can be flushed from a donor mare's uterus at 7–9 days post-ovulation. Breeding management of an embryo donor mare is essentially the same as for AI, with careful attention to determine the day of ovulation. At 7–9 days post-ovulation, the donor mare is restrained in stocks and may be sedated for the procedure because distension of her uterus with flushing fluid can result in discomfort. Her perineum is washed and dried, and sterile equipment used to deliver specialized fluid into the mare's uterus. The liquid is then siphoned out and the embryo caught in a specialized cup with a filter attached. The embryo can be seen under a stereomicroscope and is washed and graded for quality. The viable embryo can then be transferred through the cervix into a recipient mare at a similar stage of her oestrous cycle to the donor mare. Alternatively, the embryo can be cooled and transported to another location for transfer to a recipient or stored indefinitely in liquid nitrogen after a process called vitrification. The surgical transfer of embryos is now uncommon.

Oocyte retrieval and intracytoplasmic sperm injection

Oocyte retrieval and intracytoplasmic sperm injection (ICSI) are commercial techniques that allow infertile mares and those with high risks of pregnancy complications to remain in the breeding pool. These techniques also allow the use of frozen sperm from stallions with poor fertility or those that have died. Oocytes (unfertilized eggs) are harvested from the ovaries of mares restrained in stocks, using a transvaginal, ultrasound-guided approach. Mares are usually heavily sedated for the procedure to reduce movement and the risk of injury and are given pain-relieving medication. Harvested oocytes can be matured in the laboratory and injected with a single spermatozoon in the process of ICSI. The resulting embryos can be matured in the laboratory and inseminated transcervically into a donor mare.

There are no studies assessing the negative welfare effects on the donor mare, although the procedure of oocyte retrieval is likely to be painful for the mare (Campbell and Sandøe, 2015). Surgical procedures to transfer oocytes and embryos into donor mares have become less common with ICSI and improved laboratory techniques to mature ova and embryos.

Cloning

Nuclear transfusion techniques using harvested cells have been successful in producing horse clones. Due to the relatively small numbers of horse clones, there are few reports documenting the health and welfare issues in the foetus and newborn foal clones, compared with those reported for other species. Mares carrying clones do not have the placental problems reported in other species, but cloned foals may need intensive care after birth (Campbell and Sandøe, 2015).

Abnormalities and Irregularities of Mare Reproductive Behaviour

Non-oestrus mares displaying oestrus-like behaviour

Anoestrus mares and mares that have had their ovaries removed may display low-level oestrus signs in response to a stallion, presumably due to the lack of progesterone. Pregnant mares may also show signs of oestrus due to hormones produced by the foetus, that first increase at days 60–90 of gestation, then peak at day 200 of pregnancy. Mares with ovarian tumours that produce hormones may show persistent oestrus or nymphomania signs but more commonly show persistent anoestrus.

Prolonged oestrus behaviour

Erratic and prolonged periods of teasing behaviour occur during the spring and autumn transition periods. Early in the breeding season, mares will have a longer oestrus interval, which is shorter later in the breeding season. Mares with chronic uterine inflammation may have very short dioestrus intervals and appear to be in heat more often. Abnormalities of ovulation (persistent anovulatory follicles and haemorrhagic follicles) occur in up to 20% of cycles late in the breeding season (Ginther *et al.*, 2007). They may show prolonged oestrus behaviour, more commonly in older mares.

Aggression and stallion-like behaviour in mares

Aggression may occur during teasing. This is likely due to the mare's inability to show normal repetitive courtship behaviours in the breeding shed, so restraint is applied to the mare. Pregnant mares may show stallion-like behaviour or exhibit aggression in response to increases in hormones produced by the foetus. A small proportion of mares with ovarian tumours may show stallion-like behaviour.

Mares not showing signs of oestrus during the normal breeding season

Prolonged dioestrus intervals lasting up to 3 or 4 months occur in approximately 8% of cycles during the normal breeding season and up to 28% of mares in autumn (King *et al.*, 1993), and may be misinterpreted as a sign of pregnancy. Young mares with foals at foot may be reluctant to tease a stallion during oestrus and may be referred to as shy breeders. With patience and persistence, teasing these shy mares may often cause oestrus behaviour. Ovarian tumours may produce hormones that can result in mares not cycling.

Abnormalities and Misunderstood Stallion Reproductive Behaviour

Masturbation

All stallions (and geldings) show spontaneous erections and penile movements described as masturbation. This is normal behaviour, occurring every 90 minutes, and is rarely associated with ejaculation (McDonnell, 2009). The use of devices to discourage masturbation in horses has negative welfare consequences, including the risk of penile injuries, reduced libido and copulatory behaviour anomalies in stallions in the breeding shed.

Low libido

Reductions in libido, or the urge to breed, are common in domestic stallions and are considered a problem caused by humans (McDonnell, 2009). Loss of libido can occur for stallions that are bred in hand when required to breed more than twice a day. Some of these shy or slow-breeding stallions may exhibit behaviours more like a bachelor band stallion, with sneak breeding behaviours; others may be reluctant to breed due to chronic pain (McDonnell, 2016). Keeping stallions near other stallions can result in a bachelor-band type effect, where some individuals will have reduced libido. Changing housing for the affected stallion and keeping it near mares or fillies can improve its libido. Allowing more interaction with the mare, including allowing mare movement, can improve libido when combined with good handling by experienced personnel (McDonnell, 2000).

Unruly stallions

Most stallions quickly learn the appropriate in-hand breeding routine. However, inappropriate handling by humans, often in response to normal but misunderstood behaviours, including prancing and vocalization, can easily train unwanted behaviours in the breeding shed. Stallions are best retrained by the use of positive and negative reinforcement techniques by an educated handler (McDonnell, 2009).

Self-mutilation

Stallions (and geldings) can display what is normal intermale aggression but is misdirected at themselves. Behaviours that may occur include biting, kicking, stomping and lunging into objects, resulting in damage to themselves (reviewed by McDonnell, 2008). Castration may, or may not, resolve this behaviour. Self-mutilation behaviours can also result from chronic, unrelenting pain and may be resolved by identifying and addressing the source of pain.

Stallion-like behaviour in non-breeding horses

After castration

Castration is a common management procedure involving surgical removal of the testicles from a colt or stallion. This is performed so that the horse is no longer fertile, and male hormone production is reduced, making him easier to manage. However, up to half of all castrated horses continue to show stallion-like behaviours towards mares (McDonnell 2009).

Colt foals

Colts reach puberty at around 1–2 years of age. Prior to puberty, it is common for colt foals to display some stallion-like behaviours, including attempts at mounting their dam or other foals and developing erections.

Summary

Domestic horses are typically kept for breeding under human control. This reduces the ability of horses to display normal reproductive behaviours and potentially induces negative welfare states. Some stallions do not have the opportunity to interact with the mare, her urine, urovaginal secretions or faeces before breeding. Mares in AI programmes may never interact with a stallion. Misunderstanding of normal reproductive behaviour can lead to inappropriate restraint by handlers and may result in unwanted behaviours and increasing the risk of injury for humans and horses.

References

Allen, W.R. and Wilsher, S. (2012) The influence of mare numbers, ejaculation frequency and month on the fertility of Thoroughbred stallions. *Equine Veterinary Journal* 44, 535–541.

Blanchard, T.L., Thompson, J.A., Love, C.C., Brinsko, S.P., Ramsey, J. *et al.* (2012) Influence of day of post-partum breeding on pregnancy rate, pregnancy loss rate, and following rate in Thoroughbred mares. *Theriogenology* 77, 1290–1296.

Campbell, M.L.H. and Sandøe, P. (2015) Welfare in horse breeding. *The Veterinary Record* 176, 436.

Crowell-Davis, S.L. (2007) Sexual behavior of mares. *Hormones and Behavior* 52, 12–17.

Davies Morel, M.C. and Newcombe, J.R. (2008) The efficacy of different hCG dose rates and the effect of hCG treatment on ovarian activity: Ovulation, multiple ovulation, pregnancy, multiple pregnancy, synchrony of multiple ovulation; in the mare. *Animal Reproduction Science* 109, 189–199.

Fraser, A.F. (2010) *The Behaviour and Welfare of the Horse*, 2nd edn. Centre for Agriculture and Bioscience International, Wallingford, Oxford.

Ginther, O.J., Gastal, E.L., Gastal, M.O. and Beg, M.A. (2007) Incidence, endocrinology, vascularity, and morphology of hemorrhagic anovulatory follicles in mares. *Journal of Equine Veterinary Science* 27, 130–139.

Górecka-Bruzda, A., Jaworski, Z., Suwała, M., Sobczyńska, M., Jastrzębska, E. *et al.* (2017) Aversiveness of husbandry procedures for pre-weaned foals: A comparison using behavioural and physiological indices. *Applied Animal Behaviour Science* 191, 31–38.

Hanlon, D.W., Stevenson, M., Evans, M.J. and Firth, E.C. (2012) Reproductive performance of Thoroughbred mares in the Waikato region of New Zealand: 1. Descriptive analyses. *New Zealand Veterinary Journal* 60, 329–334.

Hemberg, E., Lundeheim, N. and Einarsson, S. (2005) Retrospective study on vulvar conformation in relation to endometrial cytology and fertility in Thoroughbred mares. *Journal of Veterinary Medicine Series A* 52, 474–477.

Hodder, A.D.J., Liu, I.K.M. and Ball, B.A. (2008) Current methods for the diagnosis and management of twin pregnancy in the mare. *Equine Veterinary Education* 20, 493–502.

Ille, N., Aurich, C. and Aurich, J. (2016) Physiological stress responses of mares to gynecologic examination in veterinary medicine. *Journal of Equine Veterinary Science* 43, 6–11.

King, S.S., Neumann, K.R., Nequin, L.G. and Weedman, B.J. (1993) Time of onset and ovarian state prior to entry into winter anestrus. *Journal of Equine Veterinary Science* 13, 512–515.

Lane, E.A., Bijnen, M.L.J., Osborne, M., More, S.J., Henderson, I.S.F. *et al.* (2016) Key factors affecting reproductive success of thoroughbred mares and stallions on a commercial stud farm. *Reproduction in Domestic Animals* 51, 181–187.

Linklater, W.L. (2000) Adaptive explanation in socio-ecology: Lessons from the Equidae. *Biological Reviews* 75, 1–20.

McDonnell, S.M. (2000) Reproductive behavior of stallions and mares: Comparison of free-running and domestic in-hand breeding. *Animal Reproduction Science* 60, 211–219.

McDonnell, S.M. (2008) Practical review of self-mutilation in horses. *Animal Reproduction Science* 107, 219–228.

McDonnell, S.M. (2009) Stallion sexual behavior. In: Samper, J. (ed.) *Equine Breeding Management and Artificial Insemination*, 2nd edn. W.B. Saunders Company, Philadelphia, Pennsylvania, pp. 41–46.

McDonnell, S.M. (2016) Revisiting clinical stallion sexual behavior: applying ethology in the breeding shed. *Journal of Equine Veterinary Science* 43, S18–S22.

Murphy, B.A., Walsh, C.M., Woodward, E.M., Prendergast, R.L., Ryle, J.P. *et al.* (2014) Blue light from individual light masks directed at a single eye advances the breeding season in mares. *Equine Veterinary Journal* 46, 601–605.

Osborne, V.E. (1966) An analysis of the pattern of ovulation as it occurs in the annual reproductive cycle of

the mare in Australia. *Australian Veterinary Journal* 42, 385–388.
Perkins, N.R. and Grimmett, J.B. (2001) Pregnancy and twinning rates in Thoroughbred mares following the administration of human chorionic gonadotropin (hCG). *New Zealand Veterinary Journal* 49, 94–100.
Pickerel, T.M., Crowell-Davis, S.L., Caudle, A.B. and Estep, D.Q. (1993) Sexual preference of mares (*Equus caballus*) for individual stallions. *Applied Animal Behaviour Science* 38, 1–13.
Rogers, C.W., Gee, E.K. and Firth, E.C. (2007) A cross-sectional survey of Thoroughbred stud farm management in the North Island of New Zealand. *New Zealand Veterinary Journal* 55, 302–307.
Scoggin, C.F. (2015) Not just a number: effect of age on fertility, pregnancy and offspring vigour in Thoroughbred brood-mares. *Reproduction, Fertility and Development* 27, 872–879.
Sigurjónsdóttir, H. and Haraldsson, H. (2019) Significance of group composition for the welfare of pastured horses. *Animals* 9, 14.
USDA (2016) Equine 2015, "Baseline Reference of Equine Health and Management in the United States, 2015". USDA–APHIS–VS–CEAH–NAHMS. Fort Collins, CO, #718.1216m, pp. 1–190.
Whitwell, K.E. (1980) Investigations into fetal and neonatal losses in the horse. *Veterinary Clinics of North America: Large Animal Practice* 2, 313–331.

10 Mare and Foal Dynamics

Erica K. Gee BVSc, PhD, Diplomate ACT*

Massey University, Palmerston North, New Zealand

Introduction 138
Equine Pregnancy 138
Gestation length 138
Mare behaviour during pregnancy 139
Foetal behaviour during gestation 139
Parturition 140
Prediction of parturition 140
Mare behaviour near foaling time 140
Stages of parturition 140
Stage 1 140
Stage 2 140
Stage 3 141
Dystocia 141
Mare Behaviour Post Foaling 142
Abnormal Mare Behaviour Post-foaling 142
Strong maternal protectiveness 142
Ambivalence 143
Fear of the foal 143
Nursing avoidance 143
Savaging of the foal 143
Stealing foals 143
Foster Mares 143
Foal Behaviour After Birth 143
Suckling behaviour 144
Abnormal foal behaviour after birth 146
Summary 146
References 146

Introduction

It is of vital importance to understand the normal process of parturition to optimize outcomes for mare and foal and improve welfare implications. Similarly, a good understanding of the normal mare and foal behaviour and interactions in the critical neonatal period can help to avoid outcomes that have negative welfare implications.

Equine Pregnancy

Gestation length

Equidae have the largest variation in gestation length amongst domestic animals, ranging from 320 to 360 days, with a mean of around 340 days, for delivery of a viable foal. Foetal maturation to ensure readiness for birth occurs in the very last 2–3 days of gestation. The delivery of a foal at less

*Corresponding author: e.k.gee@massey.ac.nz

 Fraser's the Behaviour and Welfare of the Horse (eds C.B. Riley, S.E. Cregier and A.F. Fraser)
DOI: 10.1079/9781789242133.0010

than 300 days gestation results in a non-viable offspring in most cases. If delivery occurs before 320 days, the premature foal may have incomplete development of multiple body systems and a greater risk of developing life-threatening complications (see Chapter 11).

Gestation length is influenced by time of year, with longer gestation lengths earlier in the breeding season (around ten days longer) and shorter gestation lengths in summer. This could indicate an adaptation to ensure foals are born when pasture supply and environmental conditions are best suited to support foal growth and viability. However, this seasonal variation occurs in both mares kept indoors (with feed supplied) and outdoors. For unknown reasons, colt foals are typically born at around three days longer gestation than filly foals. Latitude, environmental temperature and nutrition may also influence gestation length. In the lower Southern Hemisphere, mares tend to have longer gestation lengths than mares in the Northern Hemisphere (Dicken *et al.*, 2012; Rosales *et al.*, 2017). This may reflect management differences; mares in New Zealand are foaled (birthed) outdoors, while in the Northern Hemisphere, this occurs indoors. Artificially increasing daylight length can decrease gestation length by ten days (Hodge *et al.*, 1982).

Mare behaviour during pregnancy

The normal social behaviour of the mare does not change significantly during late gestation. Pregnant mares preferentially stay near other pregnant mares in mixed-class herds (Van Dierendonck *et al.*, 2004).

Foetal behaviour during gestation

By day 40 of gestation, all major organs have developed in the foetus. Foetal activity has been reviewed extensively by Ginther (1998), and here it is briefly summarized. In early foetal life, the long umbilicus of the foetus allows for extensive movement of the whole body within the spacious surrounding fluid in the membranes attached to the uterus. Head nods, neck arching and limb thrusts are observed during ultrasound examinations, with many changes in direction and location. The foetus is most mobile in the third and fourth months of gestation, decreasing over the next four months, with less space available.

Before 150 days gestation, the foetal head is positioned towards the mare's head or her cervix. From five months onwards, the foetus is most often situated with the head towards the mare's cervix, the same position for nearly all foetuses in late pregnancy. Control of the head position may be mediated by an inner ear response to maternal directional signals. Almost 99% of all foals are delivered headfirst, evidence that this orientation mechanism is very effective in the horse foetus.

As the foetus rapidly grows in mid-to-late gestation, there is relatively less room for movement within the placental fluid, but the foetus remains very active. Whole body movements can include complete rotation along the long axis of the foetus. These movements are needed to promote muscular development and proper function of joints, ensuring successful postnatal adaptation after birth (Bucca *et al.*, 2005).

At around eight months of gestation, the foetal hindlimbs are held in position within the foetal membranes attached to the uterine horn, causing the foetus to effectively lie on its back and keep the head positioned towards the mare's cervix. This hindlimb positioning ensures the foetus remains with the head presented towards the mare's cervix for the remainder of the pregnancy. The hindlimbs remain active even while trapped in the horn, with piston-like thrusts. Even with a relatively small pool of fluid around the foetus, it continues active movement of the forelimbs and hindlimbs in late gestation. In the last month of pregnancy, the foetus is most often lying on its back, with forelimbs and hindlimbs flexed.

It is believed that the foetus is capable of feelings (sentience) from around halfway during gestation. However, through the action of hormones and the uterine environment, it remains in an unconscious state until birth is completed (Mellor and Diesch, 2006). Both sentience and consciousness are required for an individual to perceive pain. Therefore, it is currently thought that the foetus cannot feel pain or suffer (Mellor and Diesch, 2006).

Monitoring the foetus and foetal environment within the uterus in late pregnancy is done to evaluate its viability (Bucca, 2006). Detection of abnormalities *in utero* means that treatment can be attempted to increase the chance of foetal survival to term. Foetal activity is used as one indicator of foetal viability and assessed by ultrasonography through the abdomen of the late pregnant mare. Periods of foetal inactivity are normal and usually last for 10 minutes or less. Foetal movement that is excessive or absent suggests a poor foetal outcome when observed on several occasions (Bucca *et al.*, 2005). Other parameters used as indicators of foetal viability include foetal heart rate and heart rate variability. As the foetus ages, the heart rate decreases with the development of the autonomic nervous system. Decreases in heart rate variability may indicate foetal stress.

Parturition

Most mares foal during the hours of darkness, perhaps so the foal is ready to run with the herd at daylight in free-ranging situations. However, more than 20% of mares on commercial stud farms foal during the day (Dicken *et al.*, 2012; Rosales *et al.*, 2017). Spontaneous parturition is driven by the foetus, with increased activity of the hypothalamic–pituitary–adrenal axis. However, the mare can prolong stage one labour, as seen when the mare is disturbed or excited. For example, some mares prefer to foal when human activity is reduced. The mechanism governing how mares prolong stage one labour is unknown.

Prediction of parturition

Foalings are attended for most commercial breeding establishments to improve the survival of the mare and foal. Predicting the time of foaling is difficult in the horse, with a highly variable gestation length. Clinical signs of impending parturition are highly variable and inconsistent. Signs include mammary gland development and filling of teats, waxy substance at the end of teats, and relaxation of pelvic ligaments that may appear as a change in the shape of the pelvis from rounded to more angular. The daily sampling of mammary secretions in the evening improves the prediction of foaling by detecting a reduction in pH or changes in electrolyte concentration (especially calcium) (Canisso *et al.*, 2013). Less predictable changes in mammary secretions include changes in colour, consistency and immunoglobulin content before foaling.

Mare behaviour near foaling time

In free-ranging herds, mares usually separate from the herd for foaling. In mares kept in stalls (loose boxes), there are changes in behaviour on the night before parturition compared to their behaviour in the stall two weeks before foaling. Behavioural changes include an increase in walking, lying on the side, lying in a sternally recumbent position and a reduction in standing. Most mares show a pronounced increase in activity 20–30 minutes before foaling.

Stages of parturition

Stage 1

The principal parturient events are outlined in Table 10.1. In the first stage of labour, uterine contractions become coordinated, increasing uterine pressure. These contractions cause the foetal membranes to push towards the dilating cervix. The foetus extends the front legs and head into the mare's pelvis and rotates so the shoulders and spine of the foal move from being close to the mare's belly to being closer to the mare's spine. The mare may show signs of mild colic and patchy sweating. She may roll, which may assist the movement of the foetus into position for birth. At the end of stage 1 the mare's waters break, and the fluid is passed as the chorioallantois ruptures near the mare's cervix.

Stage 2

In the second stage of labour, the mare shows strong abdominal contractions and coordinated uterine contractions to help push out the foetus. She usually lies on her side for labour but may get up several times, perhaps in an attempt to assist in the correct positioning of the foal. A thin white membrane (amnion) is seen at the vulval lips within five minutes of the waters breaking, and inside the amnion should be one front hoof, followed by the other front hoof, followed by the nose of the foal. The soles of the hooves should be facing towards the ground. Strong abdominal contractions push out the foal to the level of its hips; usually the mare will rest at this stage. At monitored births, the amnion should be pulled away by the attendant from the foal's head if it is still present so it can start to breathe. At this stage, the mare usually rests in sternal recumbency and may vocalize to the foal (nicker) and attempt to lick it. As the foal attempts to stand or the mare stands, the umbilicus breaks a few centimetres from the foal's abdomen. The simultaneous elastic recoil of the umbilical vessels means little blood is lost. Typically, stage 2 labour and delivery of the foal are complete within 20–30 minutes.

Table 10.1. Principal parturient events in mares. Adapted from Fraser, 2010.

Immediate prepartum period	Parturition	Postpartum period
Anatomical changes		
Filling of teats Softening of the cervix Distension of the udder Vulva becomes flaccid Waxing of teats indicating imminent foaling	Cervix enlarges and opens during first stage Chorioallantois ruptures as second stage begins (waters break) Amnion usually remains intact in this stage Rapid placental separation and expulsion in an inside-out form	Rapid resolution of any swelling, including that of the teats and vulva Uterine involution is very rapid, and is virtually completed in 8 days
Behaviour		
Avoids human interference Ceases to eat immediately before foaling Swishing of tail is shown as first-stage parturition commences Usually delays birth until night	First stage: restlessness, aimless walking, tail swishing, kicking, pawing at bedding Second stage: lies down to strain powerfully and regularly to expel foetus Break taken when the foal is delivered up to the hips Expulsion lasts 10–30 min	Lies out flat on side for about 10–20 min Does not eat foetal membranes but investigates membranes and grooms foal overall Attention directed at foal Reacts to invasion of foal's space
Miscellaneous		
Pulse rate increases (e.g. to 60) Patchy sweating on flanks begins as an early development during first stage labour	Parturition often occurs at night (80% of foalings) Patchy sweating continues throughout first stage (1–4 hours) Expulsive (second) stage lasts only 10–30 min Foal may be delivered with amnion over the head	Third stage: transfusion of blood from placenta to foal while resting Expels membranes within 3 hours Grooms foal Abnormal delay in passing complete foetal membranes may lead to metritis/laminitis Oestrus shown by ninth day (foal heat)

Stage 3

After foaling, the mare will stand, normally with the amnion and the umbilicus protruding from the vulval lips. These may be tied in a knot by the attendant, so the mare does not stand on them. These protruding membranes are attached to the remaining foetal membranes inside the uterus. In stage 3 of parturition, the foetal membranes are passed, usually within 3 hours, with further uterine and abdominal contractions that may result in signs of abdominal discomfort.

Many mares will investigate the placenta when it has passed, sniffing and displaying signs of flehmen. Eating the placenta is uncommon. The expelled foetal membranes are examined closely by staff to ensure no parts are retained inside the mare. Foetal membrane retention can lead to serious complications for the mare, including inflammation and infection of the uterus and laminitis.

Dystocia

Dystocia, or foaling difficulties that need assistance, are relatively uncommon. Only 4–10% of foalings require human assistance to deliver the foal. Some suggest that mares should not routinely be assisted to protect the foal from fractured ribs caused by excessive traction by attendants (Jean *et al.*, 1999). However, it is common practice on stud farms for trained assistants to provide pulling assistance when the mare strains. Assistance is especially given to maiden mares, when the foal is large, when stage 2 labour is prolonged, or if the mare is not making progress. Early recognition of foaling difficulties by attendants may save the life of the foal and mare and preserve the mare's breeding future (McCue and Ferris, 2012). Timeliness of assistance is vital. There is a 10% increased risk in a foal being born dead for every 10 minutes delay in resolving foaling difficulties after 30 minutes of stage 2 labour (Norton *et al.*, 2007). Stage 2 labour for greater than 40 minutes is associated with a significantly greater increase in foal death (McCue and Ferris, 2012).

Most foaling difficulties are due to the incorrect posture of the long extremities of the foal, including carpal flexion and head and neck turned back towards the mare's head. Interventions may also be required when the foetus is oversized relative to the mare's size. Most consider foetal oversize uncommon in horses, as the mare controls the size of the foal at birth (Allen *et al.*, 2002), but 44% of dystocias in commercial Thoroughbred mares are attributed to foetal oversize (Rosales *et al.*, 2017).

Mare Behaviour Post Foaling

The most intense maternal behaviour is shown in the first 30 minutes after foaling (Houpt, 2002). Licking and sniffing of the foal are a vital part of bonding. Licking also helps stimulate the foal to breathe and helps to dry the foal. The mare first interacts with the foal's head and later transfers her attention to the hindquarters (Houpt, 2002).

In free-ranging situations, the mare may move back to the herd once the foetal membranes are passed. There is an increase in activity of the post-foaling mare within a herd, mostly relating to the mare protecting and retrieving the neonatal foal. During her first postpartum oestrus (foal heat), these activities may be maximal and reduce until around 3 weeks after foaling. Mares expend more efforts in protective behaviours of the foal when there are multiple stallions in the herd or, if in a single-stallion herd, the foal is not the offspring of the stallion (Cameron *et al.*, 2003). Herd members, including the sole stallion, often assist in keeping the young foal with the dam (McDonnell, 2012).

Mares may show signs of aggression to other horses or humans in the first day after foaling. Generally, there is reduced social interaction of the dam with other herd members postpartum, although her pre-foaling mare–mare bonds remain strong. These long-lasting mare bonds are considered very important in maintaining a stable herd (Van Dierendonck *et al.*, 2004). Mares and foals tend to form separate groups from pregnant mares. Other mares with foals at foot may show ambivalent or protective behaviour towards the mare and foal. Geldings and stallions may be especially protective and tolerant of foals, although infanticide by stallions has been reported (McDonnell, 2012).

Mares that give birth to stillborn foals investigate the foal and foetal membranes but usually move away in 1–3 hours when at pasture. Allowing a stalled mare to spend time with her dead foal may reduce the signs of separation stress when the body is removed (Grogan and McDonnell, 2005).

The foal initiates and terminates most of the nursing interactions; although, in the first month of life, the mare may terminate nursing activity by walking away. In the first week of life, the mare's movement away from the foal attempting to suckle may encourage the foal to follow the mare. Mares rarely show aggression towards their foals, most often when the foal initiates nursing, but foals appear to not respond to these displays of aggression (Barber and Crowell-Davis, 1994).

The bond of the mare to the foal increases in the first two weeks after foaling and then decreases as the foal gets older (Houpt, 2002). During the first week of life, the mare and her foal spend 90% of the time at a distance less than 5 m apart from each other. As the foal matures, the mare and foal spend more time at greater distances from each other. When the young foal is in sternal recumbency or lies down, the dam either stands by it (the recumbency response) or grazes in a close circle around the foal, protecting it from other horses (Crowell-Davis and Houpt, 1986). This mare recumbency response diminishes as the foal gets older, and the foal spends less time down as it ages (Barber and Crowell-Davis, 1994).

Separation of the mare and foal leads to vocalization and distress shown by both. For veterinary procedures of the young foal requiring separation of the mare and foal, placing a wooden foal image in front of the mare's stall may reduce mare stress (Rogers *et al.*, 2012). Gradual increases in time apart acclimate both mare and foal to intervals of separation.

Abnormal Mare Behaviour Post-foaling

Grogan and McDonnell (2005) and McDonnell (2012) have reviewed aberrations of maternal behaviour; these are briefly covered here.

Strong maternal protectiveness

Strong maternal protectiveness can be misinterpreted as aggression towards the foal (McDonnell, 2012), especially in confined spaces with other horses nearby. This strong protectiveness is not usually seen immediately after foaling and may take 18–36 hours to develop. Over 3 days to 2 weeks, the strong protective behaviour usually wanes but may persist for weeks in some individuals (Grogan and McDonnell, 2005; McDonnell, 2012). Giving the over-protective mare and foal more space and reducing proximity to other horses may reduce the risk of injury to the foal.

Ambivalence

First-foaling mares and those in pain may have reduced interest in their foals and in foals who have been separated from the mare during the neonatal period or are sick (Grogan and McDonnell, 2005). Treating pain and other disorders in the dam and its offspring should be attended to first. Healthy mares may show normal protectiveness of the foal when faced with other horses or predators such as dogs (Grogan and McDonnell, 2005).

Fear of the foal

First-foaling mares may show fear responses to their foals, similar to fear responses when horses see another species for the first time. For mares that are fearful of their newborn foal or show signs of mild aggression, techniques such as separating the foal from the dam may encourage her to vocalize, become agitated, and attempt to join the foal (Grogan and McDonnell, 2005). Physical restraint of the inexperienced mare with a halter and lead rope will often allow the foal to suckle (White and Scoggin, 2014). The mare's behaviour can be modified with positive reinforcement techniques, often in conjunction with physical restraint (White and Scoggin, 2014).

Nursing avoidance

Some mares may show aggression towards the foal only when it attempts to nurse, especially if the mare is suffering from a painful udder. Positive reinforcement together with hand milking and pain relief for the mare, may assist in overcoming the mare's avoidance of the foal nursing.

Savaging of the foal

Some mares that show mostly normal maternal behaviour may intermittently attack their foal, behaving in a manner similar to when horses kill smaller mammals (McDonnell, 2012). These mares may return to normal maternal behaviour and savage the foal again at another time, so the foal should be removed from the mare for its safety. This unsafe maternal behaviour is likely to recur with subsequent foals (McDonnell, 2012). Arabian mares are more likely to reject their foals compared to other breeds (Houpt and Olm, 1984).

Stealing foals

Late-term pregnant mares may steal a foal from a recently foaled mare, especially under crowded conditions (McDonnell, 2012).

Foster Mares

Foster mares may be used for orphan foals or foals with sick dams or in some geographic locations for foals whose dams are sent elsewhere for breeding. Foster mares include dams that have recently lost their own foal and purpose-bred mares that have their own foal weaned. A small number of mares will accept another foal in addition to their own. These mares are invaluable as nurse mares on commercial stud farms. Non-pregnant mares can also be induced to lactate using drugs. Induction of lactation is best suited to mares who have successfully raised foals

Fostering foals less than 7 days old with mares foaled less than 24–48 hours earlier is usually successful (White and Scoggin, 2014). More patience and persistence are required to facilitate the acceptance of older foals with mares that have raised their own foal for several days. All early interactions of the foster mare and foal should be under close human supervision to ensure bonding occurs.

Foal Behaviour After Birth

Foals become conscious within minutes of birth. From this point, they perceive pain and suffer in response to noxious or aversive stimuli (Mellor and Diesch, 2006). Full-term foals that are born normally should be capable of complex behavioural sequences such as the ability to find the teat, suck and bond with the dam efficiently after birth. Normal foals should stand within 1 hour of birth, suckle by 2 hours, and pass meconium by 3 hours. There is an increased risk of a foal developing disease or death if the interval from birth to standing is more than an hour or the time from birth to nursing is greater than 2 hours (McCue and Ferris, 2012). Knowledge of these normal milestones can improve the welfare of the foal if treatment is sought for those that do not achieve these milestones in the expected timeframe (see Chapter 11).

The normal functions of the foal in the first three days after birth are outlined in Fig. 10.1. Normal foal behaviour includes kicking (sometimes referred to as 'kick up') when the foal backs up to the mare and kicks out with hindlegs towards the mare's udder or abdomen to stop the mare moving forward and to allow nursing (Grogan and McDonnell, 2005). Normal filly and colt foals show sexual behaviour and mounting of the dam (Grogan and McDonnell, 2005).

Suckling behaviour

The normal neonatal foal and mare will display a stepwise progression of behaviours in suckling as outlined in Table 10.2.

The nursing and suckling behaviours relate to the transfer of milk from the mare's mammary gland to the foal's stomach. Milk release is commonly termed the milk 'letdown' and is associated with a sudden rise in milk pressure in the mammary gland. The full reflex path is a neuroendocrine arc that commences with udder stimulation and passes via peripheral and central nervous systems to the hypothalamus and the posterior pituitary. In response, oxytocin is secreted into the general bloodstream and to the udder, where a sudden rise in milk pressure then occurs. With the establishment of this pressure, milk gravitates (letdown), and the foal can readily suck out the milk.

Although the principal stimulus to milk letdown is the local physical stimulation of the mammary gland, there are visual and other factors such as odour and, most importantly, conditioning. The letdown of milk can be prevented by stress factors due mainly to epinephrine release, acting directly on the mammary gland (Mason, 1975).

Suckling refers to the behaviour of the dam and her foal while feeding. The mare has a unique suckling posture, which relates to how the mammary gland located in the inguinal region is suspended close to the body. Since the mare's mammary gland is not very accessible, the foal is required to extend and rotate its head and neck to reach it while retaining its parallel-and-opposite position with the mare (Fig. 10.2). The mare soon develops a nursing posture in which she flexes the hindlimb on the side opposite to the foal. The effect of this is to tilt her pelvis slightly in such a way that her udder is directed at her foal as it sucks (Fig.10.3). It appears that this udder-tilting coincides with the milk letdown.

During suckling, the foal's orientation is not always parallel to the mare's body and not fully in physical contact with her. In these instances of neonatal disorientation, some mares have not cooperated in suckling, and the milk letdown may fail. On the first day of nursing activities, the mare may feed the neonate hourly throughout the day and night; but as the young animal becomes a few weeks old, the frequency and duration of nursing bouts lessen (Crowell-Davis and Houpt, 1986). In free-ranging herds, foals naturally wean from milk at around 9–10 months of age or until shortly after the arrival of the mare's next foal (Henry *et al.*, 2020). This nutritional weaning takes place gradually over several months, and the mare–foal bond remains for

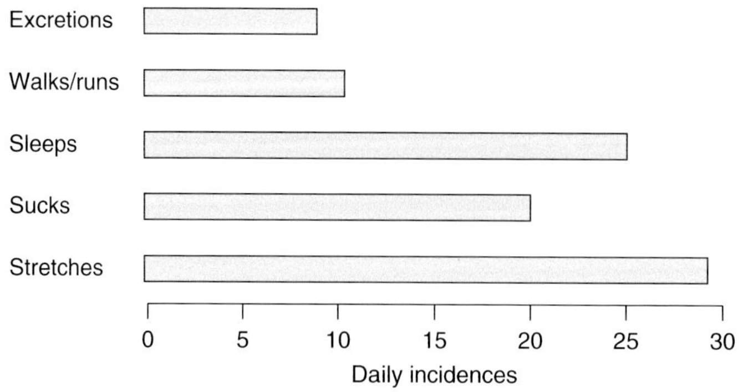

Fig. 10.1. Incidences of basic functions in foals during the first three days after birth (Fraser, 2010).

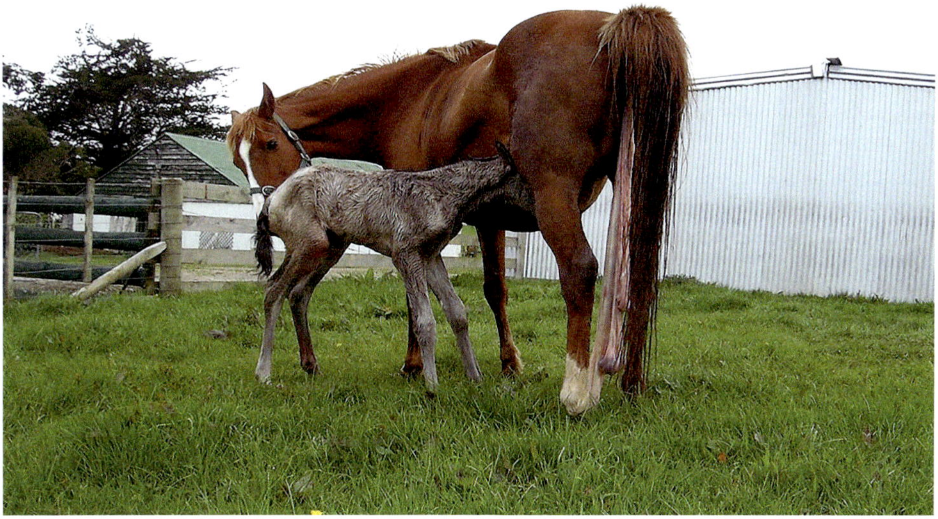

Fig. 10.2. Foal attempting to suckle mare in stage 3 of labour. Note the foetal membranes protruding from the vulva. Photo: author.

Table 10.2. Postural characteristics of equine suckling. Equine suckling requires mutual physical fitment in a combination of mare–foal postures, as listed below. Adapted from Fraser, 2010.

Principal components of foal's nursing posture	Principal components of mare's suckling and letdown posture
1. Full extension of head and neck with ears back	1. Arrest of all other activity
2. Some rotation of head towards mare's udder	2. Alignment with foal's axis
3. Stance in opposite alignment with mare	3. Muzzle to foal's rump
4. Close intimate lateral contact with mare	4. Flexion of hind leg opposite to foal
5. A slight rotation of hindquarters around mare's forequarter	5. Stationary throughout the full nursing period

some time afterwards. In contrast, under commercial conditions, foals are typically weaned at 4–6 months of age with the dam's sudden removal of nutritional and social support. Foal attachment to the mare is complete by 2 weeks of age, so early weaning may be most stressful at this point, as the mare–foal bond slowly declines beyond this age (Houpt, 2002). Weaning is discussed further in Chapter 11.

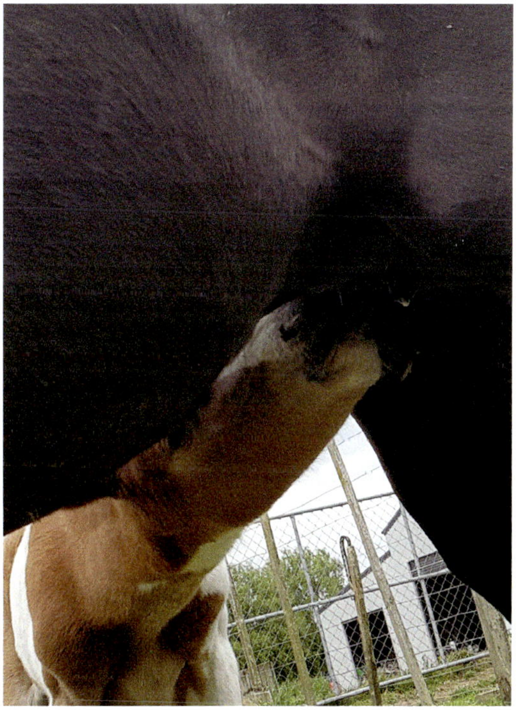

Fig. 10.3. As the foal latches on to suckle one teat, the other is dripping milk as part of the letdown response. Photo: author.

Abnormal foal behaviour after birth

After birth, abnormal foal behaviour usually indicates a medical problem that requires veterinary investigation (see Chapter 11).

Summary

Optimization of mare and foal welfare requires a good understanding of normal behaviour during the foaling and the perinatal period. Recognition and appropriate intervention for abnormalities during parturition and the periparturient period can improve the likelihood of positive welfare outcomes for the mare and foal.

References

Allen, W.R., Wilsher, S., Turnbull, C., Stewart, F., Ousey, J. *et al.* (2002) Influence of maternal size on placental, fetal and postnatal growth in the horse. I. Development in utero. *Reproduction* 123, 445–453.

Barber, J.A. and Crowell-Davis, S.L. (1994) Maternal behavior of Belgian (*Equus caballus*) mares. *Applied Animal Behaviour Science* 41, 161–189.

Bucca, S. (2006) Diagnosis of the compromised equine pregnancy. *Veterinary Clinics: Equine Practice* 22, 749–761.

Bucca, S., Fogarty, U., Collins, A. and Small, V. (2005) Assessment of feto-placental well-being in the mare from mid-gestation to term: Transrectal and transabdominal ultrasonographic features. *Theriogenology* 64, 542–557.

Cameron, E.Z., Linklater, W.L., Stafford, K.J. and Minot, E.O. (2003) Social grouping and maternal behaviour in feral horses (*Equus caballus*): The influence of males on maternal protectiveness. *Behavioral Ecology and Sociobiology* 53, 92–101.

Canisso, I.F., Ball, B.A., Troedsson, M.H., Silva, E.M. and Davolli, G.M. (2013) Decreasing pH of mammary gland secretions is associated with parturition and is correlated with electrolyte concentrations in prefoaling mares. *Veterinary Record* 173, 218.

Crowell-Davis, S.L. and Houpt, K.A. (1986) Maternal behavior. *Veterinary Clinics of North America: Equine Practice* 2, 557–571.

Fraser, A.F. (2010) *The Behavior and Welfare of the Horse*, 2nd ed. CAB International, Wallingford, UK.

Dicken, M., Gee, E.K., Rogers, C.W. and Mayhew, I.G. (2012) Gestation length and occurrence of daytime foaling of Standardbred mares on two stud farms in New Zealand. *New Zealand Veterinary Journal* 60, 42–46.

Ginther, O.J. (1998) Equine pregnancy: Physical interactions between the uterus and conceptus. In: *Proceedings of the American Association of Equine Practitioners* 44, 73–104.

Grogan, E.H. and McDonnell, S.M. (2005) Mare and foal bonding and problems. *Clinical Techniques in Equine Practice* 4, 228–237.

Henry, S., Sigurjónsdóttir, H., Klapper, A., Joubert, J., Montier, G. *et al.* (2020) Domestic foal weaning: Need for re-thinking breeding practices? *Animals* 10(2), 361.

Hodge, S.L., Kreider, J.L., Potter, G.D., Harms, P.G. and Fleeger, J.L. (1982) Influence of photoperiod on the pregnant and postpartum mare. *American Journal of Veterinary Research* 43, 1752–1755.

Houpt, K.A. (2002) Formation and dissolution of the mare–foal bond. *Applied Animal Behaviour Science* 78, 319–328.

Houpt, K.A. and Olm, D. (1984) Foal rejection: A review of 23 cases. *Equine Practitioner* 6, 38–40.

Jean, D., Laverty, S., Halley, J., Hannigan, D. and Leveille, R. (1999) Thoracic trauma in newborn foals. *Equine Veterinary Journal* 31, 149–152.

Mason, J.W. (1975) Emotion as reflected in patterns of endocrine integration. In: Levi, L. (ed.) *Emotions: Their Parameters and Measurement*. Raven Press, New York, pp. 143–181.

McCue, P.M. and Ferris, R.A. (2012) Parturition, dystocia and foal survival: A retrospective study of 1047 births. *Equine Veterinary Journal* 44, 22–25.

McDonnell, S. (2012) Mare and foal behavior. In: *Proceedings of the 58th Convention of the American Association of Equine Practitioners*, Anaheim, California, pp. 407–411.

Mellor, D.J. and Diesch, T.J. (2006) Onset of sentience: The potential for suffering in fetal and newborn farm animals. *Applied Animal Behaviour Science* 100, 48–57.

Norton, J.L., Dallap, B.L., Johnston, J.K., Palmer, J.E., Sertich, P.L. *et al.* (2007) Retrospective study of dystocia in mares at a referral hospital. *Equine Veterinary Journal* 39, 37–41.

Rogers, C.W., Walsh, V., Gee, E.K. and Firth, E.C. (2012) A preliminary investigation of the use of a foal image to reduce mare stress during mare–foal separation. *Journal of Veterinary Behavior* 7, 49–54.

Rosales, C., Krekeler, N., Tennent-Brown, B., Stevenson, M.A. and Hanlon, D. (2017) Periparturient characteristics of mares and their foals on a New Zealand Thoroughbred stud farm. *New Zealand Veterinary Journal* 65, 24–29.

Van Dierendonck, M. C., Sigurjónsdóttir, H., Colenbrander, B. and Thorhallsdóttir, A.G. (2004) Differences in social behaviour between late pregnant, postpartum and barren mares in a herd of Icelandic horses. *Applied Animal Behaviour Science* 89, 283–297.

White, M.S.E. and Scoggin, C.F. (2014) How to manage foal rejection. In: *Proceedings of the 60th Annual Convention of the American Association of Equine Practitioners*, Salt Lake City, Utah, 2014, pp. 163–169.

11 Foal Function and Welfare

Christopher B. Riley BVSc(Hons), PhD, Diplomate ACVS*

Massey University, Palmerston North, New Zealand

Introduction 148
The Normal Newborn Foal 148
Birth Trauma and Immediate Periparturient Conditions 151
Rib fractures and costochondral dislocation 151
Rupture of the bladder or urachus 151
Perinatal asphyxia syndrome 151
Meconium aspiration syndrome 152
Meconium impaction 152
Neonatal Immunity and Related Health Conditions 153
Normal transfer of passive immunity 153
Abnormal transfer of passive immunity 153
Neonatal isoerythrolysis 154
Neonatal Infections 154
Umbilical infections 155
Diarrhoea 155
Bacterial bronchopneumonia 155
Septic arthritis and osteomyelitis 155
Common Non-infectious Conditions Affecting the Limbs of the Foal 156
Cuboidal bone hypoplasia 156
Congenital flexural contracture deformities 156
Congenital tendon laxity 156
Angular limb deformity 157
Osteochondrosis 157
Activity, Behavioural Norms and Maintenance Behaviours of the Foal 158
Feeding and drinking 158
Elimination behaviours 159
Pandiculation 160
Laterality 160
Grooming 161
Play behaviour 161
Orphan Foal Care 162
Foal Behaviour and Early Training 163
Summary 164
References 164

*Corresponding author: c.b.riley@massey.ac.nz

DOI: 10.1079/9781789242133.0011

Introduction

The domesticated mare and foal are affected by the environmental, social, feed and additional management inputs imposed upon them by humans. As a result, the care of the domesticated foal frequently requires our intervention to moderate the adverse effects of an environment largely managed by people. This chapter considers the foal immediately after birth, the health and welfare challenges many experience in the first few months of life and the behavioural norms of the developing foal. Emphasis is placed on the physical welfare associated with the more common health challenges, as prevention is possible. Sensitivity to behavioural changes is more likely to assure early intervention and positive outcomes. An introduction to some of the common health concerns for the equine neonate is presented.

The health of the mare is critical for the well-being of the foal and the outcome of illness. Foal welfare starts with an appropriate nutrition and health plan for the mare during pregnancy, including increasing the energy intake during the last trimester and ensuring balanced nutrition for high-quality colostrum production. Nevertheless, the nutritional intake of the mare should not be excessive, as this too increases the risk of neonatal disease (Robles *et al.*, 2018). In areas affected by endemic infectious diseases such as equine herpes virus or strangles, vaccination should be considered. Vaccination against tetanus is a must. An appropriate intestinal parasite control strategy is recommended for the mare and social companions to minimize contamination of the pastures that may infect the foal. Foals are born curious and within a short time are exploring the environment, coming into direct contact with the mare's faecal microbiota and infectious agents such as gastrointestinal parasites. The foal may also be infected with parasites transmitted through the mare's milk, which can be reduced if the mare is preventively dewormed (Reinemeyer and Nielsen, 2017).

The Normal Newborn Foal

It is important to recognize the foal's normal behaviour and physiologic parameters in the immediate post parturient period. When there is a deviation from behavioural norms, we must investigate the possibility of a compromising medical condition and render assistance. The foal should be breathing normally, apparently active, and not displaying any evidence of compulsion (persistent and/or repetitive movement) or abnormal neurologic signs.

The newborn foal behaves in a set pattern of development. After birth, the normal foal is active, supports its head (unsteadily at first), and moves into an upright position resting on its sternum within 1–2 minutes of birth (Bernard and Reimer, 2018). In this position, the heart rate should be >60–80 beats per minute, respiration >60 breaths per minute and a rectal temperature of between 37.2 and 38.6°C. The respiration rate slows to 30 breaths per minute within an hour. Tactile stimulation of the foal's nostrils and ears by the mare generates vigorous responses such as a cough or sneeze.

The progression from recumbent foal to upright mobility follows a stepwise progression (Table 11.1). During attempts to stand, the foal may fall several times. The drive to stand is strong, with newborn pony foals stable on their feet within half an hour of birth, and Thoroughbreds within an hour (Axon, 2018) (Fig. 11.1). Some larger breeds may take a little more time, and healthy male warm-blooded foals take longer than female foals in their first attempt and success standing (Wulf *et al.* 2017).

Ideally, human intervention at this time is limited to avoid interference with the early stages of bond development between the mare and foal. Once securely standing and moving, the foal begins to explore its immediate environment and particularly its mother. The dam responds positively, and there is balanced reciprocity between mare and foal in the attention they pay to each other. Early signs of

Table 11.1. Progression of the newborn foal to the standing position in successive order.

Specific behavioural items of antigravity tonicity by sequence
Rotation on to sternum from lateral recumbency
Raising head and slight elevation of neck
Erection of ears from floppy state
Foreleg extension forward
Partial elevation of hindquarters
Head and neck upwards extension
Elevating thrust of hindlimbs
Full hindlimb extension and forward stretch of forelimbs
Initial attempt to stand on all limbs in half-up position
One, two or three falls and re-risings
Stability of stance on all limbs
Some tentative steps forward, then competent walk

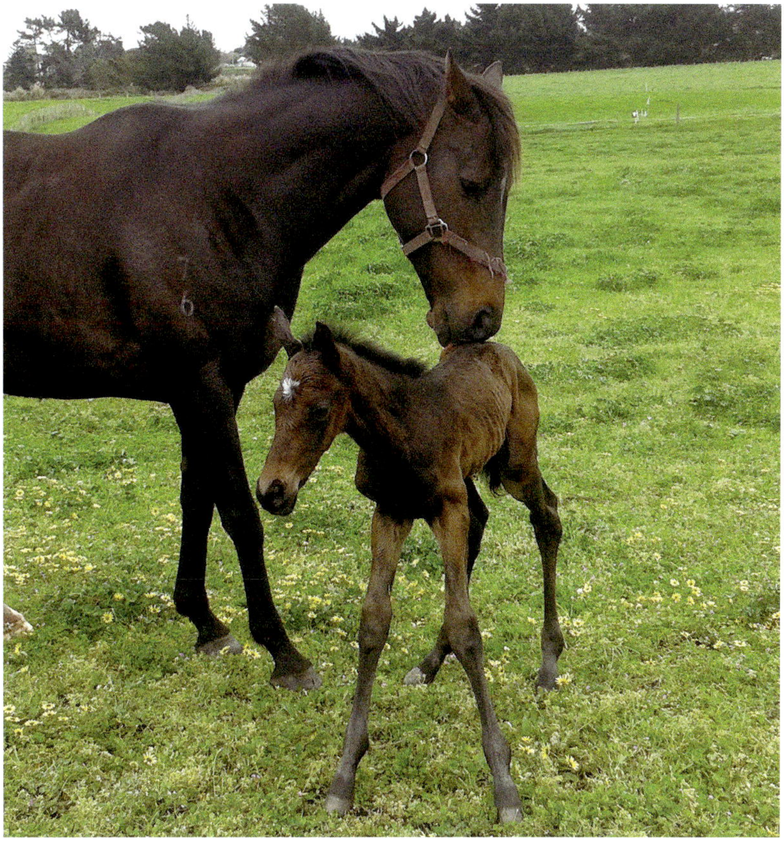

Fig. 11.1. Foal standing unsteadily for the first time while the mare continues to lick and nuzzle her new offspring. Photo: author.

neonatal weakness or illness include lower carriage of the head, no longer purposeful motions, and falling asleep while standing. Almost all the foal's activities after standing are initially concerned with teat-seeking. Its actions are initially random in their direction, and a certain amount of exploratory activity is required before finding the dam's mammary region. This requires the patience of inexperienced horse managers as the foal locates the mammary gland by trial and error (Fig. 11.2). The foal should have attempted to suckle the mare within two hours of birth (Table 11.2).

The foal should now be bright, alert and inquisitive about the mare and its environment, rising to nurse approximately every 30 minutes or when aroused. Do not assume that a foal with its head near the udder or its mouth on the teat that it is suckling. An ill or distressed foal may seek comfort from the mare in this way without ingesting milk. Closely observe that the foal is indeed nursing and that it has a good tongue seal without milk coming from the nostrils (Axon, 2018). Sick foals may have dried milk on their faces. This occurs when milk leaks from the teats of the engorged mammary gland in response to the pressure of the foal's face. A distended, uncomfortable and tight mammary gland indicates that the foal is not suckling and possibly suffering from an illness.

This is also a critical time for the social and behavioural development of the foal (Table 11.3). The norms of the foal (discussed later) depend on the newborn's most important relationship with its dam. She is the source of initial immune protection, nutrition, physical and social well-being. In order of importance to the developing foal are social relationships and accompanying acceptance: foal–dam, foal–herd mate and foal–human (and/or other species) (Beaver, 2019). Shortly after delivery of the

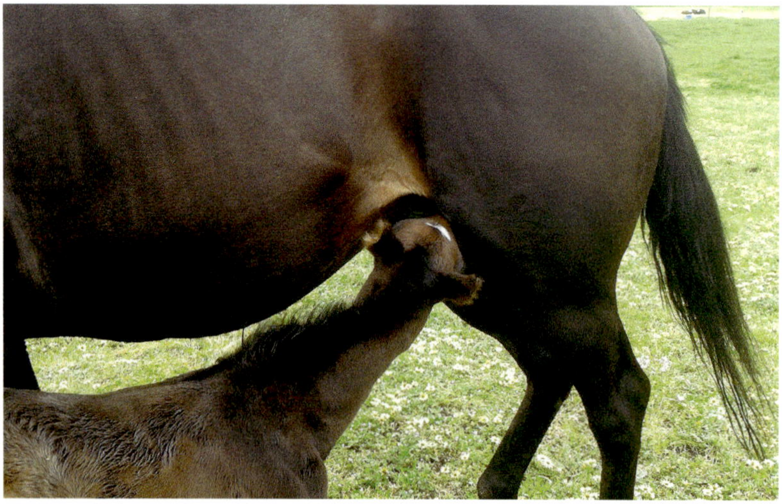

Fig. 11.2. The same newborn foal, with its coat still damp after birth, suckles for the first time. Note the foal is rearward facing with its body alongside that of the dam. Photo: author.

Table 11.2. Timing of primary neonatal functions in foals of various breeds.

Primary functions	Time (min)
Head lifting and shaking	1– 5
Sternal recumbency after chest rotation	5–10
Ear erection and mobility (ears pendulous at first)	5–10
Rising attempts (several)	10–20
Stance attained firmly	25–55
Walking	30–60
Defecation (passage of meconium)	30–60
Oral actions of a sucking nature	30–60
First successful suck and intake of milk	40–120

Table 11.3. Normal order and timing of the secondary neonatal functions in ponies.

Order	Functional activity	Features	Usual time postpartum (h)
1	Walk	Brief trot	0.5–1
2	Sleep	Session 20 min	1–2
3	Pandiculation (stretching)	After sleep	2–3
4	Saltation (sudden jumping)	Spontaneous jumps	2–4
5	Urination	After 3 or 4 feedings	4–6

newborn, the mare turns to face the foal either while recumbent or on standing. She smells and licks the foetal membranes and quickly moves to a tactile and olfactory exploration of the foal (Grogan and McDonnell, 2005). The mare's muzzle and tongue facilitate this tactile encounter, with intermittent contact with the foal's muzzle, head and body.

Touching of the foal's limbs stimulates their extension and other locomotor activity. Once standing, the foal tends to be attracted to and imprint upon the first large moving creature it encounters, which should be the mare for pair bonding to occur. Ideally, the mare permits the foal to suckle and then terminates the suckling by moving away. The foal follows and is rewarded for doing so by being allowed to suckle again. This constitutes the first lesson from the mare: teaching the foal to follow her. It is repeated during the first few days of life as part of imprinting. Licking and touching of the foal by the mare continue over 3 days, by which time the mare recognizes her own foal. However, the foal may take up to 2 weeks to form a complete attachment via frequent touching of the mare (Houpt, 2002).

Barriers to developing this important relationship include inappropriate human intervention, theft of the newborn foal by another mare close to parturition, rejection by the mare and the loss of the mare at or shortly after parturition. When stolen by another pregnant mare, the foal is later abandoned when the thief goes into labour. The biological dam often rejects the returned foal because it has not had the opportunity to bond (Beaver, 2019). Careful observation of groups of mares during foaling facilitates timely intervention to minimize this risk. A mare that rejects her foal or is otherwise hostile may need to be restrained or sedated to help the foal suckle.

If the mare has died, a foster mare within two or three days of losing her own foal should be sought. Foetal fluid or placental membranes from the adopting mare may be placed on the orphan foal to increase acceptance but should be free of evidence of infectious disease.

Birth Trauma and Immediate Periparturient Conditions

The stages of birth (parturition) are described in the previous chapter. Here we focus on possible adverse consequences of the process for the foal. Equine parturition is described as 'explosive' in comparison to the process in other domestic species. During expulsion, the foetus is subjected to powerful voluntary and involuntary contractions by the mare. Sometimes problems arise at the time of birth or shortly thereafter that compromise the physical and, in some cases, behavioural and social development of the neonate. These are more likely to occur in mares that experience a difficult birth (dystocia), increasing the risk of foetal stress and trauma (Rossdale, 1999). Human error may contribute to the risk of injury. The birth canal requires time to expand fully for delivery, so a reasonable period of labour must be permitted to prepare and dilate the cervix, vagina and vulva for foetal passage. Traction on the foal's limbs is a common form of assistance at foaling that is often unnecessary. If applied too hastily, too vigorously, or incorrectly, there will be excessive pressure on the foal's head, neck and chest as it is pulled through the birth canal. This can severely damage the foal; premature traction on the foal is potentially dangerous. Outside of that norm, assistance may be necessary, but it is not wise to interfere if the birth is progressing normally.

Rib fractures and costochondral dislocation

The horse has the strongest abdominal wall among domestic livestock, and the foaling mare's voluntary straining stems from her abdominal musculature. This pressure can cause fractured ribs or separation of the cartilage portion of the ribs in neonates. This risk is even greater with the use of forced traction on the limbs (Jean *et al.*, 2007). Fractured ribs may penetrate the chest resulting in internal bleeding with fatal results or be an incidental finding without causing significant compromise. A post-foaling examination or observation of a foal in respiratory distress includes an evaluation of the symmetry of the thorax and gentle palpation of the ribs. If a painful response occurs or the movement of part of the chest wall is abnormal, then veterinary ultrasound is better than radiographs for detecting these injuries. Ultrasound reveals rib fractures and detects blood in the chest, air leakage and rupture of the diaphragm. Each of these more serious consequences of rib fracture will require veterinary attention and support. Most are managed conservatively, but some unstable fractures that threaten the vital structures of the thorax may require surgical intervention (Williams *et al.*, 2017).

Rupture of the bladder or urachus

These conditions occur in newborns with uncomplicated births and older septic neonates. When this occurs during dystocia, the foal is firmly positioned within the pelvic canal and unable to relieve pressure within the bladder via the urethra, resulting in bladder rupture. The associated signs and behaviour of the foal are due to the complications arising from urine accumulation within the abdominal cavity (uroperitoneum). Although bladder rupture may occur at birth, it may not be recognized for 24–48 hours. Distension of the abdomen, abdominal discomfort and straining to urinate with little to no result is observed. As urine accumulates within the abdomen and is absorbed into the circulation, the foal becomes depressed, unwilling to suckle, and heart and breathing rates increase. Urgent veterinary attention should be sought, and medical treatment initiated to stabilize the foal. Once diagnosed and stabilized, surgical repair of the bladder results in a favourable recovery

Perinatal asphyxia syndrome

Perinatal asphyxia syndrome, also called neonatal maladjustment syndrome, hypoxic or ischaemic encephalopathy, dummy syndrome, 'barker' foals or compulsive foals, is usually a non-infectious problem of foals less than 3 days of age. Signs range from behavioural disturbances to neurologic abnormalities and multiorgan malfunction. Most affected foals appear normal at birth and suckle, but rapidly develop behavioural abnormalities within 6–24 hours; some do not show signs until 24 hours of age. Some foals are affected from birth with abnormal reflexes and behaviour in association with parturition or placental problems. Perinatal asphyxia syndrome is associated with conditions including dystocia, artificial induction of parturition, caesarean section, placentitis or placental insufficiency, meconium aspiration and a range of other conditions (Wilkins, 2015). The problem underpinning the syndrome is oxygen deprivation (hypoxia or ischaemia) before, during, or immediately after birth, affecting the brain and other vital organs. Hormonal abnormalities within the foal may also play a role. The range of signs is related to the degree of oxygen starvation experienced by the foal. Neurologic signs are most often seen, including loss of the suckling reflexes, poor teat searching, persistent chewing motions, aimless wandering, poor mental awareness, and reduced interaction with the mare and/or environment (Stoneham and Munro, 2011). More severe neurologic signs include hyperesthesia, the inability to remain standing, central blindness, seizures, and coma. Respiratory signs include abnormal breathing patterns, apnoea, and occasionally barking vocalizations. Evaluation by an experienced veterinarian is required to rule out other causes and initiate intensive medical therapy and nursing care. Some foals may be assisted by a technique that provides short periods of physical compression to the chest (Aleman *et al.*, 2017). The outcome depends on the severity of the hypoxia, with those affected during parturition responding well to treatment and those affected during pregnancy doing poorly.

Meconium aspiration syndrome

The meconium is the foal's first stool. It is produced in utero by glandular secretions, the residue of swallowed amniotic fluid, intestinal epithelial cells, bile and mucus. Of the perinatal conditions that occur, neonatal aspiration (inhalation) of meconium is one of the most concerning. Meconium aspiration syndrome is associated with maternal or foetal stress but is uncommon. The foetus may pass meconium and gasp, inhaling it in utero, or inhale it with the foetal fluid during its first breath. If the birth is witnessed and there are signs of foetal stress or maternal distress, the nostrils should be checked and immediately cleared. You should be concerned if a foal is born covered in liquid brown meconium and stained amniotic fluid, particularly at the nostrils (Stoneham and Monroe, 2011). If aspiration has occurred, respiratory distress is seen over the next few days, leading to perinatal asphyxia syndrome in some foals. Management is aimed at immediately removing the meconium-stained fluids from the nostrils as soon as possible. If aspiration has already occurred, then intensive veterinary care and antibiotics may be indicated.

Meconium impaction

Meconium impaction is one of the few neonatal foal problems that is usually easily managed. The meconium usually passes within 12 hours of birth. Unlike the yellow of digested milk, meconium is usually pelleted and greenish-brown or black. The behavioural signs associated with impaction include mild to severe colic that may become progressively more severe. Foals may drop and roll without seeming to become more comfortable. When standing, the foal persistently strains to pass faeces without result, there is tail switching and lifting, and occasionally crouching (Fig. 11.3). As the problem progresses, the foal stops suckling. Other more concerning conditions may result in the foal showing similar signs. Veterinary examination determines

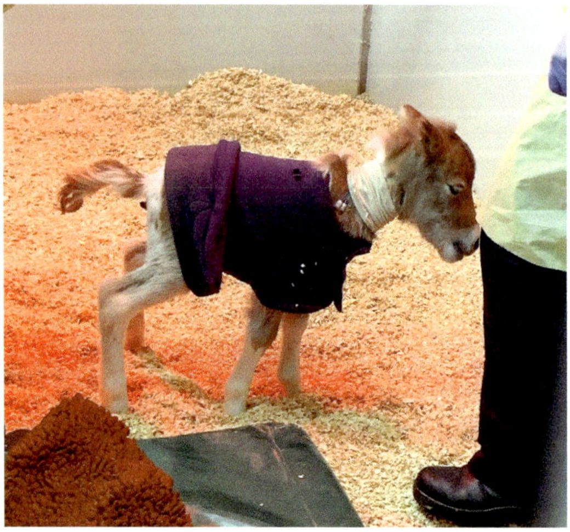

Fig. 11.3. A miniature foal strains to pass impacted meconium. Note the semi-crouched position and the elevated tail. Photo: author.

the extent of the impaction. In some foals, the condition is self-resolved by the ingestion of colostrum which acts as a natural laxative. The problem is often relieved by giving an enema administered by a trained person, using the correct products to prevent undesirable side effects. Enemas may take time to resolve the condition, and retreatment may be necessary. Occasionally foals failing to respond to an enema require surgical correction.

Neonatal Immunity and Related Health Conditions

Normal transfer of passive immunity

Equine placentation is epitheliochorial, preventing in utero immunoglobulin (Ig; antibody) transfer from the mare's bloodstream to that of the foal. After birth, the mare's antibodies derived from responses to a wide variety of organisms and vaccination are passed to the foal orally via the colostrum. Therefore, protection of the neonatal foal against bacterial and viral infections is provided by ingesting adequate amounts of immunoglobulin (Ig) containing colostrum within 24 hours, preferably within 12 hours (Perkins and Wagner, 2015). To ensure ingestion of adequate amounts of Ig, more specifically IgG, the newborn foal must suckle at least 2 L of good-quality colostrum within this narrow window of time. The adequate absorption of IgG is critical for preventing neonatal infections and foal survival. Other maternal colostrum components are absorbed, including growth factors and cytokines, further aiding foal immunity. This process of transferring maternal antibodies into the foal's bloodstream is called the transfer of passive immunity. IgG is the most abundant antibody type with at least seven different isotypes that perform different functions. For example, IgA absorbed and transferred to the mucosal lining, where it supports immunity of the gut, respiratory and urogenital systems (Jenvey *et al.*, 2012). By 1–2 weeks postpartum, IgG concentrations decline and the predominant immunoglobulins in mare's milk is IgA, providing ongoing local gastrointestinal protection while the foal starts producing its own antibodies. The quality of the colostrum (IgG concentration), and the amount of IgG absorbed by the foal may be measured (Elsohaby *et al.*, 2019). A neonatal IgG serum concentration >800 mg/dL is the minimum considered to be protective, but most foals that ingest sufficient colostrum have >1000 mg/dL.

Antibodies absorbed from the mare's milk only persist in the foal for 3–4 weeks, so the foal is required to start producing its own pathogen-specific antibodies and immune cells. The exact time the foal starts with its own antibodies is uncertain, but for IgG it may take 2–3 months to achieve detectable levels in foal serum and for IgA 1–2 months (Perkins and Wagner, 2015).

Abnormal transfer of passive immunity

Failure of transfer of passive immunity (FPT) occurs in 3–20% of foals when they fail to ingest sufficient colostrum and absorb enough maternal IgG to elevate serum levels to >400 mg/dL (Riley *et al.*, 2007). FPT is not a disease but a failure of an essential physiologic process that greatly increases the risk of neonatal infection and death.

Some mares that leak milk in the days before giving birth may have a reduced IgG concentration in the colostrum, increasing the risk that the foal may not ingest enough (Axon, 2018). This occurs with mares that have placental separation or infection or ingest certain toxic plants while pregnant. Colostrum quality also varies among different breeds, among mares, and with age. The quality of colostrum can be measured on farm. If poor, the foal is supplemented from a mare with high-quality colostrum.

Preventing FTP requires the foal to suckle a minimum of 0.5 L for a 50 kg foal, but preferably 2 L. Any condition that stops the foal standing or suckling logically prevents ingestion. Conditions such as perinatal asphyxia syndrome, dysmaturity, prematurity, orthopaedic problems, or neonatal sepsis may prevent standing and/or suckling. Some mares reject the foal or suffer from colic or other illness at the time of parturition. Their foals may therefore require colostrum administration via a bottle or stomach tube.

As described above, gut absorption is critical to prevent FPT. Foals with enteric disease or other disorders that prevent normal gut function are at risk. If oral supplementation is not possible, then intravenous plasma may be administered to achieve the benefits of transfer of passive immunity. The plasma should come from a donor horse that has a low risk of causing an adverse transfusion reaction. Laboratory testing of the blood to identify safe horse donors can be performed. Universal blood donors should be available to larger breeding establishments.

Neonatal isoerythrolysis

The antibodies contained within the colostrum do not always benefit the foal. When a newborn foal is affected by neonatal isoerythrolysis, the antibodies absorbed from the colostrum destroy the foal's red blood cells (RBCs). This occurs when the immune system of the mare has been exposed to RBC antigens (molecules that are recognized by the immune system) that differ from its own. There are 32 different blood-group antigens in the horse. In most cases of neonatal isoerythrolysis, the Aa and Qa antigens are involved, with the Aa form of the disease resulting in severe illness within 12–18 hours of birth (Stoneham and Munroe, 2011).

The mare may also develop the antibodies in response to the foal's antigenically different RBCs during parturition or after receiving tissue-based vaccines or blood transfusions. The first cause is most common, and therefore subsequent pregnancies are more likely to produce the disease in foals with antigenically RBCs different from that of their dam.

Affected foals appear healthy at birth. Then, anywhere from 12–48 hours after birth and successful ingestion of colostrum, they become depressed and lethargic and spend more time lying down and suckling less. The mucous membranes of the mouth and the whites of the eyes become markedly jaundiced (yellow) and, for severe cases, are red due to the haemoglobin pigment released from the destruction of RBCs. Less severe cases progress more slowly. Severely affected foals may collapse, become unconscious, or die (Fig. 11.4). Foals are best managed by keeping them quiet and confined with minimum handling. Careful monitoring of the RBC concentrations is required to determine if a blood transfusion is necessary. Intensive therapy with antibiotics and intravenous fluids may be required.

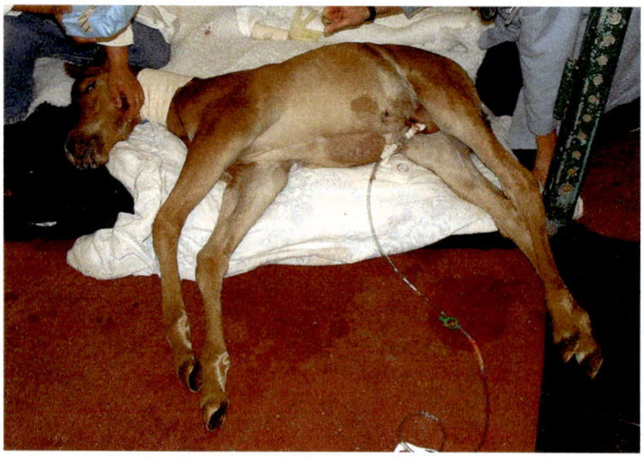

Fig. 11.4. A collapsed and critically ill Standardbred foal with neonatal isoerythrolysis. Photo: author.

Prevention is possible for mares previously identified as having had this problem. Their new foal is provided with colostrum from a suitable donor mare and muzzled for 24 hours to prevent ingestion of colostrum from its own dam. The mare is milked to aid her comfort during this time. Once the window for antibody absorption by the foal's gut has closed, it can suckle the mare freely.

Neonatal Infections

Septicaemia is the infection of the foal's blood with disease-causing organisms (usually bacteria). The bacteria are distributed throughout the body and localize in the lung, gastrointestinal tract, joints, bones, brain, and other bodily regions. It is the most frequent cause of illness and death in neonates, and many cases are linked directly with FPT. Some foals are infected before they are born if the mare has bacterial placentitis or other severe infectious diseases. Unhygienic environmental conditions and poor neonatal hygiene have been associated with these infections. In the past, the umbilicus was thought to be the major route for bacterial infection of the foal. However, most bacterial infections gain access via the gastrointestinal system, further emphasizing the importance of colostrum in preventing infection. Neonatal hygiene starts with providing a clean, quiet, safe place for foaling during the last 2 weeks of pregnancy. An open grassy area with shelter from the weather is preferred. If foaling is to occur indoors, a clean and disinfected stall is provided with ample room to prevent the mare from being cast. Clean, dry, dust-free and ample bedding should be provided. If the umbilicus is disinfected, then clean disposable gloves should be worn, and only diluted iodine or chlorhexidine used. The routine use of antibiotics is not appropriate or justified in otherwise healthy foals. Their inappropriate use increases the chance of antimicrobial-resistant bacteria affecting genuinely sick foals in the same herd or property.

The signs associated with septicaemia vary depending upon where the bacteria localize, as described below. Signs vary from dullness and decreased suckling to shock and death (Fig. 11.5). Rectal temperature is not a reliable indicator of septicaemia. It may be elevated for some affected foals but normal or below normal for others. Bright red oral mucous membranes or patchy red spots can develop. The disease is

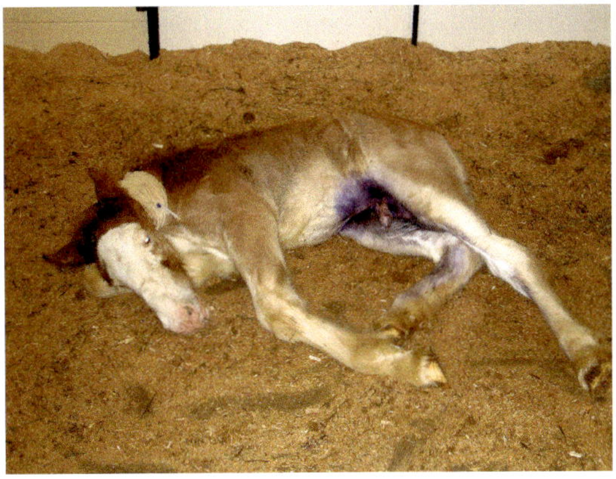

Fig. 11.5. A depressed Belgian foal moves uncomfortably with an umbilical infection that has led to septicaemia. Photo: author.

confirmed based on blood tests, bacterial culture and signs related to localization in the areas listed below (Axon, 2018).

Umbilical infections

Umbilical infections are often encountered, with bacteria invading the external and internal umbilical vessels associated with placental attachment. Environmental contamination of the external remnants or spread of bacteria in the blood to the umbilical region leads to abscess formation that may be localized or spread via the internal vessel remnants towards the bladder or liver. The bacterial species involved are the same as those most often associated with septicaemia. The most obvious outward sign is swelling in the umbilical region that is hot and painful on gentle palpation. The body wall on either side may be swollen and easily indented with the tip of a finger. The foal does not always have a fever. Pus may be drained or gently expressed for bacterial testing. There may be other structures such as joints infected simultaneously, so the entire foal should be carefully examined and all concurrent problems addressed. The condition requires veterinary treatment, including drainage, targeted antibiotic therapy based on culture results, or complete surgical resection.

Diarrhoea

Diarrhoea is one of the most common problems seen in foals and most concerning when associated with bacterial, viral, or parasitic infection. Many foals have a short bout of diarrhoea at 1–2 weeks of age, commonly called 'foal heat diarrhoea'. This type of diarrhoea is watery and profuse, but the foals are otherwise in good health and suckle normally. Diarrhoea that is associated with bacterial infection is called enteritis. Several different organisms can be involved depending upon the age of the foal. Foals with high concentrations of absorbed IgG are better able to recover, whereas those that do not tend to become gravely ill or die. Bacterial diarrhoea may cause some abdominal pain, and the foal becomes depressed and off suck. The most concerning problem is dehydration due to the loss of fluids and electrolytes in the liquid faeces. In about 50% of cases, it is impossible to determine a cause, but diarrhoea, irrespective of the cause, requires aggressive treatment for dehydration. In less affected foals, oral fluids with electrolytes and nursing support may be sufficient. However, markedly dehydrated foals will require intravenous fluids, a variety of medications, and, at times, intravenous plasma. Professional nursing care is critical to ensure the best chance of recovery.

Bacterial bronchopneumonia

Bacteria associated with septicaemia may localize in the lungs, causing bronchopneumonia. This occurs less commonly in neonatal foals in comparison with calves. Outward signs of bronchopneumonia in foals are often mild until the disease is quite advanced (Stoneham and Munroe, 2011). Because of this, they may have been infected prior to the onset of signs anywhere from 1 to 8 months of age. When the disease is more advanced, the breathing rate increases and an abnormal pattern of breathing and/or cough may occur. Other signs include fever, depression, low energy and poor appetite. Foals with these signs require a veterinary examination to determine the most appropriate medical therapy. Although many foals recover in response to appropriate therapy, some may have sufficient damage to their lungs to impair their future athletic performance.

Septic arthritis and osteomyelitis

When bacteria localize in the bones and joints of the foal, these conditions are called osteomyelitis and septic arthritis, respectively. These too may affect the future athletic performance of the foals or, in some cases, lead to humane euthanasia. The latter is more likely when multiple joints or sites are infected. The signs depend upon the joint and bones affected. Abnormalities of gait include sudden onset of lameness to severe lameness. The affected joints or bones adjacent to joints are usually swollen, warm to the touch, and painful on firm palpation. All joints must be carefully evaluated. Samples of fluid from the joints or bones are taken to culture the bacteria and to evaluate the cells within the fluid to make a diagnosis. Radiographs and ultrasound may also be required. Treatment includes the use of antibiotic therapy delivered by several different routes to ensure high levels of the drugs in the infected tissues. Flushing of the joints is a critical part of treatment and is achieved through aseptic drainage with needles or minimally invasive surgical techniques. Therapy may be prolonged and expensive, with a poorer prognosis when multiple joints are affected.

Common Non-infectious Conditions Affecting the Limbs of the Foal

Three other common perinatal conditions affect the limbs and joints of the foal. These affect their musculoskeletal health and may impair effective locomotion to keep up with the mare. Among the challenges posed by them is the requirement to suppress the foal's normal athletic and kinetic behaviour as part of treatment.

Cuboidal bone hypoplasia

The small cuboidal-shaped bones within the foetal carpus (front knee) and the tarsus (hock) do not develop from their cartilaginous precursors to bone (ossify) until the last 2–3 weeks of the mare's pregnancy. When born prematurely or not developed normally (dysmaturity), foals often have hypoplastic cuboidal bones at birth (i.e. they have failed to ossify). These hypoplastic cuboidal bones are extremely soft and malleable and prone to injury or trauma with lifelong consequences. Normal loads of standing, walking and galloping may cause a crushing injury. The signs seen include excessive laxity of the forelimb carpi, and hyperextension of the hind limbs below the hocks. Affected joints are not hot or painful on palpation. When the hind legs are affected, the foal may have a bunny-hopping gait. Radiographs and ultrasound are used to evaluate the joints and determine how far behind normal development they are. If the condition is not well managed, then the crushing of the small cuboidal bones leads to the development of osteoarthritis and lameness at a young age. Management of the hypoplastic cuboidal bones entails confinement to a stall, limiting weight bearing and activity. If the joints are highly unstable, splints or casts are used to support them as they ossify (Fig. 11.6). The foal's skin is very thin, so these need to be changed and checked several times a day to prevent pressure sores. The long-term outcome for the foals depends on the severity of incomplete ossification and management of the condition, but future athletic soundness is a concern.

Congenital flexural contracture deformities

Congenital flexural contracture deformities are observed as the inability of the foal to extend its fetlock, digit, carpus or tarsus to a normal position. The weight-bearing surface of the hoof may not be in full contact with the ground. The carpus, the fetlocks, and digits are most often affected in either one or both limbs. In milder cases, the affected limb or limbs can be readily straightened. In severe cases, the limb cannot be straightened, and the affected joints are maintained in a flexed position. Following evaluation to determine any underlying congenital deformities of the affected joints, a treatment plan is made. Foals with mildly affected carpi, fetlocks, or coffin joints capable of standing on the soles of their hooves may improve within a few days simply by allowing normal paddock exercise. Small shoes with toe extensions can be glued to the hooves to aid in the extension of the limbs. Mild to moderately affected neonates often respond well to a combination of oxytetracycline and splinting of the limbs. Severely affected foals require surgical correction. If this is not possible, humane euthanasia is necessary.

Congenital tendon laxity

Hyperextension of the limbs associated with tendon laxity is most often seen in foals that are born premature or dysmature. Most commonly affecting the fetlocks and coffin joints, the foal has weakness in the fore, hind, or all limbs. Affected foals often rock back onto the heels with their toes losing contact with the ground, and the fetlocks are dropped. Problems with bony alignment should be ruled out with radiographs. Foals that are mild to moderately affected improve within a few days as the limbs gain

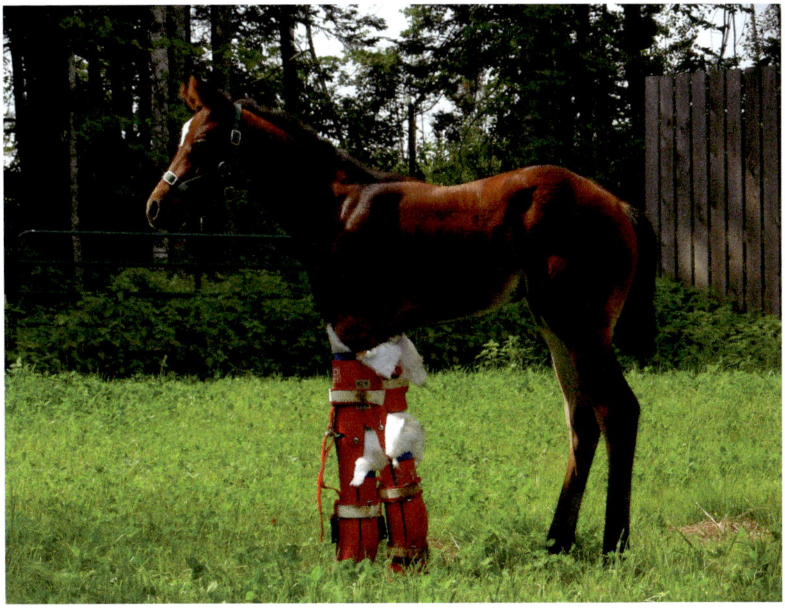

Fig. 11.6. A dysmature foal with carpal cuboidal hypoplasia is supported and stabilized with an adjustable splint system (Redboot, Buenos Aires, Argentina). Photo: author.

strength. For those that do not improve or are more markedly affected, the hooves are trimmed carefully to provide a flat weight-bearing surface, and shoes with caudal heel extensions are glued on. This encourages the foot to maintain a weight-bearing position. If the fetlocks are traumatized, a soft bandage may be applied to protect the fetlocks.

Angular limb deformity

Abnormal deviations of the limbs centred at joints towards the foal's midline (varus) or away from the midline (valgus) are called angular limb deformities. These most commonly affect the fetlocks (usually varus), carpi, or tarsi (usually valgus). This must be differentiated from other causes of limb deviation, such as cuboidal bone hypoplasia and laxity. The signs are evident by looking at the foal from the front. Deformity is observed as arising from either the carpus or the fetlock or, in some cases, both. For the hind limbs, the condition is evaluated standing behind the foal. Balancing and trimming the hooves often yields an improved appearance in mild to moderately affected foals. If this is not sufficient, then radiographs allow the evaluation of the joints and treatment planning. In mild to moderately affected foals, glue on shoes with lateral extensions (outside) for fetlock varus or medial (inside) extensions for valgus are applied. This is combined with stall confinement of the mare and foal until the limbs are straight, as excessive exercise traumatizes the affected joints, impedes improvement and risks worsening the condition. Angular limb deformities that are severe or fail to respond to conservative treatment require surgical correction. This involves bridging the growth plate of affected joints on the convex side of the joint with a surgical implant until the deviation is corrected. The timing of this intervention is critical because the techniques rely upon manipulation of the natural growth process of the limbs to correct the deformity. The window of opportunity closes within 2 months for the fetlock and 4–6 months for the carpi and tarsi.

Osteochondrosis

Osteochondrosis of the growing foal is a developmental condition affecting the joints of the limbs and vertebrae of the neck. During bone development and elongation, the cartilaginous scaffold in the growth plates is resorbed and replaced by new bone. When this process fails, the cartilage template is retained, becomes necrotic, and results in cyst-like structures that communicate with the joint, shedding inflammatory materials into the joint. Alternatively, when this occurs later in development, portions of the articular (joint) cartilage with its underlying bony attachment are sheared off and released into the joint space, causing inflammation. The consequence of the lesions is impaired limb function due to the early onset of osteoarthritis. Although the disease has its origins in the foal, it is often not diagnosed until the horse is older, when it is subjected to the demands of training and/or gains in body weight on high energy diets in preparation for sale.

Nevertheless, the disease is initiated in foalhood. Outward signs include mild to marked enlargement of the joints due to inflammation and extra fluid within the joint, and variable degrees of lameness depending on the severity of the lesions. Some youngsters show joint effusion only without lameness, whereas others have severe lameness due to instability associated with structural disruption of the joint. The most common sites for lesions are the stifle and hock, although the fetlock and coffin joints are often affected. Predilection sites vary depending on breed, and a genetic predisposition that varies among breeds. The role of over-nutrition and mineral imbalances is clear, starting with the mare. Mares that are obese with a higher body condition score are more likely to have offspring with osteochondrosis (Robles *et al.*, 2018). Therefore, appropriate nutritional management of the mare is important in its prevention (Peugnet *et al.*, 2016), as is the nutritional management of the growing foal (Savage *et al.*, 1993). In foals less than six months of age, mild lesions may respond to nutritional restriction alone. However, once signs are apparent in the yearling or older horse, surgical treatment is usually required.

Activity, Behavioural Norms and Maintenance Behaviours of the Foal

The normal series of events indicating vitality and engagement with its social and physical environment is of particular importance in the foal (Tables 11.4 and 11.5). Recognition of irregularities in maintenance behaviours indicates the need for speedy investigation and the provision of remediating procedures for foal care and welfare.

Feeding and drinking

The normal sequence of ingesting milk for the first time has been described. If the newborn foal is incapable of rising to suckle, then intervention is imperative. A foal that is weak or has a physical deformity of the limbs but can suckle, may require human assistance during its standing attempts (after it has repeatedly failed to the point of exhaustion) or to find the teat (when it has failed in teat-seeking). The root of the foal's tail can serve as

Table 11.4. Norms for quantitative functions in newborn foals.

Function	Normal frequencies (per day)
Number of urinations	4–10
Number of defecations	3–5
Number of walks	8–14
Duration of sleeps	20–25 min
Number of sucks	18–24
Duration of sucks	25–58 s
Number of pandiculations	40–60

Table 11.5. Stretching in foal behaviour (usually with eyes closed).

Position	Behaviour
Standing upright	Neck upraised and head pulled down close to the breast area, back straight
	One hind leg and then the other extended to the rear, neck arched, back straight
	Both hind legs extended to the rear, neck arched, back straight
	All four legs straight and stiff, neck arched, and head pulled in to breast, back straight
	All four legs straight and stiff with back humped and head pulled into the breast
	Both forelegs and head outstretched
	Standing with head outstretched and yawning
Lying outstretched on one side	All four limbs stiffly extended straight out at right angles to the body
	Both hind legs extended straight out with both forelegs bent at the knees
	Both forelegs extended straight out with hind legs resting flexed
	Both hind legs and upper foreleg extended straight out with lower foreleg lying flexed at the carpus
	Limbs outstretched, head and neck outstretched
	Limbs outstretched, head drawn into the breast area

a lift point that is grasped gently to support the foal's hindquarters as they are raised, and it is up on all its legs and standing steady. By holding the tail with one hand and gently steering with the other hand on one side of its chest, the foal can be guided to the mare's udder and then pressed against her side for full contact to be established. Forceful assistance must be avoided, and patience practised as repeated use of the tail in this way may result in nerve injury. A foal that is too ill or weak to suckle requires veterinary evaluation and the nasogastric tube delivery of colostrum.

Foals typically access the mammary gland from alongside the mare, facing rearwards. They follow the mare, initiating nursing several times a day and sucking vigorously with intermittent pauses. The foal ingests 15% of its body weight in the first 24 hours, drinking up to 25% within a week. Initially, foals nurse 4–7 times per hour, with each session lasting about 2 minutes. This drops to 3 times per hour by 4 weeks and then to once an hour by 6 months of age (Carson and Wood-Gush, 1983). The mare's milk provides 500–600 kcal (2–2.5 megajoules) of energy per litre, depending upon the stage of lactation. Therefore, at 15 L of milk a day, a healthy 50 kg foal consumes 7500–9000 kcal (30–37.5 megajoules).

Within a few days, foals begin ingesting small amounts of the freshly deposited faeces of its dam, continuing for several weeks and peaking at 2 months of age. This establishes the hindgut microbiota of the foal that is vital for the extraction of energy and other nutrients from the high fibre diet of horses (Quercia *et al.*, 2018). Although its nutritional needs are initially met wholly via milk, foals commence nibbling grass (if available) within a week for about 5 minutes an hour. This intake remains limited, to fewer than 15 minutes per hour by three months of age, but thereafter the foal spends more time grazing and less time nursing so that by 7 months, it spends 40 minutes per hour grazing (Tyler, 1972).

It is common to offer extra food (creep) rations to the growing foal by 3–4 months of age in the Northern Hemisphere. Commercial creep rations are started at up to 0.5–1 kg of feed per 100 kg of body weight per day. These feeds contain approximately 14–16% crude protein, 0.7–0.9% calcium, 0.5–0.6% phosphorus, 50–90 parts per million copper and 120–240 parts per million zinc. Food must be fresh and clean. If the foal is on creep rations when weaning is due at 5–6 months, the effect of weaning stress is reduced (Heleski *et al.*, 2002). In contrast, foals in the Southern Hemisphere raised on pasture alone attain similar growth rates to supplemented Northern Hemispheric foals (Morel *et al.*, 2007). Foals that are orphaned or weaned early require a milk replacement. Quantities needed range from 2 L (0.5 gal)/day, when the foal is only a few days old, to 15 L (4 gal)/day at 1 month old. Foals learn quickly to drink reconstituted milk replacer from a bucket, but a nipple bucket is needed for some. All feeding items must be rigorously cleaned with soap and water between each use.

Nursing foals rarely drink water and rely on the moisture content of the mare's milk. This has the effect of increasing the water intake of the mare in lactation, especially during the warmer months. However, as the foal grows and its milk intake decreases, it drinks water when the mare does, usually after she eats or in the afternoon in a pasture-based management system.

Elimination behaviours

Elimination behaviours expel body wastes through urination and defecation. Defecation is a vital part of the newborn foal's early functions starting with the passage of its meconium. Gastrointestinal peristalsis is initiated with the ingestion of colostrum, leading to the expulsion of the meconium. Behavioural evidence of failure to expel the meconium is tenesmus, in which the animal persists in attempts to pass it. The straining may be severe, and the foal becomes distressed and increasingly weakened. The management of meconium impaction is addressed above, but it is important to monitor the foal and intervene appropriately. Subsequently, the foal learns from the dam to defecate (and urinate) in specific latrine areas with a reducing frequency as it ages (Table 11.4). Normal defecation is accompanied by minimal postural change other than lifting the tail. Abnormal posture may accompany defecation when the foal has an impaction resulting in tenesmus, colic or diarrhoea.

Urination by the foal typically first occurs within 3–9 hours of birth. Colts tend to urinate earlier than fillies (6 hours compared with 11 hours), and thereafter foals urinate hourly for the first two weeks of life (Jeffcott, 1972). Foals that are in the proximity of their dam when she urinates will frequently smell the urine, display flehmen, and themselves urinate in the same spot (Pluháček *et al.*, 2019). The frequency of urination decreases to every 4 hours in summer and 4.5 hours in winter by the time the young horse is a yearling. Unlike defecation, prior to urination, the foal adopts a distinctive posture. The head and neck are lowered slightly, the tail raised, the rear limbs are spread apart and extend behind the body in a slightly crouched position. Fillies tilt their pelvis slightly, and the hindlimbs are not displaced as rearward as colts'. Colts extend the penis slightly from the sheath when urinating. Failure to extend the penis during urination or to withdraw it afterwards indicates a problem requiring veterinary evaluation.

Pandiculation

Systematic and symmetrical stretching is called pandiculation. In the equine neonate it relates to physical competence and well-being (Fraser, 1989). Vigorous stretching actions involving the head and neck, trunk, forelegs and hindquarters are performed numerous times daily by young foals from the first day of life onwards, using extensor and tensor muscles (Fig. 11.7). These inherent actions ensure that all major body parts of the foal are systematically extended, tightened and exercised, even without much locomotion.

Newborn foals are sometimes stiff after their restrictive period in the womb. Pandiculation assists the young foal in its orthopaedic and neurologic development. In the latter case, newborn foals are born with joint and tendon laxity, and a base-wide and unsteady posture. Stretching results in activation of stretch receptors in muscle, tendons, and joints and stimulates spinal pathways and reflex muscle contraction (Adams and Mayhew, 1984). With muscle activation and strengthening, the neonate's posture becomes more upright and steadier in the ensuing weeks. This stretching occurs as brief exercises, performed when the foal is relaxed and undisturbed. These actions need a quiet environment and are usually performed on rising after rest. Most stretching occurs as follows: flexion at the throat, arching of the neck, straightening of the back, elevation and movement of the tail, plus the full extension of the forelimbs and then the hindlimbs. Extension of each hindlimb singly or in sequence is a related exercise.

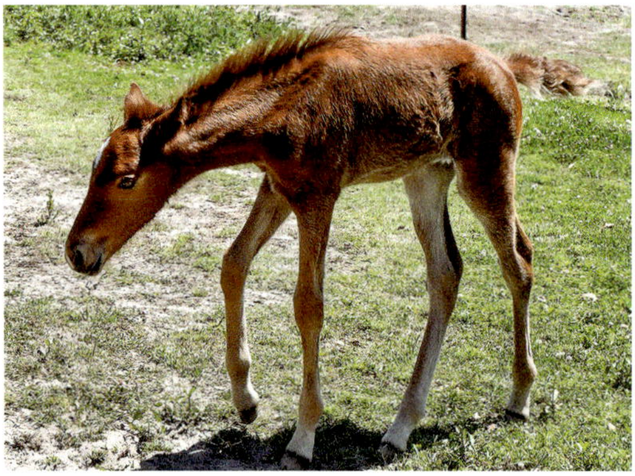

Fig. 11.7. An 11-day old foal stretches its neck. Photo: Sheba licensed under CC BY-SA 2.0.

Pandiculation is vital to a foal's growth and musculoskeletal development. It has as much effect on tendons, bones and joints as on muscles with respect to their performance. It is part of self-development in the young animal. In fast-developing foals, it is essential because with rapid bone lengthening, stretch receptors need to be reset. When these adaptations fail, tendon contracture may develop. Healthy foals perform pandiculation most often, about 50 times per day. In contrast, stressed or ill foals do not pandiculate vigorously or frequently, if at all. Pandiculation is, therefore, a clear sign of good health and a positive signal of equine neonatal well-being. Its absence may be associated with illness.

Usually, stretching occurs after the first deep or true sleep, commonly at about 4 hours of age. Before the end of the first day, foals sleep and stretch regularly. They frequently stretch during sleep and recumbency as well as in the upright position. Stretching becomes more frequent over days 2 to 4. This is when the foal's legs straighten if they have been born with mildly contracted tendons. The variety of performances is evident in Table 11.5.

Laterality

The concept of laterality or 'sideness' in horses, preference for one side over the other, is a source of some debate. However, observations support it as a maintenance behaviour (Drevemo *et al.*, 1987). For example, when foals lie out flat, most lie on one specific side, maintaining this one-sidedness throughout the first week of life. By the second week, they adopt the opposite side for lying on for a day or two, after which they alternate sides randomly. A few foals will persist in lying on one side exclusively throughout the first two weeks after birth. In these cases, the lower limbs do not get stretched to the same extent as the upper limbs. These foals may benefit from being turned over, especially if a lower leg has not perfectly straightened, as in contracted tendons. Some horses remain one-sided in their preferred actions until this is trained out of them (e.g. unable to change a lead). McGreevy and Thomson (2006) found persistent motor laterality in numerous performance horses. Although there is a strong preference for left motor laterality among many Thoroughbreds, sensory laterality also occurs in horses (Farmer *et al.*, 2018). Laterality is likely to be genetically predetermined and influenced by gender and environmental factors.

Grooming

Grooming behaviours facilitate ectoparasite removal, exfoliation of dead skin and hair, distribution of body oils and self-relief of itching. The teeth, tongue and upper lip are used on accessible areas of the body for self-grooming. Foals perform 60% of their self-grooming effort nibbling their trunk or hindlimbs at a frequency double that of their dams. The face and area around the eyes are groomed, and biting insects are dislodged by rubbing them on the forelimbs. The foal also uses its hindlimbs to remove insects from the lower abdomen and to scratch the upper forelimb, neck, and head. They self-groom about 12 times an hour at 2 months of age, decreasing to 6 times an hour at 6 months (Crowell-Davis, 1987). Although a less frequent finding than for adults, foals may also use inanimate objects, including rolling to groom the dorsal topline, back and rump (Matsui *et al*, 2009). These behaviours facilitate drying of the wet coat and shedding. The dust may contribute to protection against insect bites and the sun. Rolling is also a form of pandiculation. Mutual grooming (allo-grooming) begins within a few weeks of age, peaking at 3 months (Fig. 11.8). Fillies kept with other foals practice this almost twice an hour, and more frequently than colts. Allogrooming is a key part of the bonding that develops between mare and foal and among herd mates. A decrease in self-grooming behaviour often indicates illness or dysfunction, whereas increases are associated with stress.

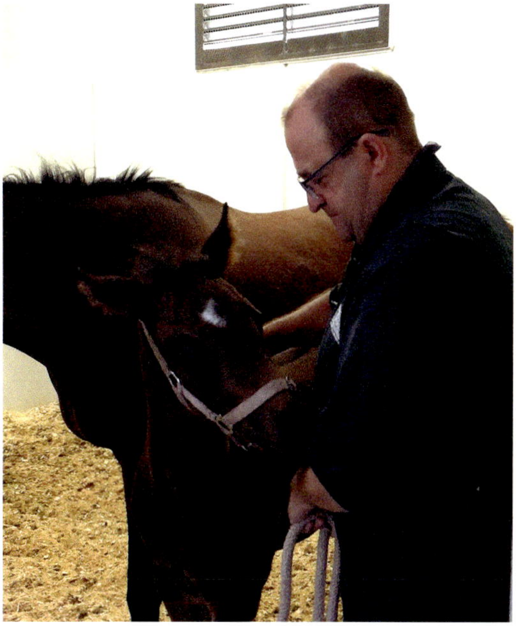

Fig. 11.8. A Thoroughbred foal is scratched on the neck, stimulating reflexive allogrooming of the handler by the foal. Photo: author.

Play behaviour

Play behaviours are complex in form and function (Table 11.6). They serve a role in the foal's social (including play fighting and sexual play), musculo-skeletal and locomotor skills development (Rogers and Dittmer, 2019). The behaviour occurs first in the foal as self-play (Fig. 11.9), and then as play interactions with the mare. This progresses to play with other foals in a herd within a few months, with fewer high-energy bouts observed by the fourth month (Fig. 11.10). During this time, play accounts for the major portion of the foal's exercise including 66% of running effort and almost all high speed turning. This includes play with inanimate objects and mounting play. Self-play (bucking and running alone) is more common in fillies whereas interactive play becomes more common for colts. Where there is opportunity, foals gradually progress to play with young animals of similar age and gender. For colts, approximately half of play activity is associated with play fighting unrelated to social order. As the capability of the musculoskeletal system to accommodate strain and stress develops, so too does the complexity, nature and range of play activities. Thus, there is an integral relationship between play behaviours and musculoskeletal development as there is with the mental and social involvement of the foal. A summary of the foal behaviours is outlined in Table 11.6 and are all considered part of the normal development of the foal. Where there is a lack of opportunity for social interaction, or environmental restrictions are placed upon the foal, these behaviours may be restricted or not observed. In some cases, abnormal behaviours may be substituted.

Table 11.6. A summary of foal and young horse behaviours. Adapted from Beaver (2019).

Nature of play	Behaviours
Social play fighting	Forelimb nipping, biting or grasping
	Head, neck, or chest nipping and biting
	Hind limb nipping, biting or grasping
	Front nipping or biting
	Evasive jumping
	Kicking or threatening to kick with the hindquarters
	Neck or mane grasping
	Wrestling or sparring with the neck
	Chest pushing
	Rearing on the hindlimbs
	Hoof stamping or striking
	Swerving or abruptly stopping in play with other horses
	Whirling or spinning evasively from other horses
Musculoskeletal/locomotory play	Bucking or kicking out
	Frolicking or gambolling
	Chasing or charging
	Jumping (pushing off on the hindlimbs into the air)
	Leaping (pushing off upwards with all limbs in the air)
	Prancing
	Galloping or running (apparently random or towards/from an object or horse)
Object play	Carrying, dragging or pulling objects
	Chewing, mouthing, lifting or holding objects, with or without dropping or tossing them
	Circling objects or the dam
	Lifting the hindquarters off the ground in a hopping motion towards or touching another horse
	Exploratory nibbling of objects
	Shaking or swinging an object
	Sniffing and/or licking objects for odour, texture and taste

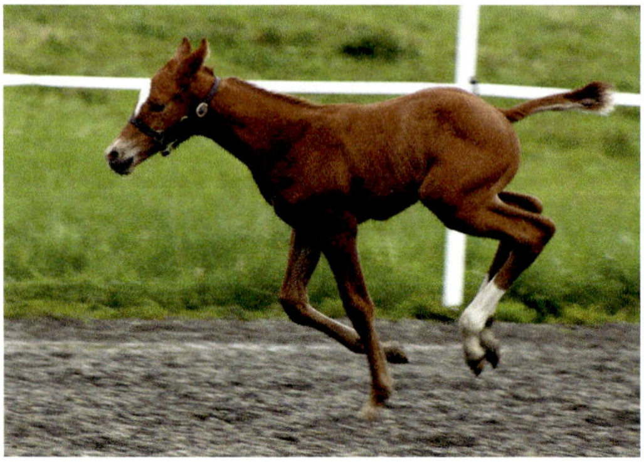

Fig. 11.9. A Quarter horse foal engages in self-play. Photo: FreeImages.com/Christine Petersen.

Orphan Foal Care

Foals may be orphaned because of death of the dam during or shortly after birth, maternal rejection, or theft by another mare close to parturition. This is a feeding crisis for the foal in the short term, requiring immediate action to ensure sufficient high-quality colostrum is delivered within 12 h. The orphaned foal should also be kept warm and comfortable. Once the immediate physical needs of the foal are met, the next challenge is to meet its social and developmental needs.

A lactating foster mare should be found for the orphan. Ideally, this is a mare with a placid disposition at a similar stage of lactation that has recently lost a foal. A milking mare suitably controlled may also be used. The foal and the foster mare must be closely supervised until a bond is formed, in some cases requiring sedation. In the absence of a nurse mare, a milking goat can be used, as horses and goats can accept each other. The goat is held on a raised surface to allow access to the goat's udder, and the foal is taught to feed. Commercial artificial mare's milk can be obtained if fostering fails, bottle feeding it warm at regular intervals of about 2 hours for the first 2 weeks of life. As the foal gets older, it can be fed at longer intervals with greater volumes of milk each time. A suitable starting

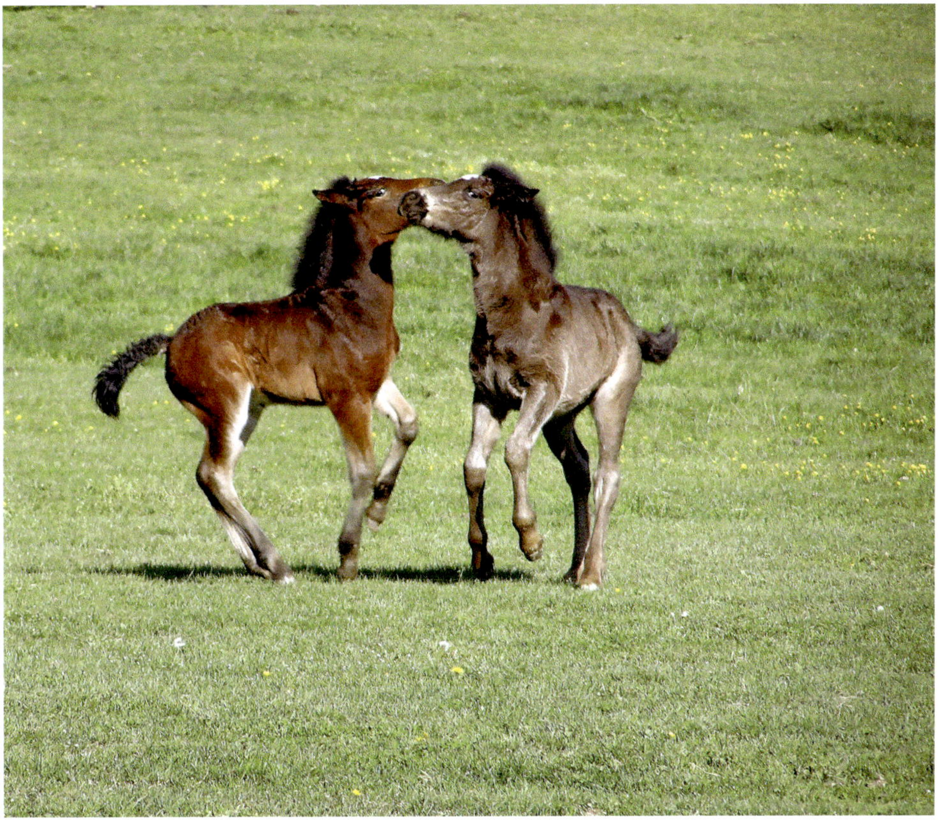

Fig. 11.10. Foals at play. Photo: FreeImages.com/Rodolfo Belloli.

quantity is 250–500 mL per feed, with the goal of increasing this to 10% of its body weight per day. By a month of age, training the foal to drink milk from a clean bucket should be attempted.

If the foal cannot be fostered, its dependence on humans may result in an improperly socialized youngster. This can result in a strong preference for human companionship and expression of play behaviours that would normally occur on interaction with the mare or herd mates. As they grow, they may become pushy and difficult to handle and resist or become aggressive during training. Such foals have impaired development of social skills with other horses and may show high levels of aggression towards others of its own age. The lack of opportunity to suckle also results in increased or abnormal object play behaviours. Therefore, human contact with orphan foals should be minimized. A companion, ideally a small pony, should be provided if a suitable companion mare cannot be found. When weaned, the foal should be kept with suitable equine company to prevent unhorse-like behaviour from developing, such as non-compliance with humans in training or use.

Foal Behaviour and Early Training

The relationship of the foal with its human carers is the second or third most important one after that with the dam, and herd mates. For many years it has been considered that very young foals, long before weaning, should be handled as much as possible until accustomed to human manipulation (Simpson, 2002). The timing of early interactions with humans and training is critical for the welfare of the horse in later life. This approach should be underpinned by the application of learning theory in horse training and an awareness of the mental, social, physical and emotional needs of the developing horse (McLean and Christensen, 2017).

Early gentling reduces the stress of training at a later age and increases the willingness of weanlings and yearlings to approach humans. When handling and educating the foal, care should be taken to acknowledge the mare's role in protecting its offspring and avoid negative verbal or physical approaches to handing. The consensus is that all foals should receive regular human contact as soon as possible. The foal can be haltered within its first days and taught to be halter-led in the company of its dam. Regardless of haltering, foals learn about directed movement by following their mares when led out for walking exercise. The foal's hooves should be picked up soon after its birth to check its legs and hooves for soundness and thereafter repeated frequently. Limb and foot handling should be done often enough to make the foal accept the procedure without reaction (Ligout *et al.*, 2008). Grooming should also be performed on foals in training, as it can have a calming effect (de Mazieres, 1993).

Foals do not always learn handling routines quickly. Every handling lesson should ideally be in the presence of the foal's mother, in which she is unable to intrude. Lessons should be brief with a single and simple learning objective in mind, with complex tasks broken down into simple steps. Once a step has been achieved, verbal or tactile positive reinforcement is given. Foals often require a few days between lessons to absorb the experience. This facilitates training without difficulty. A training session should be discontinued quickly if the foal is firmly showing negative reactions. Nevertheless, the foal must be eventually and patiently taught to accept human authority using non-harmful procedures (e.g. desensitization counter conditioning using positive reinforcement) and will learn through its developmental plasticity (Bateson *et al.*, 2004).

The essence of foal training should be steady progression. The handling of the foal's body should advance from the less to the more sensitive areas. Only when these areas can be handled without reaction can that aspect of training be considered complete. Another handling procedure is the periodic opening of the foal's mouth to inspect teeth. Of further importance are lessons in straight backing-up for several steps. While the head is controlled, gentle pushing is the means of starting the foal on this important manoeuvre. At some advanced stage in its handling education, the foal is given a girth from time to time (e.g. using stable bandages). The long-range objective is to eliminate as much stress as possible from the realities of the animal's later life. Even as a 2-year old, the young horse may find itself treated by people as an experienced adult. Conditioning is essentially what foal training is. The concept of conditioning the foal for adult life is the basic guidance for humane foal education (Visser *et al.*, 2008).

Summary

Adaptation of the foal from the protective uterine environment to that of the mare requires many behavioural and physical changes. An understanding of the normal changes and recognition and management of abnormalities are key to ensuring the welfare of the foal. Early conditioning is recommended to reduce stresses associated with husbandry and use later in life.

References

Adams, R. and Mayhew, I.G. (1984) Neurological examination of foals. *Equine Veterinary Journal* 16, 306–312.

Aleman, M., Welch, K.M. and Madigan, J.E. (2017) Survey of veterinarians using a novel physical compression squeeze procedure in the management of neonatal maladjustment syndrome in foals. *Animals* 7, 69.

Axon, J. (2018) *The Foal*. New Zealand Equine Research Foundation, Palmerston North, NZ.

Bateson, P., Barker, D., Clutton-Brock, T., Deb, D., D'Udine, G. *et al.* (2004) Development plasticity and human health. *Nature* 430, 419–421.

Bernard, W.V. and Reimer, J.M. (2018) Physical examination. In: Bernard, W.V. and Reimer, J.M. (eds). *Equine Pediatric Medicine*, 2nd edn. CRC Press, Boca Raton, Florida, pp. 1–15.

Beaver, B.V. (2019) *Equine Behavioral Medicine*. Academic Press, London.

Carson, K. and Wood-Gush, D.G.M. (1983) Behaviour of thoroughbred foals during nursing. *Equine Veterinary Journal* 15, 257–262.

Crowell-Davis, S.L. (1987) Self-grooming by mares and foals of the Welsh pony (*Equus caballus*). *Applied Animal Behaviour Science* 17, 197–208.

de Mazieres, F.C. (1993) Grooming at a preferred site reduces heart rate in horses. *Animal Behaviour* 46, 1191–1194.

Drevemo, S., Fredricson, I., Hjerten, G., and McMiken, D. (1987) Early development of gait asymmetries in trotting Standardbred colts. *Equine Veterinary Journal* 19, 189–191.

Elsohaby, I., Riley, C.B. and McClure, J.T. (2019) Usefulness of digital and optical refractometers for the diagnosis of failure of transfer of passive immunity in neonatal foals. *Equine Veterinary Journal* 51, 451–457.

Farmer, K., Krueger, K., Byrne, R.W., and Marr, I. (2018) Sensory laterality in affiliative interactions in domestic horses and ponies (*Equus caballus*). *Animal Cognition* 21, 631–637.

Fraser, A.J. (1989) Pandiculation: The comparative phenomenon of systematic stretching. *Applied Animal Behaviour Science* 23, 263–268.

Grogan, E.H. and McDonnell, S.M. (2005) Mare and foal bonding and problems. *Clinical Techniques in Equine Practice* 4, 228–237.

Heleski, C.R., Shelle, A.C., Nielsen, B.D. and Zanella, A.F. (2002) Influence of housing on weaning horse behaviour and subsequent welfare. *Applied Animal Behaviour Science* 78, 291–302.

Houpt, K.A. (2002) Formation and dissolution of the mare-foal bond. *Applied Animal Behaviour Science* 78, 319–328.

Jeffcott, L.B. (1972) Observations on parturition in crossbred pony mares. *Equine Veterinary Journal* 4, 209–2012.

Jean, S., Picandet, V., Macieira, S., Beauregard, G., D'Anjou, M.A. *et al.* (2007) Detection of rib trauma in newborn foals in an equine critical care unit: A comparison of ultrasonography, radiography and physical examination. *Equine Veterinary Journal* 39, 158–163.

Jenvey, C., Caraguel, C., Howarth, G.B. and Riley, C.B. (2012) Identification of periparturient mare and foal associated predictors of post parturient immunoglobulin A concentrations in Thoroughbred foals. *Equine Veterinary Journal* 44 (Suppl. 43), 73–77.

Ligout, S., Bouissou, M.F. and Boiviu, X. (2008) Comparison of the effects of two different handling methods on the subsequent behaviour of Anglo-Arabian foals towards humans and handling. *Applied Animal Behaviour Science* 113, 175–188.

Matsui, K., Khali, A.M. and Takeda, K. (2009) Do horses prefer certain substrates for rolling in grazing pasture? *Journal of Equine Veterinary Science* 29, 590–594.

McGreevy, P.D. and Thomson, P.C. (2006) Differences in motor laterality between breeds of performance horse. *Applied Animal Behaviour Science* 99, 183–190.

McLean, A.N. and Christensen, J.W. (2017) The application of learning theory in horse training. *Applied Animal Behaviour Science* 190, 18–27.

Morel, P.C.H., Bokor, Á, Rogers, C.W. and Firth, E.C. (2007) Growth curves from birth to weaning for Thoroughbred foals raised on pasture. *New Zealand Veterinary Journal* 55, 319–325.

Perkins, G.A. and Wagner B. (2015) The development of equine immunity: Current knowledge on immunology in the young horse. *Equine Veterinary Journal* 47, 267–274.

Peugnet, P., Robles, M., Wimel, L., Tarrade, A. and Chavatte-Palmer, P. (2016) Management of the pregnant mare and long-term consequences on the offspring. *Theriogenology* 86, 99–109.

Pluháček, J., Tučková, V., King, S.R.B. and Šárová, R. (2019) Test of four hypotheses to explain the function of over marking in foals of four equids species. *Animal Cognition* 22, 231–241.

Quercia S., Freccero, F., Castagnetti, C., Soverini, M., Turroni, S. *et al.* (2018) Early colonisation and temporal dynamics of the gut microbial ecosystem in Standardbred foals. *Equine Veterinary Journal* 51, 231–237.

Reinemeyer, C.R. and Nielsen, M.K. (2017) Control of helminth parasites in juvenile horses. *Equine Veterinary Education*, 29, 225–232.

Riley, C.B., McClure, J.T., Low-Ying, S. and Shaw, R.A. (2007) Use of Fourier-transform infrared spectroscopy for the diagnosis of failure of transfer of passive immunity and measurement of immunoglobulins concentrations in horses. *Journal of Veterinary Internal Medicine* 21, 828–834.

Robles, M., Nouveau, E., Gautier, C., Mendoza, L., Dubois, C. *et al.* (2018) Maternal obesity increases insulin resistance, low-grade inflammation and osteochondrosis lesions in foals and yearlings until 18 months of age. *PLoS ONE* 13(1), e0190309.

Rogers, C.W. and Dittmer, K.E. (2019) Does juvenile play programme the equine musculoskeletal system? *Animals* 9, 646.

Rossdale, P.D. (1999) Birth trauma in newborn foals. *Equine Veterinary Journal* 31, 92.

Savage, C., McCarthy, R. and Jeffcott, L. (1993) Effects of dietary energy and protein on induction of dyschondroplasia in foals. *Equine Veterinary Journal Supplement* 16, 74–79.

Simpson, B.S. (2002) Neonatal foal handling. *Applied Animal Behaviour Science* 78, 303–317.

Stoneham, S. and Munroe, G. (2011) The foal. In: Munroe, G.A., Weese, J.S. (eds) *Equine Clinical Medicine, Surgery, and Reproduction.* Manson Publishing Ltd., London, pp 165–994.

Tyler, S.J. (1972) The behaviour and social organization of New Forest ponies. *Animal Behaviour Monographs* 5, 87–196.

Visser, E.K., Ellis, A.D. and Van Reenen, C.G. (2008) The effect of two different housing conditions on the welfare of young horses stabled for the first time. *Applied Animal Behaviour Science* 114, 521–533.

Wilkins, P.A. (2015) Perinatal asphyxia syndrome. In: Sprayberry, K.A., Robinson, N.E. (eds) *Robinson's Current Therapy in Equine Medicine,* 7th edn. Elsevier Saunders, St. Louis, Missouri, pp 732–740.

Williams, T.B., Williams, J.M. and Rodgerson, D.H. (2017) Internal fixation of fractured ribs in neonatal foals with nylon cable tie using a modified technique. *Canadian Veterinary Journal* 58, 579–581.

Wulf M., Erber, R., Ille, N., Beythien, E., Aurich, J. *et al.* (2017) Effects of foal sex on some perinatal characteristics in the immediate neonatal period in the horse. *Journal of Veterinary Behaviour* 18, 37–42.

12 Development and Social Behaviour

Natalie K. Waran PhD[1]*, Gemma Pearson BVMS, MScR, MRCVS[2] and Andrew F. Fraser MVSc, MRCVS[3]

[1]*Eastern Institute of Technology, Hawke's Bay, New Zealand;* [2]*The University of Edinburgh, Midlothian, Scotland, UK;* [3]*Carbonear, Newfoundland, Canada*

Introduction	166
Early Locomotory Patterns	166
Play	167
General play	167
Function of play	168
General features of horse play	172
Social Behaviour	172
General social behaviour	172
Social structure and communication	173
Avoidance behaviour	174
Social Groups and Housing	175
Welfare One Welfare: the Horse–Human Dyad	176
References	178

Introduction

At about half a day old, the newborn foal will have completed its normal biological timetable by achieving ambulatory and feeding competence, maternal attachment, the performance of excretory functions and deep sleep. Its achievements also include the passive acquisition of the mare's immunities in her colostrum. The eponychial footpads (which protected the intrauterine environment from sharp fetal limb actions) will have been removed from the hoof soles by the abrasions from walking. This removal of the large under-hoof pads helps with stability. The articulation of all its skeletal joints will have occurred, and the foal now walks with distinct strides, going to its mother and inspecting its immediate surrounding.

When it is one day old, the foal can perform running gaits, particularly if it has outdoor freedom or sufficient space with its mother. Such runs can be fast and lengthy. It also exhibits the early natural preferences of a social species, being closely bonded with its dam. The mare reciprocates, going where the foal goes, tilting her udder towards the suckling foal, and often places herself over it as it lies flat out in its numerous, short sleeping sessions (Fig. 12.1). In addition to visits to its mother, the neonatal foal's essential musculoskeletal exercises in its first days stem mostly from the high frequency of stretching while it is laying down and from short episodes of activity.

Early Locomotory Patterns

The foal's early locomotory behaviour occurs about 2 h after birth (Fraser, 1992). Forms of movement include kicking, hopping, trotting, and running. Some of these actions are later included in bouts of play when space permits. Games develop between foals as such mutual activities lead to exchanges and contests. Physical activity has a significant effect on the neonate's vascularization and strength. The phenomenon counters the arrested activity in the foal's numerous sleep sessions between sucklings. Since

*Corresponding author: nwaran@eit.ac.nz

  Fraser's the Behaviour and Welfare of the Horse (eds C.B. Riley, S.E. Cregier and A.F. Fraser)
DOI: 10.1079/9781789242133.0012

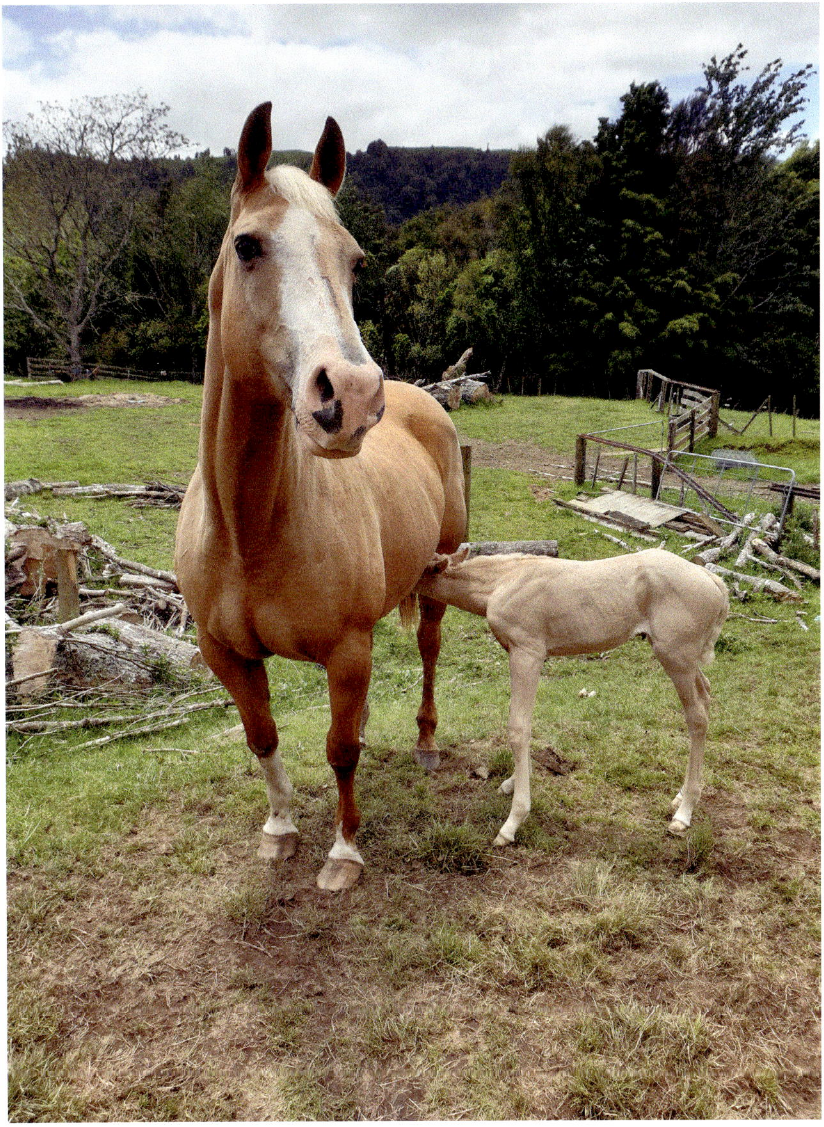

Fig. 12.1. A mare tilts her udder towards her foal. Photo: C.B. Riley.

these early locomotory activities are functional for the foal's growth and health, their absence is likely to relate to poor health and, therefore, should be used to monitor the foal's well-being.

Play

General play

Play behaviour is widespread amongst animals and takes many forms (McDonnell, 2003). Play in horses is taken to be any substantial activity occurring spontaneously or reactively in horses that does not have relevance to basic maintenance or reproductive behaviour (Fig. 12.2). It occurs as solitary play with or without objects and in social groups of varying numbers. It is typically an activity of juvenile or young horses that is essentially kinetic in nature, usually taking the form of fast, short runs in which vigorous kicking and head waving may be expressed. There are also competitive activities when playing in pairs, particularly in young subjects. These competitions

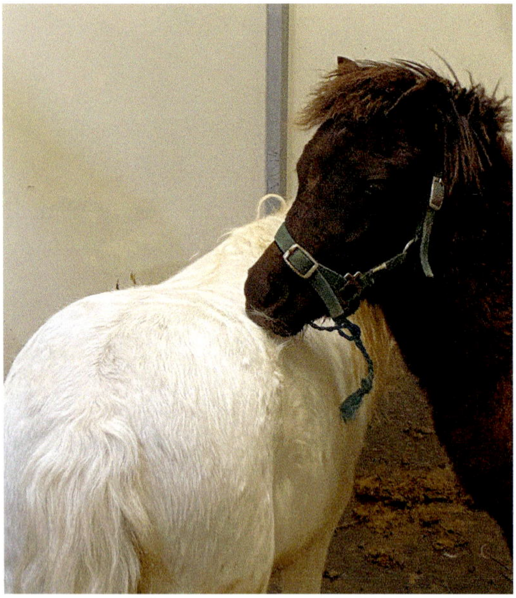

Fig. 12.2. Playful partnership. Photo: C.B. Riley

include mock fights, with pushing, head-to-head rearing, and biting. Competitive racing also occurs in pairs and sometimes in larger numbers (Fig. 12.3). In young foals, mounting each other is shown by both sexes in bouts of social play. Foal gender doesn't affect the frequency of play behaviour, but male foals will initiate more of their play bouts than females (Cameron *et al.*, 2008). Play evidently has a role in social development (Hall, 1998).

The day-old foal will show locomotory play in the form of jumping upwards, suddenly running about alone or in groups, chasing with much head tossing, sudden stops and starts, and kicking of the hind legs in the air. Foals play increasingly socially as they mature. Social play often begins with the foal nibbling at the legs of its main companion, its mother. However, in addition to grooming with their dams, foals maintained in groups will also groom one another. Grooming bouts often initiate play. An oral snapping action that appears to act as a submissive signal can also be observed during play initiation. Play is an important business and is a necessary part of maturation. As they grow, play becomes important as a form of exercise. It functions as a means of practising and perfecting adult behavioural skills necessary for a wide range of actions in later life. Play is clearly valuable for the development of normal behaviour. It occurs most often in healthy animals when there are no other competing motivational factors, such as the need to escape or find food. In concise terms, it can be stated that play is the appearance in the behavioural repertoire of a motivating force concerning movement and social development and maintenance. It possesses evident conation (Bruner *et al.*, 1974). Therefore, an absence of play forms should be considered an indication of a problem with the animal's internal or external environment, but a presence of play activity could be seen as an indication of good welfare.

Function of play

Certain parts of the neuromuscular system, such as those concerned with the change of posture and walking, are adaptive in the newborn foal. An adaptive role for other parts of the neuromuscular system is not so evident. These latter parts are precisely those concerned with the phenomenal activities collectively called play. Play is composed of patterned behaviours. Similar patterns are typical traits of the species, not of a breed. Acts of play are simulations, and although non-serious in nature, they are strongly motivated. It can be seen that horse play is the projection into behaviour of a motivating force concerning action. Play facilitates the capability of the individual horse as a mobile and social unit. It has a major role in the behavioural, social, and physiological development of all horses. The 'serious' adult activities of fight and flight are not functional in the foal, as the dam provides food and protection. The juvenile normally does not need to fight, nor does it need to initiate flight. Yet, although these serious activities are not needed, the neuromuscular requirements are already in existence and are thus included in playful practice. The development of dynamic skills begins in play and is kept through the whole life of the animal in many situations. Each component skill is characterised by its own rate of development and by its susceptibility to environmental influence. In addition, play can be seen as a release of strain or stress and an outlet for positive expression and as such, can be used as an indicator of a state of good welfare.

Some learning is required by foals for their play. Although play movements are basically innate and patterned, they are not perfectly performed on the first occasion. Proficiency in play is attained remarkably quickly after foals learn the attributes of associates and environment and gain their strength. Play is evidently one major method of

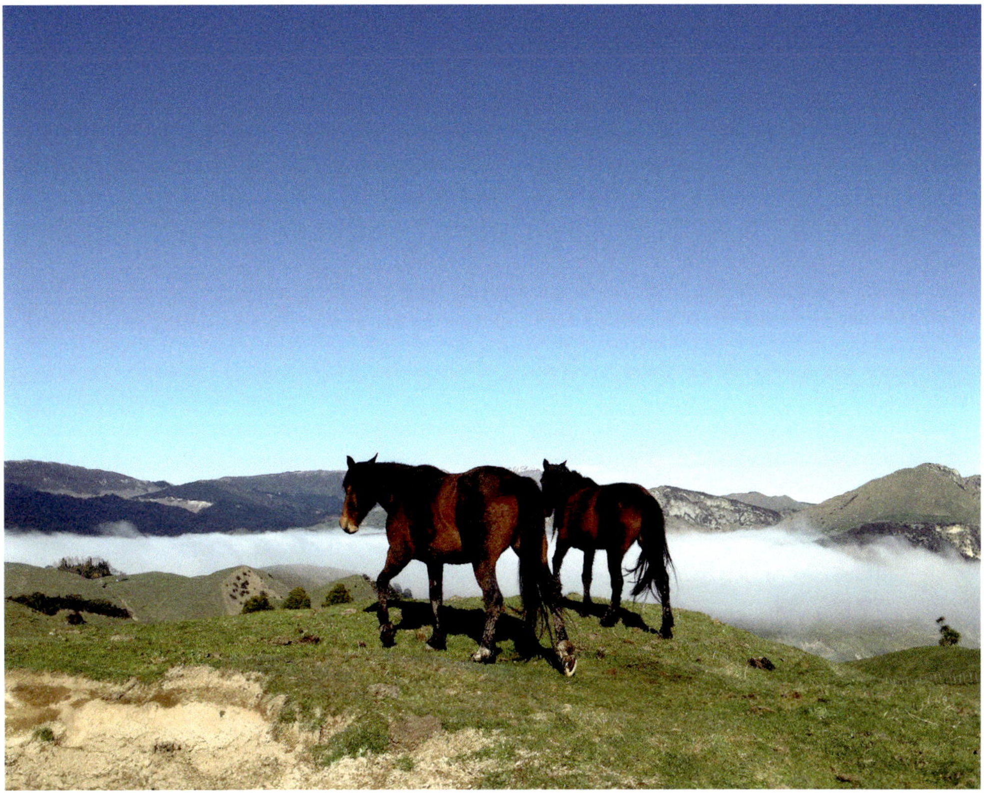

Fig. 12.3. Activities such as play may be useful as an indicator of good welfare: Photo: N.K. Waran.

harmonious integration between the foal and its ambience. It can therefore be presented as a system of particular importance to the equine species, which is so very reactive, kinetic, and social. Play-fighting is a notable component of general play (Pellis and Pellis, 1998). Play is beneficial in the early social integration of the foal in its group. Social play is common as pursuit and mock fighting. Pairs become formed as a result of a series of playful episodes and exchanges by two individuals. Neck overlapping is often shown by the pair, as well as joint scampering, and when the playful partnership has become established, a close bond is formed between the two. This binds them together in all circumstances. When the pair is part of a larger group, the twosome arrangement operates dynamically in their interests.

Interactive play is displayed in the form of chasing and reverse chasing and includes body contact in the form of pushing, biting, neck-wrestling, mutual rearing, or riding (Fig. 12.2). This form of play is especially frequent in group-living young horses and may merge into low-intensity agonistic fighting. Social interactions involving physical contact between young males can sometimes combine structural and functional characteristics of play with low-intensity agonistic fighting. This may determine position or rank in young horses just entering sub-adult society. The characteristics of fearfulness can emerge at this time (Lansade *et al.*, 2008). Foal play has certain rules that distinguish between these activities and the analogous ones that can occur in serious adult circumstances in later life. For example, the various play activities differ from the 'serious' counterpart activities in their accompanying emotions and in the duration of action. In the 'serious' situation, when an animal has fled beyond the reach of its opponent, flight ceases; again, when an animal has repelled its opponent, flight ceases. Equine play is a good demonstration of play as a purely kinetic activity, and 75% of the kinetic activity of foals is in the form of play.

Social play among foal groups usually increases with age. In social pairs or groups, foals groom one another. Grooming bouts often initiate play, and oral snapping actions are also seen in foals when they are initiating play. The commonest form of social play between foals involves nipping of the head and mane, gripping of the crest, rearing up towards one another, chasing, mounting and side-by-side fighting. Play tends to be more frequent in male than female foals; sex differences can be observed, with colts mounting more frequently and generally engaging in play more vigorously than fillies. A response of fillies to colt play is often withdrawal or aggression. Foals initiate play bouts with each other more frequently as they mature and leave the mare, with foals of 3–4 weeks of age often having play bouts lasting 10–15 minutes. Such bouts are usually initiated by one foal developing the bout from a mutual grooming episode by changes to acts of nipping. A bout may be ended mutually by the two foals separating or, more often, by the withdrawal of one foal.

As the foal develops into a more competent juvenile horse, play continues to be a prominent part of its behaviour. In juvenile play, the same locomotor or manipulative behaviour is often repeated, with slight variation, at a given stage of mastery. Such behaviour involves jumping vertically and running away from the mother, and then back to her suddenly. In addition, various repetitive manipulations of objects occur in solitary play. This persists in lone foals, with their social play being directed towards other species of animals and humans. This can become problematic if the play behaviour involves unchecked aggressive behaviours, and as such, should not be encouraged. Providing foals and youngsters with appropriate outlets for their natural curiosity and need to play is important for the development of a well-adjusted horse, and consideration should be given to this when designing the equine housing and management system.

Play is central to behavioural development, both as a set of social rules and as a mechanism for modifying these rules in response to individual play experiences (Fagen, 1976, 1981). The phenomenon of play could become a basic factor in the assessment of welfare, particularly as it relates to the development and life experience of the athletic horse (Fig. 12.3). The sudden increase (the so-called 'rebound effect') that occurs after long term deprivation of social contact in horses (Christensen *et al.*, 2002) demonstrates the significance of the behaviour to the animals' well-being. When voluntary muscles are deprived of optimal blood flow by the absence of play activity during prolonged confinement, there is usually an outburst of such activity on the release of the affected animal. This can be presumed to indicate lasting tension in play motivation, which may relate to physiological as well as behavioural needs. It could be suggested that the kinetic motivation of the horse has been diverted in domestication into forms of work and recreational activities. For the modern horse, these activities could be viewed as analogues to natural play, which, incidentally, ensures the integration of the animal's use and its welfare under domestication. For example, running and chasing (Fig 12.4) could be replaced by the locomotory requirements in racing; excitable animated movements horses perform when free to do so (Fig. 12.5) may be recreated in the elevated movements at high-level dressage. However, whether this fulfils the animals' needs for free play is yet to be understood. It may be that juvenile experiences of play determine the best racehorses, providing they are organically sound in all respects. Play motivation is valuable since it can override physical fatigue, to a point. The level of this in an animal may be subject to mood and to the self-image of social status among the field of runners. Those further psychological features, therefore, add greater variability to racing success in horses. Even the best bred, best fed, and best trained could have their prospects influenced by early play-related and handling factors, which have lasting effects on physique and psyche (Ligout *et al.*, 2008).

What we do know is that play between horses facilitates the development and maintenance of social cohesion and, as such, is essential for group survival (van Dierendonck and Spruijt, 2012). Several authors have indicated that endogenous opioids are involved in key behaviours such as reproductive behaviour, play, and grooming, ensuring that these are maintained due to the pleasure the animals experience during performance activities (van Ree *et al.*, 2000). There is a suggestion that play behaviour is not motivated by the consequence of the behaviour, but by its actual performance.

Play has a number of survival functions including (Caanitz *et al.*, 1991):

- promotion of development rates in the physique.
- experience yielding awareness and behavioural adaptability.
- development of physical strength and endurance.
- establishing and strengthening social bonds.
- providing the exercise that is essential for health.

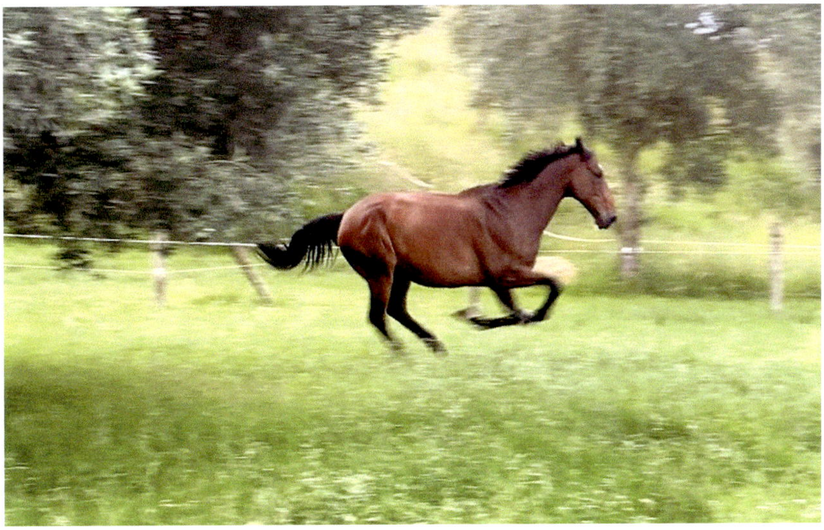

Fig. 12.4. Racing in play. Photo: N.K. Waran.

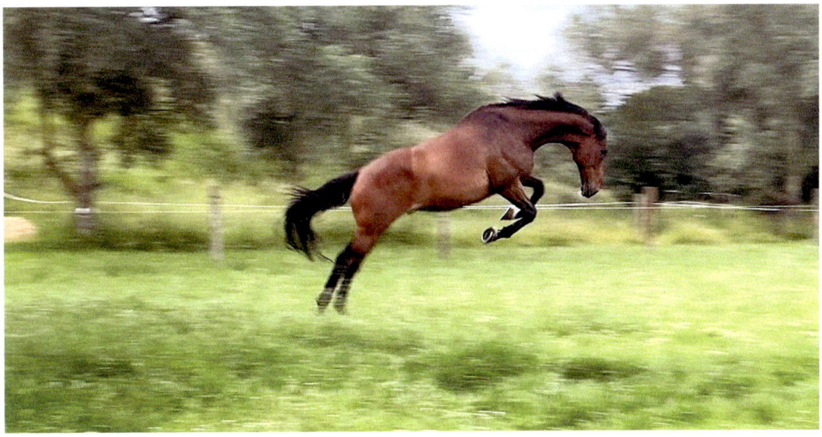

Fig. 12.5. Leaping upward in play. Photo: N.K. Waran.

Social play reflects biological adaptation in the service of fitness. Because of this, it is clear that play is neither essentially cooperative nor necessarily competitive since partners are usually evenly matched and bonded. Typical activities are non-injurious and do not harm social relationships. It may help to establish lasting cooperation for individuals remaining in one group. Even when an older animal plays cooperatively with a young one, special communicative signals and stabilizing techniques ensure that play is fair to both participants, and the non-serious nature of play ensures that real injury is seldom inflicted. For example, no escape is truly achieved in a playfight since real aggressive intent is absent.

Play also has an emotional component. In particular, neuromuscular activity is evidently emotionally satisfying in foals when this factor is activated in playful sessions. The animals seem emotively reinforced in playing, as they play repeatedly and spontaneously. When play is denied, as in chronic confinement of the adult, an outburst of play activity is usually observed when these animals are released from work and put on pasture. Although the kinetic manifestations of play simulate those seen in the 'serious' activities of fight and avoidance, the evident emotions in these various activities differ between the 'serious' situation and play. In a serious fight, there is anger and in serious flight there is fear, whereas in play there is only one very evident emotion of pleasure.

Finally, the benefit of repeated and extended play sessions on physical health is also of consideration. Improved blood flow throughout the body and specifically to the voluntary musculature involved is the chief physical benefit. Vascularization is markedly influenced by the activities of vigorous play. In the foal, with the onset of postpartum life, a new situation arises regarding vascularity. Each system of the body is liable to make its own demands on an essentially limited blood supply. Blood supply is influenced by the work of the heart. Without the existence of play, the neuromuscular systems would be denied the heart's optimum activity, with consequent failure to obtain optimal blood supply for the foal. The physiological role of play is apparent because play does not occur in cold wet weather when haemodynamic factors are being fully used to maintain body temperature. As a result of increased blood circulation during play, there is physiological benefit in general somatic development, creating, temporarily, generalised hyperaemia. This contributes to the physio-behavioural development of the individual animal

General features of horse play

Play sessions often follow a similar pattern with horses joining and leaving at different stages.

The twelve features that most exemplify the various criteria describing horse play are listed below:

1. When ready to play, horses show a play appetite by looking for an opportunity to play and then initiating it.
2. Inhibitions control horse play and these avoid injuring the play partner.
3. Use of inanimate objects or individuals of other species as substitutes in play indicates a need for this activity.
4. A horse repeatedly returning to the stimulus source indicates that play has the character of habit.
5. Bouts of play are typically preceded by a signal of playful intent, such as nipping or pushing. These signals may recur during the bout to keep it continuing. This transmission of a playing mood to other individuals, particularly playmates, shows social facilitation as a play facilitator.
6. Short sequences and repetitious motor patterns are characteristic of brief bouts.
7. Sequences of play bouts may involve jumping and bouncing actions. Repeated actions in an exaggerated manner are very characteristic. These may be relatively unordered in sequence from one time to another.
8. Playful movements within the sequence may be repeated more often than they would usually be in 'serious' situations.
9. Movements within the sequence may not be completed and incomplete elements may be repeated, indicating that behavioural units in play are not essentially linked in a chain.
10. Play lacks a consummatory act as an endpoint. It usually winds down.
11. Horse play stops when a stronger stimulus or an important event becomes the focus of attention.
12. Play occurs in a relaxed motivational setting when it is not displaced by events or essential maintenance. The activity appears 'pleasurable' to the participants.

Social Behaviour

General social behaviour

One of the main functions or purposes of social behaviour relates to group cohesion which in turn contributes to the survival of the herd. This makes good evolutionary sense since a prey species such as a horse relies upon the many eyes approach to detecting potential dangers, and social connectedness ensures that information relayed to the group members can be trusted (Waran, 2001). Further, sociality is associated with increased reproductive success being essential for the survival of the offspring. The population strategies of horses are implemented by systems of collaborative behaviour, as in the 'group effect', also termed 'social facilitation', which influences communal activities. The various forms of association between individuals permit the organization of numbers of horses into social units and herds.

Social force brings discipline to all the individuals of a horse group, ensuring the mutual pursuit of tactics required for living, while social motives are manifestly related to common survival (Hamilton, 1964). Among horses, the phenomena of social behaviour are found to be pursued with particular vigour. The evident need of the horse for the company of its own kind makes it a very social animal and social features compose much of its ethos. The ability to develop social bonds is one of the main reasons for its success as a domesticated species and is certainly essential to its efficient manipulation in husbandry. In the use of horses, their readiness to accept human association is a vital quality. It has been stated that domestication has had little if no effect on sociality (Waran, 2001).

Horses readily form and maintain a social structure. When they live in bands a social order becomes established, in which the older and larger animals are usually found to be higher in the order. Stallions can easily dominate geldings or mares, but do not always do so. A leader dictates the movement of the herd through the grazing area and maintains a vigilant role. As has been recognized down through the ages, socially dominant horses are sometimes found to have very aggressive temperaments. Individual mares are found to associate closely with certain individuals serving as close friends. Colts and fillies tend to separate from the mares and stallions. and herd stallions will round up mares on the periphery of his herd or 'harem' but will ignore or repel the fillies. Among free-living ponies, close groups of various sizes are formed comprising family groups, with fillies remaining with their mothers for two or more years. Once they leave their mothers at the end of the mare–foal bond (Houpt, 2002), young mares tend to change groups, often joining older mares with foals. Typically, young stallions join bachelor groups in a loose social organization. Some members will leave to form other groups for a period and then may rejoin their original group. Thus, demonstrating the fluid nature of the social organization under natural conditions.

Social structure and communication

Various features of social behaviour are observed in domesticated horses, and the development of strong and sometimes specific social bonds are most notable among them. Even under free-range conditions in extensive territory, there is such group bonding that horses maintain visual contact with each other continually. Very modified social behaviour is seen in the domesticated horse's ability to develop positive relationships with people. Other interspecies affiliations can occur in remarkable forms between horses and dogs, goats, and pet animals of various kinds, even chickens. Being able to be social is essential for horse survival and well-being. Horses appear sensitive to the intra-species transfer of information, and the phenomenon of social facilitation has evolutionary significance for a herd species such as the horse. This group effect, depending on space, serves as a basis for the strategies of group behaviour (Rifa, 1990). Social facilitation in a herd or group may be a motivating force in the daily movements of horses, as in occasional running and marching from place to place. Being able to respond quickly to the behaviour of others, to do the same thing at the same time, can also be seen in the domestic horse when under saddle where a horse may respond rapidly and in the same way to another's reaction to a novel object that it hasn't actually seen. This means that where horses are kept in isolation, they will not show the same stability in maintenance activity, such as ingestion, as shown within groups. It appears that optimum group size aids homeostasis in horses (Søndergaard and Ladewig, 2004) and housing them in groups is recommended for normal behavioural development and positive horse–human relationships (Søndergaard and Ladewig, 2004; Bourjade *et al.*, 2008).

Social structure is determined by the type and quality of the relationships between individuals within the group. Frequency of mixing, space restrictions and limited feed resources will all constitute a social challenge for domestic horses as compared with more natural conditions and these may account for the higher rates of aggression often reported for horses under modern domestic husbandry conditions (Waran, 2001). In their affiliative movements, horses often respond to the initiative of a lead animal by following. Such leadership, in socially stable groups of horses, is often provided by an older mare or gelding. Age is likely to affect leadership, and the status of the animal in the social hierarchy may not be a determinant factor. In fact, the lead role is often taken by horses from the middle of the group hierarchy. Leadership may be shared but the following order tends to be similar from event to event. Types of leadership in grazing horses can be observed in the way specific horses initiate movement and the way in which groups move between locations for feeding, drinking, and resting.

Communication through body language is used to convey information about potentially dangerous situations, intentions, and feelings, through a wide array of highly sophisticated visual signals. Some body postures or outlines are more obvious than others to the human observer, such as the flattened ears indicating aggressive behaviour. Others are more subtle, such as facial movements; relaxing or tensing of the muscles around the nostril, mouth, and chin. It is interesting to note that humans tend to be more focused on overtly aggressive behaviours and are generally better at interpreting them. This applies to horses where aggressive displays are well researched and documented. Although horses appear much more reactive than many of the larger domesticated species, the purpose of the displays is generally to ensure that individual space is maintained, and damage is limited. The horse, like other social animals, shows escalating warnings of aggression, which are often ritualised. Mild bite threats are displayed by laying back both ears and moving the mouth suddenly towards the stimulus, in some cases, and if the desired response does not occur, the horse lunges with an extended head and neck and will bite. Bite threats have been shown to account for 74% of all agonistic interactions in a group of horses. Another social signal is the tail swish, which seems to indicate irritation, and if ignored can lead to escalation such as a lift of the hind leg and finally a 'turn and kick'. In addition to the ears and tail, there are whole-body postures that act as social signals communicating emotional state. Horses in a high state of arousal exhibit elevated postures with head raised and tail held up, and often animated paces. This posture makes the horse appear much bigger and is often seen in stallions. By contrast, a drooping head and tail in a horse showing a low body posture are usually indicative of pain, distress, or depression.

By far the most common behaviour that occurs within a social group of horses, is affiliative in nature. Although comparatively less research has been carried out to identify the postures and signals that are used for this type of communication. Horses will have preferred grooming partners, and grooming is extremely ritualised with one horse signalling its desire to be groomed by approaching in a walk, standing sideways on and head towards tail, with ears forward, mouth slightly open and lower lip dropped to show the incisors. Handlers and trainers can take advantage of this form of communication by providing a pleasurable experience that may have some important social meaning. There are some studies (Thorbergson *et al.*, 2016) that show that scratching the horse in the wither region, such as occurs during horse or horse (allogrooming), can lead to a lowered heart rate or de-arousal effect. This can be used when the horse is under saddle and in situations where it may experience mild stress such as during veterinary examination.

Like many social animals, horses employ techniques for ensuring that they can live as a cohesive unit. This means that they signal their displeasure with another individual in order to avoid getting into a full-on disagreement that might lead to injury or worse. These warnings escalate if the receiver is not behaving accordingly. You often see this with horses in their interactions with humans, for example when people get kicked or bitten. Often these horses will be labeled aggressive. However, there is often a good reason for the horse's response. It is usually due to the horse's original subtle signal to communicate that it would rather be left alone being inadvertently ignored and so the horse ends up increasing his negative response to try to protect himself from what he perceives as a threatening situation. For example, many stabled horses have little control over their personal space, especially in commercial yards where different people can enter the horse's stable and where the horse has nowhere to escape. In this situation, you will often see horses developing a defensive response and will often turn their rear-end towards the door, so that they can avoid interaction and defend themselves if necessary. Frequently this signal does not have the desired effect for the horse, and the handler will either ignore it and invade the space anyway or will be aggressive with the horse to try to frighten it into turning around. Both responses can potentially lead to problem behaviour, with the horse being unable to communicate effectively, feeling stressed and then escalating the behaviour more rapidly the next time someone enters the stable. It's worth noting that a direct attack with no warning is usually a learned response directed towards a human after they have failed to respond appropriately to more subtle signals.

Avoidance behaviour

Whilst there are many research papers describing dominance hierarchies in horses, it is now considered more accurate to discuss sociality in terms of social order, affiliative relationships, and avoidance. Horses generally have a clear unidirectional social order, which may not be linear from end to end. The group order can therefore be complex while quite stable. Access to desired and/or limited resources is where the place within the social order will be observed. Horses who are lower in the social order (sometimes referred to as subordinate) will deliberately avoid moving too close to those higher in the order (so-called dominant individuals). Horses are peaceful creatures who would far rather avoid conflict. They have a range of submission signals that serve to convey a non-threatening message or deference to another horse. For example, the 'snapping' or 'mouthing' behaviour that a foal will often display to another herd member characterized by its extended neck and head, ears forward, lips drawn back, and mouth opening and closing, is used by the foal to inhibit aggression. It is often retained in the juvenile horse and used to greet new horses, or towards more 'dominant' individuals suggesting that it may be used to signal deference when the young horse wants to make contact but is unsure of the outcome. Most adult horses signal submission or appeasement by simply 'moving away' from a threatening gesture or giving up space in relation to a desired resource such as a bucket of food, so avoiding an aggressive response.

The performance of avoidance behaviour is therefore the chief social tactic involved in maintaining social stability in a permanent herd of grazing horses. The 'avoidance order' is maintained chiefly through the behaviour of the subordinates. They perform the necessary acts of behaviour, mainly submissive and flight behaviour. In view of this, the avoidance order is a better description of the equine social system. Appropriate ethological methods of husbandry for horses, by use of adequate space in grazing, allow a stable social order to be established and keep energy-wasting and stress-inducing aggression within groups of horses under control. Within housing systems that provide security of position at feeding and secondary space for resting, it is possible for a constantly settled avoidance order to exist continuously. Avoidance as a general strategy calls for specific behavioural tactics, and these tactics demand space for their effective operation.

Being of a higher status does not require a horse to be overtly aggressive to be effective. A mature animal, very sure of its status at any time, can be placed in a strange group and be immune from the usual attention given to a newcomer. Such a horse employs a quiet authority, occasionally reinforced with a few discrete kicks or indignant squeals. A set of eye, ear, mouth, neck, and head positions can compose a meaningful display and signal that a self-assertive individual has entered the herd. It's important when handling horses to be familiar with the behaviour of horses of different status, and the way in which these can be used to ensure horse and human safety. Some trainers have identified licking, chewing, and head lowering as submissive signals and utilize these in their training techniques. However, there are alternative explanations that do not involve submission, and it is more likely that these are what are termed by ethologists as 'displacement activities', or behaviours that an animal will exhibit when they are in a situation where they are experiencing conflicting motivations. In this case, the horse will perform a normal behaviour out of context, leading to a reduction in arousal or stress. We often see these sorts of oral behaviours in horses who are expecting to be fed, but where they are thwarted by the stable door and the slowness of the human arriving with the food. Studies of free-living New Forest ponies have shown that head lowering appears to be a behaviour that is more about reducing distances between individuals, and in Grevy's Zebras, head lowering occurs during the approach phase of social interaction.

Social Groups and Housing

Among horses and ponies, most aggressive reactions occur when first introduced to one another. Much of the restless activities are exercises determining the status of each animal in the group. Two ponies encountering each other for the first time show much mutual exploration (Fig. 12.6). This exploratory behaviour involves an investigation of the other's head, body, and hindquarters by smelling. In a typical encounter between two animals of different social status, one will often reach out to snap at the skin around the shoulders and neck of the adversary. If the adversary then recognizes that it is of lower status in the social hierarchy to the animal attacking it, its response would be one of quick avoidance. At this point, the aggressive exchange between the two animals ceases since its purpose has been fulfilled.

However, horses are generally very gregarious, and although they act like a typical herding species, they show a marked preference for close contact with certain individuals in their group. The maintenance of such preferred partnerships eliminates much social aggressiveness for the 'preferred' individuals (van Dierendonck *et al.*, 2009). At pasture, pairs of ponies spend long spells in affiliative behaviours such as mutual or allogrooming, and the pairs are usually matched for age and size. It is for this reason that it is suggested that social or group housing of horses is recommended for stable

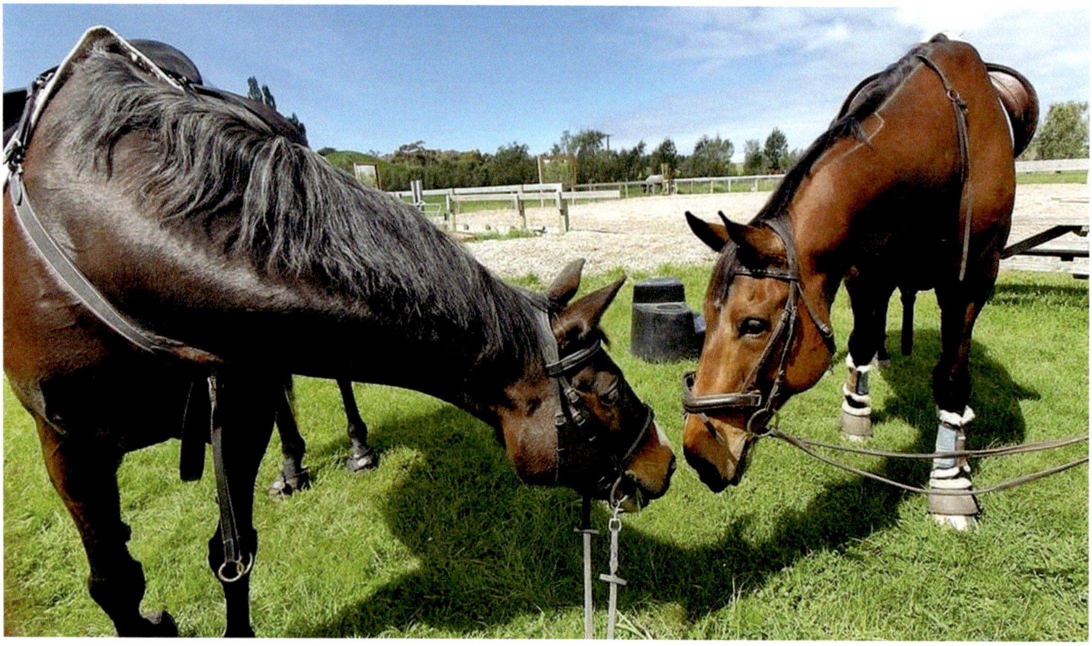

Fig. 12.6. Mutual exploration between unfamiliar horses. Photo: N.K. Waran.

groups. Studies involving horse owners in Nordic countries (Hartmann, *et al.*, 2015) show that group-housed horses have the ability to freely socialize with conspecifics and the majority of horse owners believe that horse welfare is improved as a result. Housing animals socially reduces the levels of stress; however, a main concern relates to increased chance of injury due to aggressive interactions in a smaller space. Sectioning the living accommodation and consideration of functional elements such as feed troughs, water, and lying areas along with consideration of feeding frequency not only influence the activity levels of the animals but also their tolerance of one another.

Welfare One Welfare: the Horse–Human Dyad

The ethics of animal use compel animal carers to operate in good conscience. The horse's fundamental behavioural needs must be met if its welfare is to be positive (Keeling and Gonyou, 2001). It is clear that the social needs of a herd animal cannot be met if it is kept in isolation and its behavioural needs suffer when its environment is restricted in terms of space and quality as well as choice (Fig. 12.7).

Equine 'Quality of Life' is highly influenced by human management and horses have very limited control over their environment and limited choices. In addition, improving the emotional health of a horse is beneficial for the welfare of the human caretaker. Frightened, stressed, painful, and poorly adjusted animals will show defensive and protective behaviours that can be dangerous for humans. This is particularly pertinent for equine veterinarians who carry a high occupational risk of injury because of the behavioural responses of their patients whilst they are trying to treat them. Often the problem relates to a lack of adequate training, the horse being unclear about what is being required of it, and the handler's lack of knowledge about how to train the horse to behave appropriately when being examined for treatment. Advancing veterinarians' understanding of the application of learning principles for horses would improve safety, increase ease of handling and restraint during clinical procedures, and increase clinical efficacy (Fig. 12.8). It is for this reason that it is now strongly suggested that all veterinarians become familiar with the effective application of learning theory in a practical context, recognising indicators of fear and stress in their patients and how to reduce these emotional

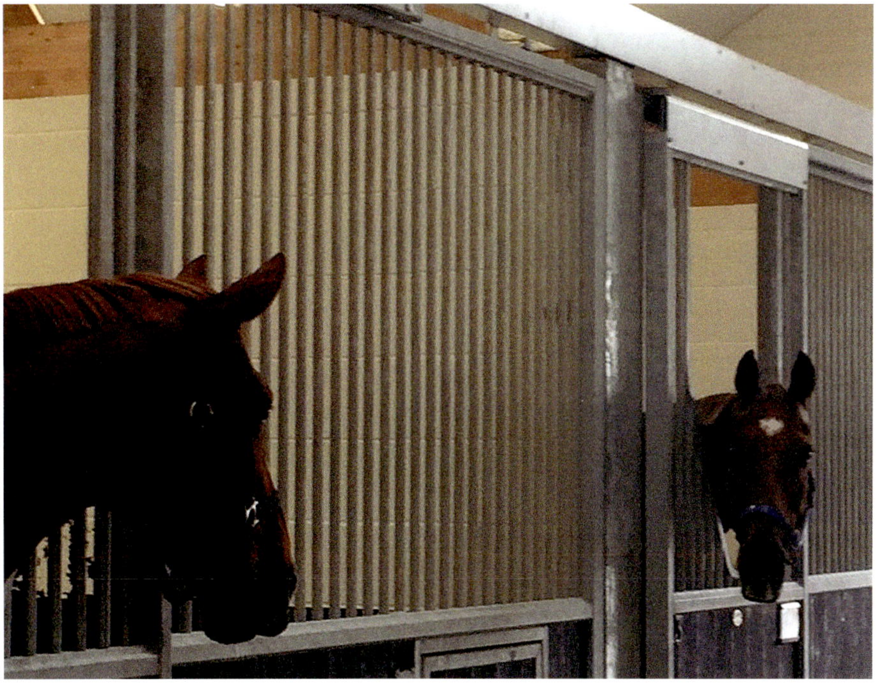

Fig. 12.7. Horses need social interaction and should not be kept in isolation. Photo: N.K. Waran.

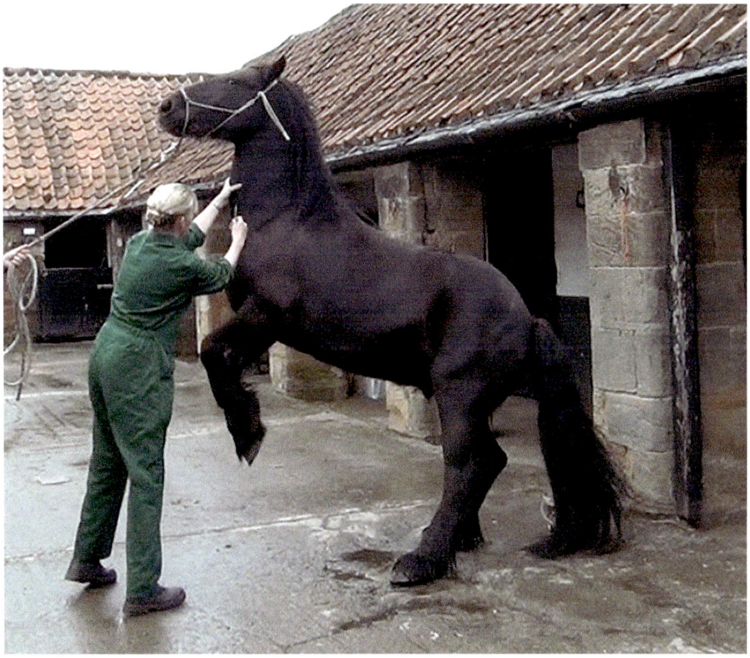

Fig. 12.8. Learning theory should be applied by veterinarians to improve horse welfare. Here, a horse displays needle aversion, putting the veterinarian and horse at risk. Photo: G. Pearson.

responses through their own behaviour towards the horse. Improving equine welfare through consideration of the social nature of the species is also shown to be beneficial for its performance. Horses reared in a group situation were easier to train and handle than those reared singly and showed less aggressive behaviour overall and less biting and kicking during training. It is for this reason that for horse and human welfare, it may be better to consider how horses can be provided with quality social experiences from an early age.

References

Bourjade, M., Moulinot, M., Henry, S., Richard-Yris, M.A. and Hausberger, M. (2008). Could adults be used to improve social skills of young horses, *Equus caballus*? *Developmental Psychobiology* 50, 408–417.

Bruner, J.S., Jolly, A. and Sylva, K. (eds) (1974) *Play: its Role in Development and Evolution*. Penguin, Harmondsworth, UK.

Caanitz, H., O'Leary, L., Houpt, K., Petersson, K. and Hintz, H. (1991) Effect of exercise on equine behaviour. *Applied Animal Behaviour Science* 31, 1–12.

Cameron, E.Z., Linklater, W.L., Stafford, K.J. and Minot, E.O. (2008). Maternal investment results in better foal condition through increased play behaviour in horses. *Animal Behaviour* 76(5), 1511–1518.

Christensen, J.W., Ladewig, J., Søndergaard, E. and Malmkvist, J. (2002). Effects of individual versus group stabling on social behaviour in domestic stallions. *Applied Animal Behaviour Science* 75(3), 233–248.

Fagen, R.M. (1976) Exercise, play and physical training in animals. *Perspectives in Ethology* 2, 189–219.

Fagen, R. (1981) *Animal Play Behaviour*. Oxford University Press, New York.

Fraser, A.F. (1992) *The Behaviour of the Horse*. CAB International, Wallingford, UK.

Hall, S.L. (1998) Object play by adult animals. In: Bekoff, M. and Byers, J.A. (eds) *Animal Play: Evolutionary, Comparative and Ecological Perspectives*. Cambridge University Press, Cambridge, pp. 455–460.

Hamilton, W.D. (1964) The genetical evolution of social behaviour II. *Journal of Theoretical Biology* 7, 1–16.

Hartmann, E., Bøe, K.E., Christensen, J.W., Hyyppä, S., Jansson, H. *et al.* (2015). A Nordic survey of management practices and owners' attitudes towards keeping horses in groups. *Journal of Animal Science* 93:4564–4574.

Houpt, K.A. (2002) Formation and dissolution of the mare–foal bond. *Applied Animal Behaviour Science* 78, 319–328.

Keeling, L. and Gonyou, H. (eds) (2001) *Social Behaviour in Farm Animals*. CAB International, Wallingford, UK.

Lansade, L., Bouissue, M.F. and Erhard, H.W. (2008) Fearfulness in horses: a temperamental trait, stable across time and situations. *Applied Animal Behaviour Science* 115, 182–200.

Ligout, S., Bouissou, M.F. and Boiviu, X. (2008) Comparison of the effects of two different handling methods on the subsequent behaviour of Anglo-Arabian foals towards humans and handling. *Applied Animal Behaviour Science* 113, 175–188.

McDonnell, S. (2003) *The Equid Ethogram: a Practical Field Guide to Horse Behaviour*. Eclipse Press, Lexington, Kentucky.

Pellis, S.M. and Pellis, V.C. (1998) The structure–function interface in the analysis of playfighting. In: Bekoff, M. and Byers, J.A. (eds) *Animal Play: Evolutionary, Comparative and Ecological Perspectives*. Cambridge University Press, Cambridge, pp. 115–140.

Rifa, H. (1990) Social facilitation in the horse (*Equus caballus*). *Applied Animal Behaviour Science* 25, 167–176.

Søndergaard, E. and Ladewig, J. (2004) Group housing exerts a positive effect on the behaviour of young horses in training. *Applied Animal Behaviour Science* 87, 105–118.

Thorbergson, Z.W., Nielsen, S.G., Beaulieu, R.J. and Doyle, R.E. (2016). Physiological and behavioral responses of horses to wither scratching and patting the neck when under saddle. *Journal of Applied Animal Welfare Science* 19, 245–59.

van Dierendonck, M.C., De Vries, H., Schilder, M.B.H., Colenbrander, B., Goran, A. *et al.* (2009) Interventions in social behaviour in a herd of mares and geldings. *Applied Animal Behaviour Science* 116, 67–73.

van Dierendonck, M.C. and Spruijt, B.M. (2012) Coping in groups of domestic horses – Review from a social and neurobiological perspective. *Applied Animal Behaviour Science* 138, 194–202.

van Ree, J.M., Niesink, R.J.M., van Wolfswinkel, L., Ramsey, N.F., Kornet, M.L.M.W. *et al.* (2000) Endogenous opioids and reward. *European Journal of Pharmacology* 405, 89–101.

Waran, N.K. (2001) The social behaviour of horses. In: Keeling, L.J. and Gonyou, H.W. (eds) *Social Behaviour in Farm Animals*. CAB International, Wallingford, UK, pp. 247–274.

13 Undesirable Behaviour and Stress

Gemma Pearson BVMS, MScR, MRCVS[1]*, Natalie K. Waran PhD[2] and Andrew F. Fraser MVSc, MRCVS[3]

[1]*The University of Edinburgh, Midlothian, Scotland, UK;* [2]*Eastern Institute of Technology, Hawke's Bay, New Zealand;* [3]*Carbonear, Newfoundland, Canada*

Introduction 180
Stereotypical Behaviours 180
Crib-biting and windsucking 181
Weaving 182
Stall-walking/box-walking 182
Pawing 182
Head-tossing or nodding 182
Crib-whetting 183
Tongue-dragging 183
Abnormal Ingestion 183
Bruxism 183
Quidding 183
Chewing 183
Eating faeces 184
Litter eating and other forms of pica 184
Bolting food 184
Psychogenic polydipsia 185
Abnormal Behaviours in Stabled Horses 185
Chronic standing 185
Tail rubbing 186
Self-mutilation 186
Conflict Behaviour 187
Aggression 187
Crowding, barging and crushing 188
Bolting 188
Shying 188
Jibbing, baulking or napping 188
Stress 189
Autonomic nervous system response 190
Neuroendocrine responses 190
Behavioural responses 191
Chronic stress and subsequent consequences 191
Minimizing the stress response 191
Clinical Behavioural Expressions 191
Pain and suffering 192
Depression and learned helplessness 193

*Corresponding author: Gemma.Pearson@ed.ac.uk

DOI: 10.1079/9781789242133.0013

Welfare 193
Summary 193
References 193

Introduction

Many horses exhibit behaviours that we find undesirable. These responses include those that are part of a horse's normal behaviour but that we find undesirable, and those that are considered abnormal. Normal behavioural responses that we may find undesirable include conflict behaviours such as rearing, napping, bargy or pushy responses. Conflict behaviours are a normal, adaptive response to resolve a stressful situation (McLean and Christensen, 2017). For example, a horse that is aversive when approached by people may demonstrate agonistic behaviours such as threatening to bite and kick. These behaviours may result in the person retreating, removing the source of stress. This is an example of an adaptive response to stress.

Abnormal behaviours include stereotypical behaviours, redirected behaviours such as wood-chewing, altered levels of arousal and self-mutilation. These represent a failure of the horse to resolve stressors, resulting in a maladaptive stress response. Commonly, the stressor results from its environment and/or training protocols that do not meet the physical and psychological needs of the horse. Once developed, they can persist, even if the underlying stressors are removed. As well as demonstrating poor welfare, horses with stereotypies are of reduced economic value due to the perception that they impair performance and are contagious to other horses on a yard (McBride and Hemmings, 2009). Animals with established stereotypies are cognitively less flexible due to sensitization of their basal ganglia compared to controls with no known stereotypical behaviours.

By contrast, research has also shown that horses demonstrating stereotypies have increased motivation for reward, resulting in them being faster to acquire new behaviours but also persistent in their expression of them (i.e. they are more resistant to extinction) (Hemmings *et al.*, 2007). Cognitive underperformance may occur in stereotypic horses if they are prevented from crib-biting during testing (Briefer Freymond *et al.*, 2019). Interestingly, stereotypic behaviour is valued by some riders due to its association with trainability, to the extent that at least one Olympic event rider actively seeks horses that crib.

Stereotypical Behaviours

Stereotypical behaviours are apparently functionless, repetitive behaviours performed as a consequence of frustration, repeated attempts to cope, or dysfunction of the central nervous system (Mason, 2006). Although never documented in wild or feral populations, the prevalence of stereotypies in domesticated horses is common. In some populations, rates are as high as 26% (Kiley-Worthington, 1987). Despite the variety of these behaviours, it is notable that they occur in identical forms worldwide. This is due to their common underlying neural framework plus the same changes in brain chemistry and especially that of dopamine physiology of the basal ganglia (McBride and Hemmings, 2009). With increasing awareness of the influence of adverse childhood experiences on the neurophysiological development of children and the effects of suboptimal weaning protocols on neurophysiological development across species, this subject deserves further research in the horse (Poletto *et al.*, 2006). Extrapolating from other species, it is likely that optimizing early life experiences guards against developing stereotypies by building resilience. Regardless, this should not detract from the importance of providing an environment that meets the horse's basic needs. Most stereotypical behaviours in horses are oral stereotypies, strongly associated with feeding concentrated grain-based diets, or locomotor stereotypies associated with frustration due to barriers to free choice movement such as the stable door or fence (Table 13.1).

Traditionally, horses may have been prevented from exhibiting stereotypies, as they were considered to be vices. This would usually involve some form of physical intervention, such as a leather anti-cribbing collar to prevent horses from arching their neck or placement of a metal grill over a horse's door to prevent weaving over the stable door. Although these methods may reduce the amount of time the horse spends participating in stereotypical behaviours, they fail to address the underlying cause. McGreevy (1995) demonstrated that, following prevention, once the horse had the opportunity to perform stereotypical behaviours again, it did so with markedly increased prevalence, an example of

Table 13.1. Abnormal oral activities in horses.

Activity	Characteristics
Crib-biting or Windsucking	The affected individual typically grasps a fixed object in its stall with its incisor teeth. The upper incisors are often used alone to press down on the fixture. Air is then swallowed into the upper oesophagus with a grunt. Inspection of the upper incisors may reveal abnormal wear, although in others they appear completely normal.
Crib-whetting	The affected horse repeatedly draws the tongue slowly across the crib or manger in the stall. During this activity, the horse holds the tongue in a firm and fixed manner that does not resemble normal licking.
Tongue-dragging	This condition is revealed when the horse is bridled and being ridden, or it may be performed in the stable. It rarely occurs when the affected horse is turned out. The tongue is displaced out of the side of the mouth.
Bruxism	Also known as teeth grinding, it is indicative of pain that may be related to the oral cavity or elsewhere.

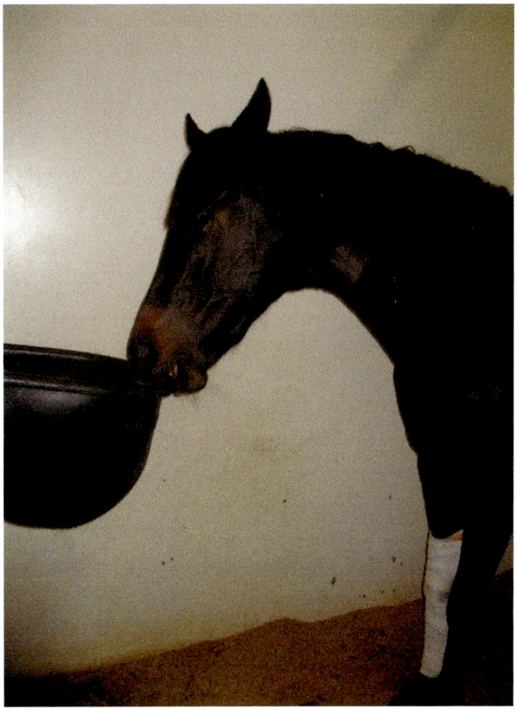

Fig. 13.1. A horse confined to a stall to recover from injury displays crib-biting on its feed container, despite the ready availably of the feed contained within. Photo: C.B. Riley.

post-inhibitory rebound. There is also the suggestion that stereotypical behaviours are coping mechanisms. Therefore, preventing them from occurring is contraindicated. Instead, preventing the development of stereotypies should be prioritized by focusing on providing an appropriate environment and optimizing early life experiences, particularly around weaning. Once developed, it is much harder to limit their occurrence because dopamine-driven feedback mechanisms are so strong that the behaviours persist, even in an appropriate environment. Providing horses with an appropriate environment and a feeding regime more in line with the horse's natural environment will minimize their occurrence and promote general well-being.

Crib-biting and windsucking

Crib-biting, also known as cribbing, is an oral stereotypy that involves the horse grasping a fixed object with its incisor teeth and then, with an arched neck, rocking its weight back onto the hindquarters (cribbing) (Fig. 13.1). Often a grunting sound is emitted as air is passed into the upper oesophagus (windsucking) (McBride and Hemmings, 2009). Contrary to what was previously believed, fluoroscopic studies have revealed that air does not actually pass into the stomach (McGreevy *et al.*, 1995). Windsucking may also occur without grasping a fixed object. For example, the chin may be rested on an object, or the behaviour simply performed in mid-air. This may result when attempts have been made to prevent cribbing, for example, by smearing unpalatable substances on surfaces that are normally grasped. These oral stereotypies are usually most prevalent when stabled, yet over time become habitual even when at pasture. An increase in frequency is always associated with the provision of concentrate feed. Early weaning combined with the introduction of a grain-based diet to foals has been linked with the development of abnormal oral behaviours and, as such, it is suggested as a practice to be avoided. The consequences of cribbing include extensive wear of the incisors. Horses with abnormal oral behaviours may have poor weight gain and increased susceptibility to colic, especially entrapment of the small intestine in the epiploic foramen (Archer *et al.*, 2008).

Weaving

The behaviour has the horse standing in one position but weaving from side to side or rocking back and forth. The main feature is swinging the head, neck and forequarters from side to side. Weight is taken alternately on each forelimb. The forefeet usually remain on the stable floor during the behaviour. In some cases, each foot is raised in turn as the weight passes on to the other foot. It occurs most commonly in riding horses that have been stabled in single stalls without adequate exercise after a phase of active use It is commonly expressed with the head and neck over the stable door, again consistent with barrier frustration. Turning the horse into a paddock provides daily freedom and exercise that allows them to express many of the behaviours they cannot show when confined in a stable. Intense exercise can be beneficial, and this can be supplemented by lunging or using a mechanical horse walker. If paddock space and a facility for exercise are not available, the horse's basic locomotory needs are unlikely to be met, and there is more risk of abnormal behaviour occurring. Making mirrors available so that the horse can view its reflection has been found to reduce weaving (McAfee *et al.*, 2002). It is considered a temporary measure in cases where confinement is necessary for a period of weeks on veterinary grounds. In stabled horses, the provision of an enrichment device that requires the horses to work to extract food with the aim of extending foraging time (Equiball™) has also been shown to reduce stereotypic behaviour (Henderson and Waran, 2001). It may also prevent the development of unwanted locomotory behaviours.

Stall-walking/box-walking

In stall-walking, the horse moves side to side or back and forward, turning sharply, in a repetitive, precise type of movement, as is consistent with stereotypies. This may be sustained for such long periods that the continuous drain on the animal's energy becomes significant. In affected horses, their physical condition deteriorates noticeably.

Stereotyped pacing is the essence of stall-walking. In this disordered behaviour, the horse constantly paces or circles around its box. The behaviour occurs when the basic needs of sufficient exercise are unmet, resulting in chronic confinement stress. The condition resembles weaving with the stereotyped precision and repetition in which the horse performs its rhythmic movements. As distinct from weaving, the stall-walker makes use of the larger area afforded by a loose box. The greater space allows the horse to perform slightly more elaborate ambulatory actions than in weaving. The quantity of work performed in stall-walking is often considerable. In many cases it leads to weight loss through energy depletion. Since the amount of the area available to the horse is limited, much spinal flexion is required in circling and turning. This can lead to painful back conditions that adversely affect the horse's performance and well-being when ridden or worked.

Pawing

It is normal for horses to paw at a recumbent foal or in activities like clearing snow from herbage. If outside the horse's usual behaviour, it is usually indicative of abdominal pain. Pawing becomes an abnormal activity when it is performed with vigour in a persistent and stereotyped manner. Minor episodes of pawing do occur very commonly and normally when horses are in a state of high arousal, such as frustration while awaiting food. This form of pawing ceases when the horses are fed. This is a good example of inadvertent positive reinforcement training of a behaviour as, from the horse's perspective, the behaviour of pawing results in the provision of food. The horse can be retrained by rewarding the behaviour of standing calmly with food as an alternative. Continual pawing on a hard stable floor can result in abnormal hoof wear and foot imbalance. When the stable floor sometimes gets dug up in one spot, it is of minor consequence. This merely serves as a diagnostic sign that the horse's basic needs are not being met.

Head-tossing or nodding

Horses can show a nodding of the head in a variety of circumstances, including various clinical conditions causing pain, frustration or confusion. When head-tossing becomes frequent and stereotyped in manner, it can be identified as such. The activity should be studied from some distance for an extended period to determine if it conforms to stereotyped characteristics such as exact regularity, precise repetition, continuing performance, and the animal's apparent concentration on this one action. The condition is often seen in horses with their heads held over the closed, lower part of the box stall door, again indicating barrier frustration. As with weaving, the provision of mirrors may alleviate the disorder but does not address the underlying problem (McAfee *et al.*, 2002).

Head shaking describes the sudden onset of vertical movement of the head in response to a stimulus that is often unknown. It is usually accompanied by guarding of the nostrils, and the horse commonly attempts to rub its muzzle on its forelimbs, in the bedding or against a wall. This is a clinical condition currently associated with neuropathy of the trigeminal nerve and is distinctive enough in appearance to differentiate it from other forms of head-tossing.

Crib-whetting

Some horses in chronic confinement show disordered oral behaviour in which the tongue is slowly and repeatedly drawn across the edge of the crib. The affected horse holds its tongue very firmly in this action so that the behaviour does not represent true licking. The repetitious nature of this disorder and its regular form make it stereotyped. As with other stereotypies, this condition is difficult to eliminate. Along with excessive licking, it may be a precursor to cribbing.

Tongue-dragging

Tongue-dragging, tongue-over-the-bit and tongue-waving are modified forms of the same condition. The affected horse puts its tongue over the bit or out of the side of its mouth repeatedly. The horse may show the activity during work, riding or at rest in the stable. Tongue-dragging at rest is an example of an oral stereotypy, whereas when ridden it represents a failure to correctly train the horse using negative reinforcement via the bit. Initially, this behaviour is offered to alleviate bit pressure. Eventually, it becomes habitual and almost impossible to resolve. As it may result in the rider losing marks in a competition and is considered unsightly, some riders resort to excessively tight nosebands to try and maintain the tongue in the mouth.

Abnormal Ingestion

Just as with stereotypical behaviours, redirected behaviours are symptomatic of an inadequate environment. In contrast, they are not exhibited with the same precise, repetitive and intensive focus. This is most likely as they do not release dopamine in the same way that stereotypical behaviours do, the reason for which they become so intense and resistant to extinction. Resolution again revolves around meeting the horse's ethological needs of turn out, social companionship with other horses, and prolonged access to fibre.

Bruxism

The abnormality of bruxism in the oral behaviour of horses was formerly unrecognized, although it is well known in human medicine as the dysfunctional habit of teeth grinding, often during sleep in the persons affected. Bruxism is usually taken to be stress related. Severe teeth grinding can be heard in some livestock when subjected to such stressors as being crated for the first time. As an anomalous condition, bruxism is an established habit and way of coping with an otherwise unresolved stressor. Bruxism in stabled horses is ordinarily indicative of pain, and further veterinary investigation is warranted before it is considered stereotypical. Bruxism may be exhibited in the ridden horse because of discomfort associated with being ridden, especially excessive bit pressure or an overly tight noseband, but may also indicate confusion regarding the aids. In this context, the horse uses it to cope with the consequent unresolved stressor.

Quidding

Quidding is a well-recognized sign of oral pain, in which partially chewed food, such as hay or grass, drops periodically from the horse's mouth. Quidding is almost invariably secondary to a fractured molar tooth or periodontal disease resulting from food entrapped and rotting in diastemata (abnormal spaces between the molar teeth).

Chewing

Abnormal chewing and eating of wood (lignophagia) are common in horses in restricted quarters or paddocks. Of all the oral ingestive disorders in the horse, wood-chewing is the most common. It is not limited to indoor horses and is as frequent in horses in outdoor enclosures. Even in pastures, wood-chewing may take the form of severe de-barking of trees. Limited paddock space clearly aggravates the condition. Although wood-chewing horses do not usually ingest most of the wood they chew, they do ingest enough to risk splinter damage to the alimentary tract. Lack of cellulose roughage in the diet undoubtedly contributes to wood-chewing. Horses fed on high sugar-concentrate diets with a low supply of roughage show the condition much more frequently than horses fed hay in abundance. A wood-chewer may chew half a kilogram of wood a day. Although a degree of wood chewing may be considered normal for a browsing species, excessive wood chewing reflects a failure to meet the horse's foraging needs and is a precursor to cribbing (Nicol, 1999).

The true eating pattern of the horse is almost continuous consumption of roughage. Its digestive tract is unsuited to rapid food processing. At pasture, the horse will graze 70% of the day and night. Chewing coarse fibres takes extra time, fulfilling the equine need for chew time and fibre filling. Much roughage is needed by the horse's alimentary system for proper digestive fermentation. The modern trend is to feed less hay and increase concentrates accordingly. All of this may satisfy the horse's need for energy, but it neglects the horse's basic need for fibre. Quality hay, such as lucerne, can be fed *ad libitum* to wood-chewers. In turn, they will show the disorder less. Modern concentrate feeds are moving towards being fat and fibre based rather than sugar based.

Eating faeces

The ingestion of faeces (coprophagia) is typically a problem of confinement in adults. It is so often seen in foals under good management that it is considered normal while they are learning to chew and ingest roughage. It most likely makes an important contribution to the development of the microbiome. Coprophagia in the adult horse is a different matter. It is typically a problem of confinement in a box stall with insufficient roughage in the diet in affected animals. Adult horses practising coprophagia are typically under chronic restrictions. Affected animals consume their own faeces in substantial quantity. In some cases, most of the faeces are regularly consumed. Although coprophagy in adults is unlikely to result in any physiological harm, it still represents a failure to meet the horse's basic needs and so should be addressed. Roughage can be given *ad libitum*. In many cases, such a diet maintained for a period of at least two months is found to stop this behaviour. Turn out, ideally with other horses, is an essential requirement of any horse.

Litter eating and other forms of pica

Horses confined on sawdust litter may eat their bedding, even after it has become soiled. Almost every horse in the confines of a stable can be observed to eat soiled litter on occasions, but with a litter-eating disorder, this activity is habitual. The habit can develop in horses that are well fed. Several causes of litter-eating in horses have become recognized. Horses at pasture graze most of the day, fulfilling their psychological need for prolonged mastication. Within stables, this occupation is curtailed, and grain or compounded food is often consumed quickly. If such food is accompanied by the provision of adequate hay (for ingestive occupation as much as balanced nutrition), horses may seek other available cellulose materials to eat. Pica describes the consumption of abnormal items not normally considered food. In horses it involves consumption of soil or even the hair of other horses. All forms of pica are symptomatic of a failure to meet the horse's basic needs. The consequences may include a predisposition to sand colic or liver disease if sand or iron are consumed in excess respectively. Provision of adequate forage and turn out are again integral to resolution.

Bolting food

The disordered eating behaviours of overeating and rapid eating are forms of hyperphagia (bolting food). Many horses have a prodigious appetite and will rapidly consume concentrate feed, but bolting takes this further. In some horses, the bolting of food puts it at risk of choking (oesphageal obstruction). The food is not fully masticated, resulting in attempts to swallow larger boluses insufficiently moistened with saliva. Such horses may consume excessive quantities if they have access to an open feed bin containing concentrated rations. In turn, this could lead to a serious digestive illness, with potentially fatal consequences.

As always, it is important first to address any potential underlying causes such as lack of roughage, turnout, social access to conspecifics, or even poor training regimes that result in a chronic stress response. The treatment of bolting involves the tactical feeding of affected horses. Spreading the grain in a thin layer in the trough and placing large, smooth stones in the bottom of the trough are methods used to make grain difficult to eat rapidly. There are many slow feeding devices, such as balls that can be filled with feed; pushing the ball around results in feed dropping out of holes in the side and can help replicate the horse's natural grazing behaviour. Supplying concentrate feed several times during the day and mixing it with larger quantities of fibre such as chaff (chopped hay) may help. Feeding hay prior to concentrates can help in the partial control of the eating disorder. It may be impossible, however, to eliminate this behaviour entirely.

Psychogenic polydipsia

Over drinking (psychogenic polydipsia) is an ingestive disorder in some horses isolated and confined to stalls with water supplied *ad libitum*. Some may consume up to 140 L daily, or about three to four times the normal quantity required. This excessive consumption can be spread over time or concentrated within a relatively short time of 2–3 hours. It is recognized with increased prevalence in countries with high relative humidity and ambient temperature. Associated polyuria may be the disorder's first sign, with caretakers noting excessively wet bedding. In some instances, polydipsia has been noted among overtrained horses. Once developed, medullary washout can result, where the cells in the kidney become depleted of salts and incorrectly signal further thirst. Slowly reducing the ration of water can resolve medullary washout. However, this must be conducted under strict veterinary supervision as restriction of water in other causes of polydipsia may have fatal consequences. Addressing the underlying cause is essential to prevent a recurrence. Table 13.2 summarizes the ingestive disorders that have been discussed.

Table 13.2. Abnormal ingestion in horses.

Abnormality	Characteristics
Wood-chewing	Regular and persistent biting, chewing and consuming wood on fence tops, doorways of stables, the bark of trees, etc., is seen mostly in horses kept fenced in or closed up. This often diminishes when fed roughage.
Eating faeces	Breaking up faecal piles and eating into the content is common and normal in young foals, especially eating the mare's dung. This is abnormal in an adult.
Litter-eating	Eating their own bedding, especially if it consists of wood particles or chaff (chopped hay). The litter may be clean or soiled.
Hair-eating	Chewing off and then eating the tail hairs of another horse. The eaten hair may rarely accumulate and remain in the gut.
Soil-eating	Persistent eating of quantities of earth or sand, depending on whatever is available.
Bolting food	Eating quickly and swallowing prior to full mastication may be a regular occurrence or a single event in a state of high arousal (e.g. trailer choke).
Psychogenic polydipsia	Frequent drinking and excessive consumption of water will result in polyuria. This disorder may or may not relate to a disease process. Abnormal water intake can occur in confined horses with an *ad libitum* water supply.

Abnormal Behaviours in Stabled Horses

Chronic standing

Chronic standing in horses kept stabled is common, particularly among older animals and individuals of heavy breeds such as Belgians and Clydesdales. They can continue to stand in stalls without lying down for months on end. Some individuals never lie down in the stall. It can be speculated that the reason for chronic standing is the horse's fear of the consequences. However, it could simply be the case that the horse is physically unable to lie down in a confined stall through such orthopaedic conditions as spinal or limb pathology. Insufficient space to easily lie down is currently considered one of the most common reasons in stabled horses.

Remaining upright and still is a natural behavioural tactic of many large quadrupeds in uncertain times regarding potential intrusion into their space. Some horses demonstrate the ability to get down, roll and rise without difficulty, and a complete physical evaluation by a veterinarian fails to reveal an underlying cause. These cases often present with injuries, especially to the knees, hocks or face sporadically. Video footage of the horse overnight usually reveals the horse appears to be lightly sleeping (slow-wave sleep, which can be achieved standing) followed by some buckling of the limbs before their sudden collapse. These cases are termed recumbent sleep deprivation. This occurs as the body needs rapid eye movement (REM) sleep for which the horse must be recumbent to achieve. Although horses may go up to three months without REM, they do collapse eventually, with electromyography studies suggesting they achieve a few seconds of REM during this process. These horses may also be seen to buckle and almost collapse before rapidly standing during grooming or tacking up procedures.

Historically, during times when heavy horses were used widely, chronic standing in the stable was well recognized as a problem by workers on the streets or the farm. Some horsemen dealt with this matter by putting a resting fixture across the heel posts of the affected horse's stall for the animal to lean its rump on. One such fixture was a strong chain slung from post to post at the height of the horse's thighs, which was secured at night. At times, the chain was inside a rubber sleeve for the horse's comfort, while at others, a heavy rope was used. Horses soon learned to lean heavily on such supports when they were resting. Following a complicated limb fracture repair horses may be restrained in a sling, allowing them to lean into it to achieve slow-wave sleep. Provision of a large, well bedded box, and resolution of any physical underlying causes or turnout with conspecifics may resolve this problem in some cases.

Tail rubbing

In many instances of tail-rubbing, it is the horse's rump that is rubbed. The action of tail-rubbing can be related to an endoparasitic infection by *Oxyuris equi* (pinworm), external parasites (lice and mites), or hypersensitivity to midge saliva (sweet-itch). In the latter case, the mane is usually involved as well. In addition, it is an element of maintenance behaviour: a normal action in the horse's own body care. Tail-rubbing is included here since the persistent performance of this action can be shown by some horses without a clinical condition of parasitism, such as rectal helminth infestation, fungal disease, or louse infestation of the tail head region. By itself, tail-rubbing is a non-specific action, also relating to certain hindlimb pain.

Little doubt exists that parasitism aside, persistent tail-rubbing can occur as an item of abnormal body-based activity. Although it is not characteristically a stabled horse problem, it is placed among them because of its behavioural kinship with self-mutilation and pawing. It can, of course, be exhibited in the stable. Tail-rubbing is often observed with the horse backing up to a tree, fence or wall, and pressing its rump against the upright surface while it rubs its tail and hindquarters rhythmically from side to side. The persistence of the action gives it a stereotyped appearance in extreme cases. The hairs on the tail against the dock become worn away, leaving a bristly look on the tail head; this sign characterizes the tail rubber. Stress-induced pruritis is recognized in a variety of species and so should also be considered. Every case should be given a clinical examination and any necessary curative therapy to differentiate between a clinical sign and stereotypy.

Self-mutilation

The horse can self-traumatize its skin by biting at it or rubbing itself on a fixed object such as the side of the stall. The severity can vary from mild skin irritation and hair loss to deep wounds. The chest, flanks, and sides are most affected, although any region of the body may be involved. Complex regional pain syndrome, although not widely documented in horses, should also be considered. Complex regional pain syndrome often occurs following an injury and results in persistent severe and debilitating pain long after the initial injury has resolved.

Affected horses are usually those that are permanently enclosed and isolated. Since this is a common scenario for breeding stallions, the condition occurs most often in these horses. However, mares and geldings can also suffer from the condition. Conceivably, the condition may be analogous to the sudden attack of widespread itching that can occur in people. An affected animal should promptly be turned outdoors to rescue it from itself. A wide pasture is an ideal place for emergency accommodation. Allowing social access to conspecifics is again important, even in stallions. The Swiss national stud has demonstrated that managing stallions in social groups turned out together (outside of the breeding season) or via social housing is possible (Briefer Freymond *et al.*, 2013; Zollinger *et al.*, 2016). Self-mutilation does not occur acutely, and these horses will have demonstrated many other signs of being unable to cope with their environment that have been missed before reaching this point. Table 13.3 summarizes the abnormal actions discussed.

Table 13.3. Abnormal actions in stabled horses.

Action	Characteristics
Weaving	Affected horses stand in one position and weave from side to side in the stall. Some move back and forth, with the head, neck and forequarters swaying side to side rhythmically.
Stall-walking	The affected horse continuously walks side to side or in circles around a box stall. This is associated with deficient exercise or chronic confinement. The walking is precise, rhythmic and repetitive.
Pawing	Vigorous and persistent pawing at the stall floor in a stereotyped action, with the pawing directed at one spot. This is different from short spells of pawing when waiting to be fed.
Tail-rubbing	Persistent rubbing of the tail head in a side-to-side action of the hindquarters against a stable wall, tree, or fence, etc. This action is also a sign of parasitism and needs differentiation.
Self-mutilation	Self-injury by vigorous biting of the flanks or excessive rubbing of the neck or body against an available structure. The action is typically intense and repetitive with vocalization.
Head-tossing	Usually occurs as a continuous bobbing of the head up and down. This can occur in a stable as a stereotyped action. The tossing of the head is also shown in various conditions of pain and requires differentiation.
Chronic standing	The subject will not lie down, and there is no sign of soil or bedding on the quarters or back in the morning. This can continue for many months. It can be taken as a sign of orthopaedic disease in some that are aged and/or infirm or may be related to an inadequate environment in others.

Conflict Behaviour

Conflict behaviours represent a horse's attempts to cope with a stressful situation. The stressor usually induces a state of fear or pain, and, consequently, the horse attempts to maintain its homeostasis by removing the stressor. It is important to recognize that, although these behaviours are unwanted and often dangerous, they are a normal part of the horse's behavioural repertoire to remove stressors and certainly do not indicate inherent naughtiness or attempts to be dominant. At least initially, they are characterized by high arousal, active responses. Over time, if the horse is unable to resolve the stressor, it may displace into a state of negative valence, but low arousal such as conditioned suppression and learned helplessness (Hall *et al.*, 2008). Resolution revolves around identifying the underlying stressor and retraining the correct response using a working understanding of learning theory. Differential reinforcement describes training a behaviour that is incompatible with the unwanted behaviour. Thinking along this approach helps people to identify how to retrain the horse to overcome a problem behaviour without resorting to punishment-based techniques. Commonly recognized forms of conflict behaviour are described below.

Aggression

When in proximity to people or other horses that they perceive to be aversive, horses normally attempt to increase the space between the individual and themselves to a more comfortable distance by withdrawing. Of course, if they are restrained as a result of the size of their enclosure or by equipment such as a head collar and lead rope, they may instead use aggression to move the stressor further from them. Aggressive responses often start with ears back posture with or without bared teeth or swinging of the hindquarters (Fig. 13.2). It can develop into lunging or charging at the person and either threats or actual attempts to kick with a hindlimb, biting or striking with the forelimbs. Aggression is seen more commonly when concentrate feed is involved as the horse may strive to guard a valued resource. Varying degrees of this disorder range from vigorous to mild. Resolution involves firstly understanding the underlying cause and then counter conditioning the horse to tolerate the previous stressor when it is in close proximity.

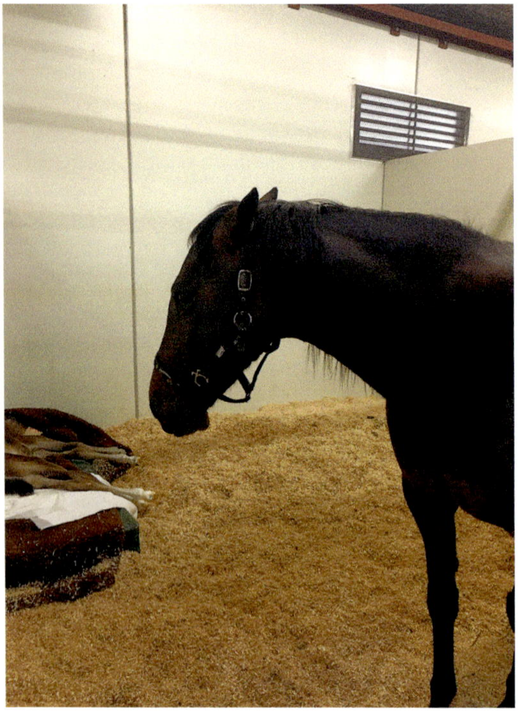

Fig. 13.2. Exhibited annoyance at people approaching her foal. Note: (i) head extended and tilted; (ii) ears turned back; (iii) watching with one eye; and (iv) jaw clenched. Photo: C.B. Riley.

Crowding, barging and crushing

Some horses may use their physical size to displace a person or crush them against a solid object such as a wall (Fig. 13.3). This has nothing to do with dominance or respect for personal space but instead results as a consequence of (1) the horse has never been trained to yield to pressure on its body, or (2) the horse perceives the person or their actions to be a stressor and so tries to displace the person from its proximity or stop them proceeding with an activity. A good example would be a horse that crushes a veterinarian against the wall when they attempt to inject them. Rather than being wilfully disobedient, the horse is simply attempting to prevent the aversive procedure. Almost invariably undertaken with faster movement than is normal for the individual, it highlights the state of increased arousal. Resolution involves retraining the basic operant responses so that the horse yields to pressure on any part of its body, working to ensure appropriate levels of arousal for the situation and addressing any underlying aversions.

Bolting

Bolting is a manifestation of the flight response, where the horse suddenly and rapidly accelerates despite cues for deceleration from the rider or handler. It is characterized by a state of high arousal. Hence the rider's deceleratory cues become less salient to the horse and ineffective. In a blind bolt, the horse also becomes less aware of its surroundings to the extent that it may gallop into objects such as fences or trees, making this scenario very dangerous. Thorough retraining, using negative reinforcement, of the halt response via rein pressure is essential. Possible underlying physical reasons such as back pain should be investigated. As with all behaviours associated with fear, the adverse response can be learned in a single trial and even after retraining, can be subject to spontaneous recovery. This highlights the importance of correct basic training that avoids fear.

Shying

A startle response is a perfectly normal reaction to a stimulus that appears suddenly or is novel. In a startle response, the horse rapidly flexes and then hyperextends all limbs and enters a state of increased arousal and hypervigilance. In contrast, shying, also known as spooking, occurs when the horse deviates from the line they were taking and may involve acceleration away from the area. Occasional shying, especially because of the sudden appearance of a novel or aversive stimulus is normal. Provided the horse is well trained to the basic responses, it can be controlled by the rider or handler. In contrast, regular shying, in which the rider or handler cannot gain control again quickly represents deficits in the horse's basic responses, especially signalling a lack of self-carriage for speed and line. It can also indicate that the horse's basic ethological needs for turnout and social companionship have not been adequately met or represent poor training regimes. Both result in a horse that is exposed to regular stress, maintains a state of high arousal, and becomes hyper-vigilant.

Jibbing, baulking or napping

Here, the horse suddenly refuses to continue forward when being led or ridden (Fig. 13.4). It may involve

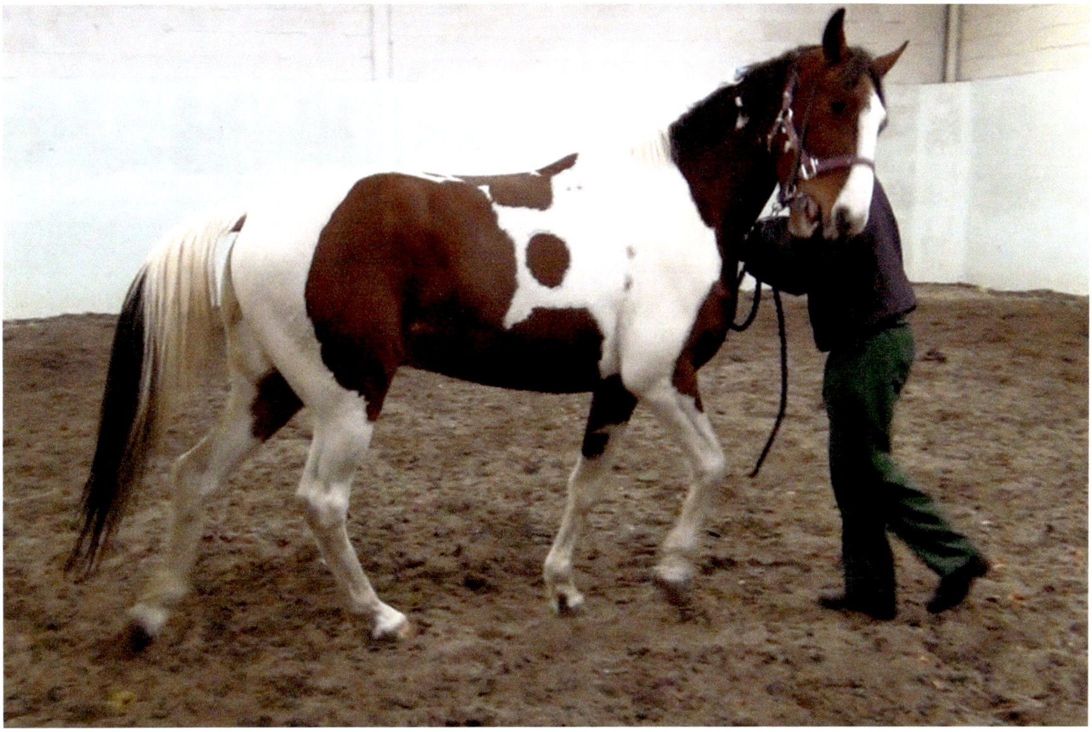

Fig. 13.3. Bargy horses will use their strength to displace people when stressed or conflicted. Note how the horse flexes its head and neck vertically and laterally in response to pressure on the lead rope rather than slowing down its legs. Photo: G. Pearson.

deviations sideways, representing loss of line, or the horse may become motionless, best described as a freeze response. Although sometimes it simply represents a conflict of interest in the direction taken between horse and human, there is usually a degree of increased arousal manifested as muscular tension. Retraining the horse's basic response to cues for acceleration utilizing negative reinforcement is key. The response can then be shaped so that it remains under stimulus control in various situations, including the place where the original episode occurred. Positive reinforcement training, in addition, will accelerate the rate at which the horse learns and establishes positive associations with the response, thus reducing the likelihood of negative emotional associations. Table 13.4 summarizes the abnormal reactions that have been discussed.

Stress

Any environmental stimulus that leads to an imbalance of homeostasis in an animal is described as a stressor and the reaction of the animal as the stress response (Möstl and Palme, 2002). This consists of both behavioural and physiological responses aimed at re-establishing homeostasis. The physiological responses are broken down further into those of the autonomic nervous system, neuroendocrine and immune systems. A stressor can be anything that has the potential to disrupt the homeostatic balance of the horse, from thermal stress in extremes of temperature to physical stress undertaken in training, to allow the horse to adapt to exercise. In the context of behaviour, people tend to refer to psychological stressors inducing pain, fear or frustration. Regardless of the type of stressor, pain, thirst, frustration, etc., the physiological response is similar and has been termed the standard stress model (McGreevy *et al.*, 2018). The first component of the stress response is the perception of the central nervous system that there is a threat to its homeostasis. It is important to emphasize that it is the perception of a threat that results in the subsequent response as opposed to an actual threat (Moberg and Mench, 2000). Many

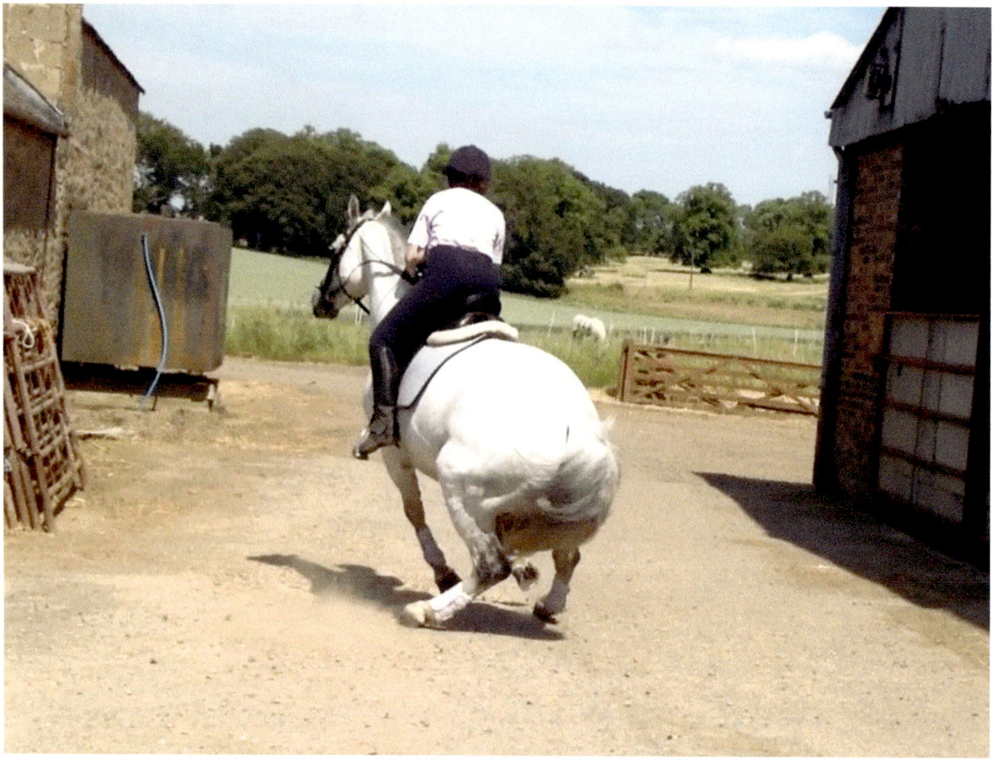

Fig. 13.4. Napping. The horse suddenly refuses to move forwards. As seen in this image, most horses prefer to push off their right foreleg and so spin to the left. Photo: G. Pearson.

people will judge a horse for appearing fearful of a stimulus that the rider considers they should have habituated to, following many exposures without any harm resulting. For example, the horse may repeatedly spook at the dustbin they walk past daily. This would be analogous to a person who fears spiders, despite many decades of exposure to them without any resulting in actual harm.

Autonomic nervous system response

The autonomic nervous system has two component arms: the sympathetic and parasympathetic branches. Although the parasympathetic is responsible for regulating basic control of internal organs, including blood pressure and digestion, the sympathetic acts agonistically and diverts focus away from daily maintenance tasks such as digestion to provide energy for the fight or flight response (Moberg and Mench, 2000). More specifically, sympathetic stimulation increases heart rate and force of contraction. The increased flow of blood is directed to the skeletal muscles and brain, preparing the horse to perform to a greater physical and mental ability than it would otherwise (Korte, 2001).

Neuroendocrine responses

The predominant response of the neuroendocrine system to a stressor is activation of the hypothalamic–pituitary–adrenal axis (Moberg and Mench, 2000). When a stressor is detected, neurons within the hypothalamus release corticotrophin-releasing hormone and vasopressin, increasing the production of adrenocorticotropic hormone from the anterior pituitary gland (Guillemin and Rosenberg, 1955). The stimulating effect of adrenocorticotropic hormone on the adrenal cortex results in increased secretion of glucocorticoids including cortisol (Merl *et al.*, 2000). Subsequently, glucose mobilized from storage in the liver and muscles again prepares the body for increased physical and mental ability in a flight-or-fight response. Endorphins, which blunt the pain response, are released. Pathways responsible

Table 13.4. Conflict behaviour in horses.

Reaction	Characteristics
Aggressive approach	Typically, the horse reacts aggressively to intrusion into its individual space or visual field with a threat charge. Some cases may show as aggressive approach at feeding.
Crowding	The horse deliberately squeezes or crowds a person against the stall when it is approached.
Bolting	The horse shows excessive alarm with a slight stimulus and will take the opportunity to run away out of control.
Threatening	The horse readily shows a threat display when approached. The display is a fight or flight reaction, with the animal showing the white of the eye and a raised head.
Kicking	Striking aggressively with one or both hind feet. Horses may also strike forward with a forefoot.
Shying	The individual tends to react readily to avoid novel items or situations by raising the head and turning away sharply from the source of fright.
Jibbing	The horse arrests its forward movement, throws up its head and refuses to go on.
Baulking	The subject effectively freezes and refuses to move regardless of coaxing, urging or punishment.

for regulating reproduction, growth and energy storage are downregulated, again promoting survival in the short term (McGreevy *et al.*, 2018).

Behavioural responses

The responses of the neuroendocrine and autonomic nervous system prepare the body to respond optimally and are standard responses regardless of the stressor. In contrast, the behavioural response aims to remove or resolve the stressor directly. For example, in the case of thermal stress where the horse is beginning to overheat, the behavioural response would be to seek shade. Avoidance of the stressor is the usual response to one that induces anxiety or fear, which, in the horse, may range from walking away from, spooking or bolting from a novel object. As already discussed in the section on conflict behaviour, if a horse perceives the cues given by the rider to be aversive, it will trial different behavioural responses to remove them. The response that removes the cue will be trialled more readily next time, whether it involves moving forward from leg pressure or rearing.

Chronic stress and subsequent consequences

The stress response evolved to increase the likelihood of survival under an acute threat to homeostasis, such as extreme weather or attack from predators. The response prioritizes short-term survival by preparing the body for fight or flight at the expense of normal maintenance, which can resume after the threat is removed. If the stressor remains or frequently occurs over a longer period, then the response becomes maladaptive (McGreevy *et al.*, 2018). The suppression of the reproductive and immune systems leads to poor fertility, increased susceptibility to disease and weakness as more energy is mobilized from the body than is stored. Chronically elevated glucocorticoids also impair learning and memory (Morris, 2007).

Minimizing the stress response

Instead of attempting to treat the behavioural element of the unwanted behaviour exclusively, remedial measures should be applied to the circumstances that initially caused the effect. The stress response can be minimized by providing predictability, controllability, outlets for frustration, and social support from conspecifics (McGreevy *et al.*, 2018). Regarding training and riding horses, adhering to the International Society for Equitation Science ‘Principles of Training’ minimizes stress and promotes optimal training. As discussed earlier, optimizing early life experiences and providing an environment that meets the horse’s physical and psychological needs generates resilience, allowing an individual horse to cope better when exposed to a stressor than it otherwise might. Prevention of unwanted behaviours through chemical, surgical, or physical restraint is unethical. It cannot be overemphasized that the stressful causal circumstances are the true problem and not the disorder. Treatment should be directed at their elimination through changed husbandry (McGreevy *et al.*, 1995).

Clinical Behavioural Expressions

Clinical behaviour in the horse contains certain major features and conditions, notably pain, suffering and depression (McEwen, 2001). These are indicated by behavioural features such as posture, over-activity, under-activity and altered ingestion or excretion. Future research should focus on the alterations in time budgets as horses are exposed to stressors. We know from other species that although the time dedicated to essential maintenance behaviours, such as eating, remain unaltered, those that are considered less essential, such as sleeping, grooming or play, are reduced. The monitoring of positive affective states, and not just an absence of negative ones, is needed to optimize welfare.

Pain and suffering

As a form of stress, pain generates a similar physiological response to that of other stressors such as hunger or confusion. It can be challenging to differentiate between horses in pain and those experiencing psychological forms of stress (Fig. 13.5). Changes in the horse's behaviour are key, particularly from normal behaviours. Pain scales, often based on facial expression (grimace scales), have been developed in an attempt to standardize pain levels for horses suffering from laminitis, colic and following castration (Sutton *et al.*, 2013; Dalla Costa *et al.*, 2014; Dalla Costa *et al.*, 2016). More recently, work has been undertaken to develop an ethogram for ridden horses that may help detect pain in horses with subtle lameness and confirm a positive response to diagnostic local anaesthesia (Dyson and van Dijk, 2018; Dyson *et al.*, 2018). Many caretakers recognize certain behavioural expressions that appear pathognomonic for pain localized to certain areas. Examples include altered gait and limb positioning indicating lameness, pawing and rolling indicating abdominal pain or quidding (dropping of partially masticated food) with pain originating from the oral cavity. Care should always be taken, and veterinary advice sought to confirm localization. A horse that stands but is reluctant to move and has altered forelimb posture may be consistent with laminitis when it is actually suffering from pleuropneumonia. Suffering because of pain associated with clinical conditions or due to their management and handling is a welfare concern. Timely recognition and management of pain using appropriate analgesia will ensure that suffering is minimized, healing is enhanced, and recovery is enabled.

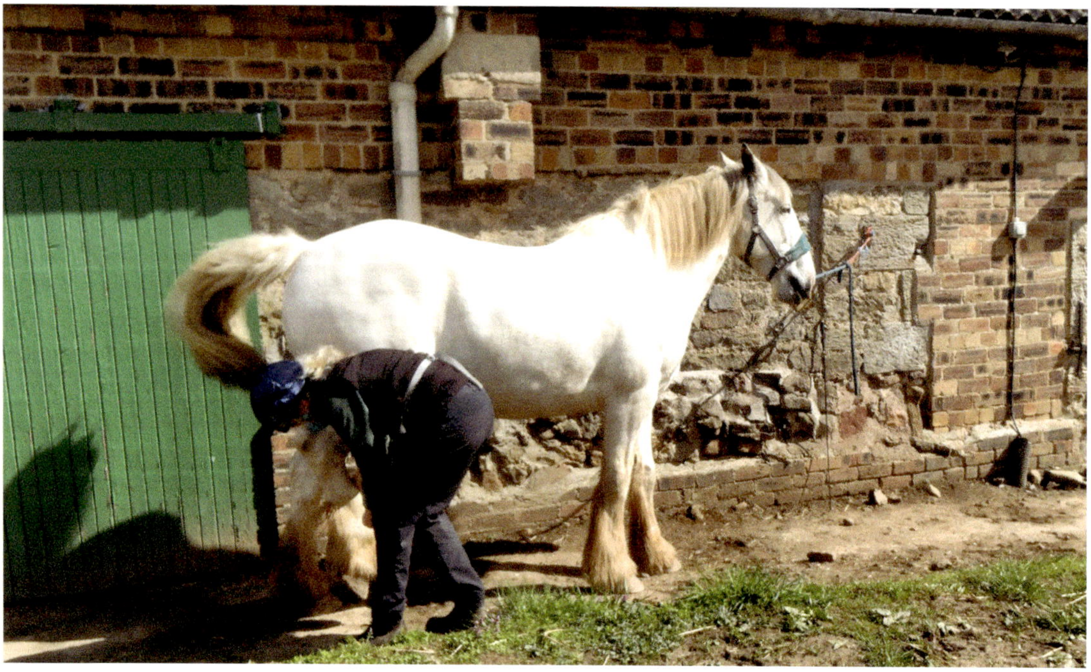

Fig. 13.5. Pain. This horse was reluctant to lift either hind leg for the farrier and would become bargy if a person persisted. Note the tail swishing, ears back posture and strained facial expression, all of which are indicators of potential pain. Treatment of the underlying hock pain along with a behaviour modification programme resulted in a successful outcome. Photo: G. Pearson.

Depression and learned helplessness

Among the observed signs of many clinical conditions in domestic animals, mention is made of depression in standard veterinary literature (Beaver, 1994). Animal depression is defined by Blood and Studdert (1988) as 'decreased interest in surroundings and decreased response to external stimuli'. The depressed animal's activity is likely derived from repeated aversive stimulation rather than through spontaneous relationships with the environment. In depression, the suffering animal shows a marked depletion of the behavioural repertoire characteristic of the normal animal. The principal features of maintenance behaviour such as trophic activities and restorative functions, together with collateral social behaviour, become significantly diminished, adding to the picture of suffering in the depressed state. Loss of maintenance homeostasis appears to be an essential criterion of that general aspect of animal illness referred to as depression in clinical terms. The established concept of adjunctive depression in animal illness recognizes the behaviour of the animal as globally changed rather than regionally modified. In this, the main significant measure is behavioural frequency. It shows most often in the reduced frequency of maintenance activities.

Of particular concern in horses is the potential for learned helplessness. This was discovered through experimental exposure to aversive stimuli in rats and dogs, namely electric shocks, over which they had no control (Seligman and Maier, 1967; Rosellini and Seligman, 1975). Although initially they attempted to escape the shock, they gave up trying and appeared dull once they realized this was not possible. Even later, when escape was possible, they remained dull and did not attempt it. These animals suffered from depression; motivational, emotional and cognitive deficits; and anhedonia, which continued after the experimentations ceased. More worryingly, several animals died during experimental treatments. Learned helplessness is of particular concern to equine welfare, as there is the potential to repeatedly expose horses to aversive stimuli over which they have no control. For example, pain through the misuse of tack and equipment or fear through punishment-based training. This leaves the horse at increased risk of learned helplessness compared to some other species (Hall *et al.*, 2008). In contrast, animals that have previous experience of escaping aversive stimuli are less likely to suffer from learned helplessness when exposed to inescapable aversive stimuli (Rosellini and Seligman, 1975). From this McGreevy *et al.* (2018) suggest training with the correct use of reinforcement. Cognitive bias testing has the potential to minimize the risk of learned helplessness developing in horses.

Welfare

Welfare involves the physical, psychological and behavioural experience of an animal. There are several risks to welfare for horses kept intensively for human purposes. For horses, constant confinement without a broad visual field and with restriction of activity can have adverse effects. Horses need access to move freely through regular turnout, social companionship and prolonged foraging time. Although a horse's physical condition may be managed in the stable, its emotional condition is likely to be adversely affected by the restricted environment. In many cases, if the restrictive husbandry is constant, the animal's natural activities become redirected, so to speak, into anomalous action patterns known as stereotypies, or the horse develops other learned behaviours that are not conducive to a positive horse–human association. These may persist even when a more suitable environment is provided. Equine quality of life involves a balance between the positive and negative emotions experienced by the horse, best demonstrated through assessing everyday behaviour, including general behavioural patterns and responses to training.

Summary

As we move from an era where good welfare was considered to relate to the absence of negative states to one in which we are actively looking for evidence of positive ones, and the use of the horse for recreation is increasingly scrutinized, the outlook for improved equine welfare looks increasingly positive.

References

Archer, D.C., Pinchbeck, G.L., French, N.P. and Proudman, C.J. (2008) Risk factors for epiploic foramen entrapment colic: An international study *Equine Veterinary Journal* 40, 224–230.

Beaver, B.V. (1994) *The Veterinarian's Encyclopedia of Animal Behaviour.* Iowa State University Press, Ames, Iowa.

Blood, D.C. and Studdert, V.P. (1988) *Baillière's Comprehensive Veterinary Dictionary*. Bailliere Tindall, London.
Briefer Freymond, S., Briefer, E.F., Niederhäusern, R.V. and Bachmann, I. (2013) Pattern of social interactions after group integration: A possibility to keep stallions in group. *PLoS ONE* 8, e54688.
Briefer Freymond, S., Ruet, A., Grivaz, M., Fuentes, C., Zuberbühler, K. *et al.* (2019) Stereotypic horses (*Equus caballus*) are not cognitively impaired. *Animal Cognition* 22, 17–33.
Dalla Costa, E., Minero, M., Lebelt, D., Stucke, D., Canali, E. *et al.* (2014) Development of the horse grimace scale (HGS) as a pain assessment tool in horses undergoing routine castration. *PLoS ONE* 9, e92281.
Dalla Costa, E.D., Stucke, D., Dai, F., Minera, M., Leach, M.C. *et al.* (2016) Using the horse grimace scale (HGS) to assess pain associated with acute laminitis in horses (*Equus caballus*). *Animals* 6, 47.
Dyson, S. and van Dijk, J. (2018) Application of a ridden horse ethogram to video recordings of 21 horses before and after diagnostic analgesia: Reduction in behaviour scores. *Equine Veterinary Education* 32 (Supplement 10), 104–111.
Dyson, S., Berger, J., Ellis, A.D. and Millard, J. (2018) Development of an ethogram for a pain scoring system in ridden horses and its application to determine the presence of musculoskeletal pain. *Journal of Veterinary Behavior* 23, 47–57.
Guillemin, R.A. and Rosenberg, B. (1955) Humoral hypothalamic control of anterior pituitary: A study with combined tissue cultures. *Endocrinology* 57, 599–607.
Hall, C., Goodwin, D., Heleski, C., Randle, H. and Waran, N. (2008) Is there evidence of learned helplessness in horses? *Journal of Applied Animal Welfare Science* 11, 249–266.
Hemmings, A., McBride, S.D. and Hale, C.E. (2007) Perseverative responding and the aetiology of equine oral stereotypy. *Applied Animal Behaviour Science* 104, 143–150.
Henderson, J.V. and Waran, N.K. (2001) Reducing equine stereotypies using an Equiball™. *Animal Welfare* 10, 73–80.
Kiley-Worthington, M. (1987) *The Behaviour of Horses in Relation to Management and Training.* J.A. Allen and Company Publishers, London.
Korte, S.M. (2001) Corticosteroids in relation to fear, anxiety and psycopathology. *Neuroscience Biobehaviour Review* 25, 117–142.
Mason, G. (2006) Stereotypic behaviour in captive animals: Fundamentals and implications for welfare and beyond. In: Mason, G. and Rushen, J. (eds) *Stereotypic Animal Behavior: Fundamentals and Applications to Welfare.* CABI International, Wallingford, UK, pp. 97–118.
McAfee, L.M., Mills, D.S. and Cooper, J.J. (2002). The use of mirrors for the control of stereotypic weaving behaviour in the stabled horse. *Applied Animal Behaviour Science* 78, 159–173.
McBride, S. and Hemmings, A. (2009) A neurologic perspective of equine stereotypy. *Journal of Equine Veterinary Science* 29, 10–16.
McEwen, B.S. (2001) Protective and damaging effects of stress mediators: lessons learned from the immune system and brain. In: Broom, D.M. (ed.) *Coping with Challenge: Welfare in Animals Including Humans*. Dahlem University Press, Berlin, pp. 229–246.
McGreevy, P.D. (1995) The functional significance of stereotypies in the stabled horse. PhD thesis. University of Bristol, Bristol, UK.
McGreevy, P.D., Richardson, J.D., Nicol, C.J. and Lane, J.G. (1995) Radiographic and endoscopic study of horses performing an oral based stereotypy. *Equine Veterinary Journal* 27, 92–95.
McGreevy, P.D., Winther Christensen, J., Konig von Borstel, U. and McLean, A. (2018) *Stress and Fear Responses. Equitation Science,* 2nd edn. John Wiley and Sons Ltd., Chichester, UK.
McLean, A.N. and Christensen, J.W. (2017) The application of learning theory in horse training. *Applied Animal Behaviour Science* 190, 18–27.
Merl, S., Scherzers, S., Palme, R. and Möstl, E. (2000) Pain causes increased concentrations of glucocorticoid metabolites in horse feces. *Journal of Equine Veterinary Science* 20, 586–590.
Moberg, G. and Mench, J.A. (2000) *The Biology of Animal Stress: Basic Principles and Implications for Animal Welfare.* CAB International, Wallingford, UK.
Morris, R. (2007) Stress and the hippocampus. In: Anderson, P., Morris, R., Amaral, D. *et al.* (eds) *The Hippocampus Book.* Oxford University Press, New York.
Möstl, E. and Palme, R. (2002) Hormones as indicators of stress. *Domestic Animal Endocrinology* 23, 67–74.
Nicol, C. (1999) Understanding equine stereotypies. *Equine Veterinary Journal,* 31, 20–25.
Poletto, R., Steibel, J.P., Siegford, J.M. and Zanella, A.J. (2006) Effects of early weaning and social isolation on the expression of glucocorticoid and mineralocorticoid receptor and 11 beta-hydroxysteroid dehydrogenase 1 and 2 mRNAs in the frontal cortex and hippocampus of piglets. *Brain Research* 11067, 36–42.
Rosellini, R.A. and Seligman, M.E. (1975) Frustration and learned helplessness. *Journal of Experimental Psychology: Animal Behavior Processes* 1, 149–157.
Seligman, M.E. and Maier, S.F. (1967) Failure to escape traumatic shock. *Journal of Experimental Psychology* 74, 1–9.
Sutton, G.A., Paltiel, O., Soffer, M. and Turner, D. (2013) Validation of two behaviour-based pain scales for horses with acute colic. *The Veterinary Journal* 197, 646–650.
Zollinger, A., Wyss, C., Bardou, D., Ramseyer, A. and Bachman, I. (2016) The 'social box' offers stallions the possibility to have increased social interactions. *Journal of Veterinary Behavior: Clinical Applications and Research* 15, 84–84.

14 Humane Control, Training and Husbandry

Christopher B. Riley BVSc(Hons), PhD, Diplomate, ACVS*

Massey University, Palmerston North, New Zealand

Introduction	195
Background	196
Learning Principles	196
Non-associative learning	196
Associative learning	199
Training Principles	200
General	200
Round pen (ring) breaking	201
General Handling and Restraint	201
Overview	201
Leg restraint	203
The upper lip twitch	203
Stocks	204
Chemical restraint	205
Recumbent restraint	205
Preventative Health and Welfare Programmes	205
End-of-life Welfare	206
References	208

Introduction

Effective restraint reduces the horse's mobility for short periods to allow the safe completion of necessary procedures. Minimum discomfort to the horse and maximum safety to the operator are the criteria. This goal is best facilitated by training that utilizes equine learning theory to reduce the effects of negative or painful stimuli that engender responses that put both at risk of injury (Starling *et al.*, 2016). Such procedures should not cause harm or incapacitate the animal but only briefly limit its freedom of movement for its well-being. Control or training involving unnecessary pain and suffering is unethical and publicly inadmissible. Older practices such as casting a conscious horse with ropes and hobbles are objectionable, resulting in marked distress, and increasing the risk of severe injuries (Fig. 14.1) (Hayes, 1889). Electric shock devices for crib-biting and other painful devices in training are abusive and, in many jurisdictions, illegal. Harsh restraint by any means for any significant period is regarded as cruelty under modern animal welfare codes. It is not a substitute for careful training or, if necessary, the use of sedatives and analgesics for more painful or invasive procedures.

*Corresponding author: c.b.riley@massey.ac.nz

DOI: 10.1079/9781789242133.0014

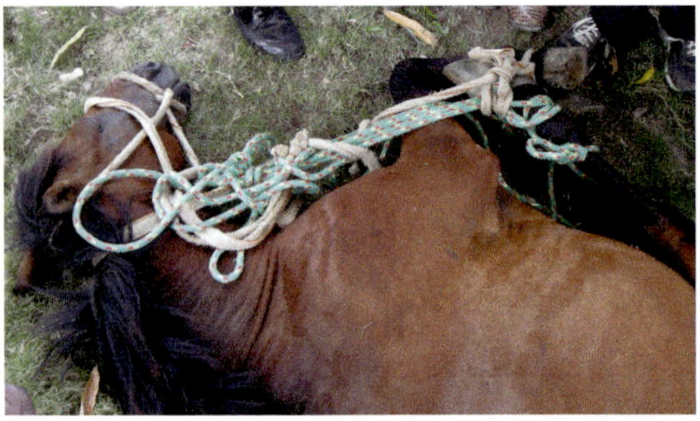

Fig. 14.1. A horse tied for castration after injection of anaesthetic agents. Restraint of a horse without marked sedation and analgesia or general anaesthesia is inappropriate and risks injury, pain and distress. Photo: author.

Background

To maintain our social license, we must recognize the exercise of control that is humane and beneficial to the horse from that which is inhumane and detrimental. To that end, the International Society for Equestrian Science (ISES) has developed principles of ethical equitation that seek to manage and train horses in ways that avoid initiating and reinforcing behaviours that endanger it and the handler (Table 14.1) (ISES, 2018). If a form of control is questionable (e.g., prolonged use of the lip twitch), the horse should be given the benefit of the doubt. Understanding the horse's ethology and cognition should be borne in mind as a guiding principle (McGreevy *et al.*, 2018b). Formerly, the first step towards control of an untamed horse was breaking, quickly imposing mastery over the animal's natural sense of self. In principle, this approach ropes the horse, forcibly puts on a bridle and bit, fixes on some harness and a girth, then firmly restrains it while directed in various ways within an enclosure. This enforcement is continued until the horse's resistance is diminished with fatigue. Although still practised in many regions, this approach is giving way to a more sympathetic one that emphasizes the application of scientific and ethically based principles (Visser *et al.*, 2009).

The domesticated horse is taught comprehensively to accept all the controls imposed upon its life. Lessons are given in the form of training. A horse must learn to respond acceptably to a variety of unnatural tasks and circumstances, including stable control (Fig. 14.2). The instruction needed to implant the desired lessons in the horse calls for knowledge and aptitude from the handler.

Learning Principles

To adapt to its environment, the horse makes continuous modifications to its conduct. Much of training is dependent on this modification process and underlying factors intrinsic to the horse (Fig. 14.3). A domesticated horse is required to learn to perform numerous acts that are not intrinsic to its nature. There is a great deal of anecdotal information about equine learning and training and, until recently, substantial resistance to and suspicion of scientific approaches to the education of horses (Thompson and Haigh, 2018; Beaver, 2019). In many ways, the ISES training principles are a product of cooperation between equestrians and equine scientists. At first glance, these principles appear to be straightforward. However, their implementation requires the reader to have an in-depth understanding of equine behaviour and learning theory as well as the practical ability to apply them to the horse. There have been substantial gains in the scientific underpinning of some of these principles, but further advances in knowledge are needed in some fields such as equine emotion (Hall *et al.*, 2018). Such advances require collaboration across research disciplines and effective communication strategies that will ultimately advance equine welfare (King *et al.*, 2018; Randle and Waran, 2019).

An extensive review of learning theory and its application to the training of horses is beyond the scope of this book. Nevertheless, some key concepts are introduced here. For more in-depth coverage, readers may consult other useful texts (McGreevy *et al.*, 2018b). Where possible, training builds upon the pre-existing motivations and responses of the horse. Tasks must be within the horse's behavioural, sensory and physical capacities to perform the activities desired of it (Beaver, 2019). Training is most effective when it uses the associative and non-associative learning processes of the horse.

Non-associative learning

Non-associative learning occurs when a single stimulus results in habituation or sensitization. Habituation is a form of learning where the subject has a progressively decreasing response to the same repeated sensory stimulation. This allows natural adaptation to dynamic environments in which many stimuli are not consequential and can therefore

Table 14.1. 2018 International Society for Equestrian Science Training Principles. Adapted from ISES, 2018

Principles
1. Regard for human and horse safety
Acknowledge the size, power and flight behaviour of the horse
Recognize flight, fight and freeze behaviours early
Minimize methods or equipment that risk causing pain, distress or injury
Avoid provoking aggressive/defensive behaviours (e.g. kicking, biting)
Ensure recognition of the horse's dangerous zones (e.g. hindquarters)
Recognize the dangers of being inconsistent or confusing
Use tools, equipment and the environment safely
Ensure horses and humans are appropriately matched in skill and temperament
2. Regard for the nature of the horse
Ensure welfare needs: foraging, equine social, freedom of movement
Avoid aversive management practices (e.g. ear-twitching)
Avoid assuming a role for dominance
Recognize signs of pain and distress
Respect the social nature of horses (e.g. touch, effects of separation)
Avoid movements horses may perceive as threatening or predatory
3. Regard for horses' mental (cognitive) and sensory abilities
Avoid overestimating the horse's mental abilities
Avoid underestimating/undervaluing the horse's mental abilities
Acknowledge that horses see and hear differently from humans
Avoid long training sessions (minimize repetitions to avoid overloading)
Avoid assuming the horse thinks as humans do; they do not
Avoid implying mental states when describing and interpreting horse behaviour
4. Regard for current emotional states
Avoid the use of pain or constant discomfort in training
Avoid triggering flight, fight or freeze reactions
Maintain minimum arousal for the task during training
Help the horse to relax with stroking and voice
Encourage the horse to adopt relaxed postures as part of training (e.g. head lowering)
Avoid high arousal when using tactile or food motivators
Don't underestimate horse's capacity to suffer
Encourage positive emotional states in training
5. Correct use of habituation/desensitization calming methods
Gradually approach objects that the horse is afraid of or, if possible, gradually bring such aversive objects closer to the horse (systematic desensitization)
Gain control of the horse's limb movements (e.g. step the horse back) while aversive objects are kept at a safe distance and gradually brought closer (overshadowing)
Associate aversive stimuli with pleasant outcomes by giving food treats when the horse perceives the scary object (counter conditioning)
Ignore undesirable behaviours and reinforce desirable alternative responses (differential reinforcement)
Avoid flooding techniques (i.e. forcing the horse to endure aversive stimuli)
6. Correct use of operant conditioning
Understand how operant conditioning works: i.e. the performance of behaviours become more or less likely as a result of their consequences
Tactile pressures must be removed at the onset of the correct response (e.g. from the bit, leg, spur or whip)
Minimize delays in reinforcement because they are ineffective and unethical
Use combined reinforcement (amplify pressure-release rewards with tactile or food rewards where appropriate)
Avoid active punishment
7. Correct use of classical conditioning
Train the uptake of light signals by placing them before a pressure-release sequence

Continued

Table 14.1. Continued.

Principles
Precede all desirable responses with light signals
Avoid unwanted stimuli overshadowing desired responses (e.g. the horse may associate an undesirable response with an unintended signal from the environment)
8. Correct use of shaping
Break down training tasks into the smallest achievable steps and progressively reinforce each step toward the desired behaviour
Plan training to make the correct response as obvious and easy as possible
Maintain a consistent environment to train a new task and give the horse the time to learn safely and calmly
Only change one contextual aspect at a time (e.g. trainer, place, signal)
9. Correct use of signals and cues
Ensure signals are easy for the horse to discriminate from one another
Ensure each signal has only one meaning
Ensure signals for different responses are never applied concurrently
Ensure locomotory signals are applied in timing with limb biomechanics
10. Regard for self-carriage
Training the horse to maintain gait, tempo, stride length, direction, head, neck and body posture
Avoid forcing a posture or maintaining it mechanically or by relentless signalling

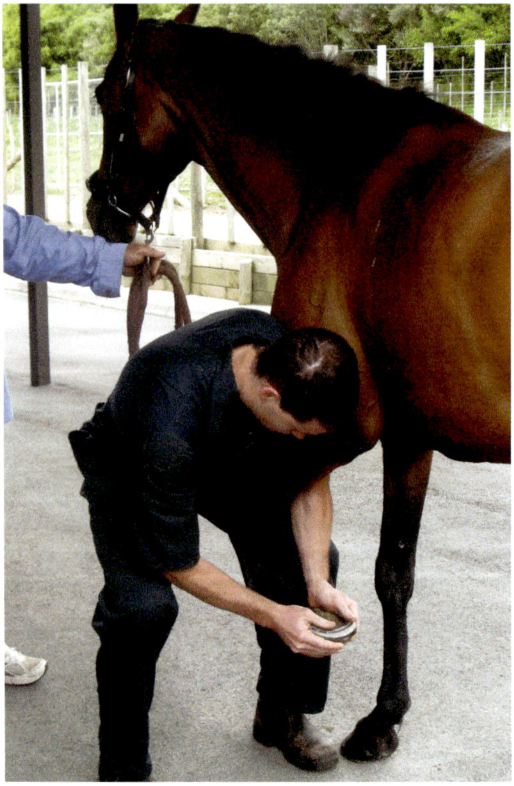

Fig. 14.2. The horse must become accustomed to many routine husbandry procedures such as hoof examination. Photo: author.

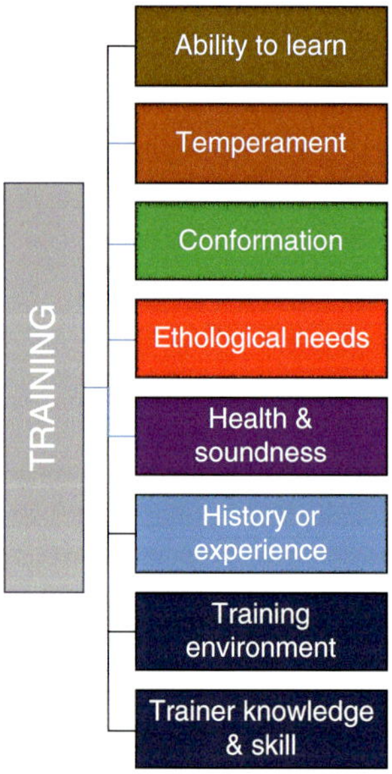

Fig. 14.3. Training considerations. Diagram: author.

be ignored. For example, a horse may adapt to trailer loading by placing it in the paddock and feeding the horse in it repeatedly (Houpt and Wickens, 2019). Habituation can result from a range of training techniques to moderate responses to novel objects (Leiner and Fendt, 2011). These approaches exploit the investigative behaviours of the horse (McLean and Christensen, 2017).

Techniques include systematic desensitization, counterconditioning, overshadowing, response prevention (flooding) and negative reinforcement (Christensen, 2013).

Systematic desensitization provides gradual habituation to the stimulus in a controlled situation. The horse is introduced to the stimulus at a low level and then rewarded for remaining unresponsive or showing an appropriate (trainer desired) response. The level or frequency of the stimulus is progressively increased when the horse does not react to the previous level of exposure.

Counterconditioning trains the horse to show the desired behaviour that differs (i.e. counter) from the one to be eliminated. Often used with systematic desensitization, the horse learns that our desired behaviour is more rewarding, and the stimulus that initiates the counter behaviour is an indicator of a positive and not an aversive event.

Overshadowing describes habituation to the least salient stimulus when two or more stimuli competing for the same response are presented simultaneously (McLean, 2008). It uses mobility responses such as stepping back and forward to modify undesired or fearful responses to noxious stimuli such as needles or clippers (Pearson, 2015).

Response prevention (flooding) is aimed at having the horse learn an appropriate alternative response to the stimulus by inhibiting reinforcement of the fear response. Briefly, the horse is restrained to remain in the situation it fears until resistance ceases. The situation or stimulus is not withdrawn until the horse ceases to respond. However, if the horse is still in a state of heightened arousal at the time the stimulus is removed, the undesired response may be reinforced. The use of flooding as a desensitization technique may result in learned helplessness, and its incorrect application is a welfare concern (Preshaw *et al.*, 2017).

Approach conditioning exploits the exploratory tendency of the horse for novel objects in unison with systematic desensitization (Christensen, 2013). In this situation, the horse is brought towards the fear-inducing stimulus while the latter is simultaneously withdrawn. The horse's approach is stopped when it slows or shows other evidence of approaching its fear threshold. The process is repeated until the horse is comfortable when it is as close to the object as possible. The method is used for horses fearful of vehicles and mechanized equipment.

Stimulus blending involves the gradual exposure of the horse to a fear-inducing stimulus concurrently with a known stimulus that it does not fear. This is repeated systematically with increasing exposure to the fear-inducing stimulus. The sensory characteristics of the fear-inducing stimulus are gradually blended with the habituated one, impeding recognition of the aversive stimulus. Slowly, the non-fear-inducing habituated stimulus is withdrawn and replaced by habituation to the novel stimulus.

Contrary to habituation, sensitization is a process whereby the response intensity is increased. In this situation, there is an increase in the response associated with repeated presentations of the stimulus so that, eventually, the stimulus is perceived as noxious by the horse (McLean and Christensen, 2017). If the horse is prevented from avoiding or fleeing the stimulus, it may become increasingly more sensitive to that stimulus. A horse thus sensitized often shows heightened awareness and increased responsiveness to a range of other stimuli in addition to the one to which it has been primed.

Associative learning

Associative learning (conditioning) is any learning process in which a new response becomes associated with a particular stimulus in close association with time or space (McGreevy *et al.*, 2018b). Learning that involves links between two or more signals results in classical conditioning. Learning that establishes links between signals or a horse's actions and outcomes develop as a result of operant conditioning (McLean and Christensen, 2017).

Classical conditioning is the development of an association between two stimuli. A stimulus that originally has no meaning for the horse (i.e. neutral) is associated with an unconditioned stimulus that has a clear meaning for the animal (e.g., food, pressure). The association develops more rapidly when the frequency and consistency of the neutral and unconditioned stimulus pairing increases. An example of classical conditioning occurs when handlers take a horse into a box to urinate after a race to collect urine for medication testing. The handler first conditions the horse as part of its race training preparation by whistling each time the horse urinates. Once the association is established, the handler whistles when the horse is placed in the box, and it responds by urinating. A common application is pairing a food reward with verbal praise (McGreevy *et al.*, 2018b).

Operant conditioning is a type of associative learning in which its antecedent and consequence modify a voluntary behaviour. It works by giving or taking away a reward (attractive) or discomfort (aversive) stimulus when the horse performs a wanted or unwanted behaviour through the following chain: stimulus–behaviour–reinforcement or punishment (McLean and Christensen, 2017). A reinforcer is used as a consequence that increases the future likelihood of the wanted behaviour. Punishment is used as a consequence that decreases the future likelihood of the unwanted behaviour. Reinforcers and punishers may be external or internal to the horse; there are positive and negative forms for both.

Positive reinforcement is the addition of an appetitive (e.g. food), verbal, or tactile stimulus in response to the occurrence of the desired behaviour. The higher the perceived value of the positive reinforcement to the horse, the stronger the reward. The delivery of the reward should occur immediately after the desired behaviour to enable the horse to learn the association rapidly. In the case of tactile rewards, neck scratching is more rewarding and reassuring to a horse than patting or slapping its neck and is associated with affiliative grooming behaviour (Hancock *et al.*, 2014; Thorbergson *et al.*, 2015). Auditory cues may be used as secondary positive reinforcers. For example, clicker training uses a primary positive reinforcer, usually food, to develop an association via classical conditioning. Thereafter, the clicker is used to reward horses for displaying the desired behaviour. Compared with negative reinforcement training, horses trained under a positive reinforcement schedule are more motivated to participate in training sessions and exhibit more exploratory or trial-and-error type behaviours in novel situations (Innes and McBride, 2008).

Negative reinforcement is associated with the removal of an aversive stimulus (e.g. pressure) as soon as the wanted behaviour is offered. It is the most commonly used approach to horse training, riding and handling (McLean and Christensen, 2017). The stimulus may be frightening, painful or merely uncomfortable. For example, a rider applies leg pressure (discomfort), and the pressure is released as a horse moves forward. Other aids such as reins, whips, spurs and seat pressure utilize the same principle. However, great care is required in the application of this approach, as negative reinforcement may result in an undesired outcome. For example, a horse inadvertently left tied inside a trailer while the handler vocalizes and agitates for it to back out may have its fear of being transported reinforced.

Positive punishment uses a negative consequence (aversive stimulus) to eliminate or lower the frequency of undesired behaviour. The application, timing and intensity of any punishment influences its effectiveness. Poor judgment on the part of the trainer increases the risk of it becoming abusive. Exploration of an electrified fence may result in a negative consequence for what is otherwise a natural behaviour. Unfortunately, positive punishment can compromise the horse's welfare. Undesirable responses to positive punishment include learned helplessness in response to habituation to punishment; learning deficits; fear of, or aversion to the punisher; ingrained fear reactions; lowered motivation for natural behaviours or exploring new ones; and psychosocial distress (Lansade *et al.*, 2008; McGreevy and McLean, 2009).

Negative punishment is the withdrawal of a positive stimulus (e.g. food) in response to unwanted behaviour. It is less frequently used in equine training. For example, when a horse flattens its ears and extends its neck in an aggressive posture at feeding time, the handler may stop moving towards the horse or retreat (Beaver, 2019). There are no benefits to using this approach to reprimand a horse for poor competitive or race performance. The horse cannot establish an association between performance and the withdrawal of a positive stimulus.

Combined reinforcement is when positive reinforcement is used in conjunction with negative reinforcement to enhance training outcomes. When both types of reinforcement are combined, the aversive effects of negative reinforcement are reduced (Warren-Smith and McGreevy, 2007).

Training Principles

General

A good trainer has practical or intuitive knowledge of horse behaviour. This was thought sufficient to give the trainer the ability to understand a particular horse. Whereas this approach still applies in many jurisdictions and within the racing industries, during the last ten years, there has been a progressive move to the training of horses for equestrian activities based on the ISES principles underpinned by a knowledge of equine learning theory and the five domains (Baragli *et al.*, 2015; McLean and Christensen, 2017; McGreevy *et al.*, 2018a).

Ideally, the training of any horse takes place in a step-by-step progression (Visser *et al.*, 2009). The first step is to observe and evaluate the horse's temperament. The trainer should get to know the horse by studying it and watching it under various circumstances. The first impression of a horse should indicate whether the horse's temperament or individuality is one that is appreciated and within the trainer's capabilities.

A simple initiating method commonly used with a young horse is to catch the animal, halter it and attempt to control it for a short period with the aid of the halter rope. This procedure is repeated at subsequent times (i.e. habituation) with intervening intervals of a few days. Three-day intervals are suitable for the horse to learn to accept this form of human control (Schomber *et al.*, 2018). This approach is not considered horse breaking since the animal is given considerable time to adapt to the situation and modify its reactivity. All of this can be helped by promptly rewarding the horse when the desired behaviour occurs. It is a time-consuming method. Haltering regularly from early foalhood obviates the need for this part of initial training. The training of foals often starts with close proximity to the mare and the introduction of directional or other cues (Christensen, 2016). The ISES principles have been applied successfully to the training of foals on busy commercial breeding farms (King *et al.*, 2018)

Round pen (ring) breaking

In the modern form of humane breaking or taming of the untrained horse, the animal is placed in a wide-ringed area (i.e. round pen or lunging yard) that preferably has high, solid sides. The trainer occupies the central area and carries a whip or rope, using arm waving or vocal cues as aversive stimuli (Kydd *et al.*, 2017). In a manner that resembles lunging, the horse is chased so that it runs (i.e. is in flight) around the inside perimeter of the circle. The trainer moves slightly towards the rear of the horse, implying a threat, but remains in the central area while constantly turning to face the horse's location. Without touching the subject, the stimulus is used to keep the horse running at a steady trot after it ceases to gallop. With an occasional change of direction, the horse's running is maintained by the continuing show of pursuit created by the trainer. The animal, in its flight, can only run close against the circular barrier and usually maintains its flight for an extended period. Practitioners claim that this simulates the natural behaviour of the mare chasing young stock, but this assumption is questionable (Warren-Smith and McGreevy, 2008). The aversive stimulus is removed as soon as the desired response emerges, which is generally approaching, remaining close, and following the trainer. This constitutes negative reinforcement. Some trainers recommend a specific duration, from 0.5–2 hours, depending on the horse's basic temperament and the time taken for the stimulus to lose its charge. However, a better approach is to set a stepwise learning objective and then stop the training once each learning step has been achieved (i.e. shaping). The stepwise approach introduces each aid separately, and patient habituation results in reduced fear and stress-related behaviours for the horse (Visser *et al.*, 2009).

Nevertheless, round-pen training results from habituation, operant and classical conditioning. The appropriateness of this form of training continues to be questioned because horses are placed in a situation where they cannot escape from or avoid aversive stimuli (Henshall and McGreevy, 2014). A highly fearful horse poses an injury risk for the trainer.

However, a natural horsemanship approach is considered a less agonistic means to accustom an untamed horse to human management than forceful or domineering methods of breaking. It is used while conditioning animals to the general husbandry procedures to follow (Marlborough and Knottenbelt, 2001).

General Handling and Restraint

Overview

Any form of restraint to immobilize or limit the movement of a horse in training and handling should only be in effect briefly and carried out by experienced handlers. The criteria in early handling are minimum discomfort to the horse and maximum safety for people. No handling procedure should be based on the infliction of pain on the animal. The principal objective is to limit the horse's movement for its own well-being while receiving some form of attention. In a paddock system, it is useful to have a catchment facility to reduce the risk of human injury. Horses at pasture do not readily give up their freedom when a trainer attempts to catch them in the middle of an open field.

Special care must be taken when handling a horse in a narrow and confined space. Where possible, provide the horse with some room to move and reduce its fear of being trapped and explosive escape or aggressive defensive behaviours (McDonnell, 2017). Remove obstacles and loose items such as buckets to prevent fearful or aversive behaviour, particularly if an item is knocked over and creates an auditory stimulus. Horses should be spoken to in a quiet and reassuring tone. They can differentiate between human laughter and growling, with the latter being more likely to cause horses to freeze and adopt vigilance behaviours (Smith *et al.* 2018). Louder vocal reprimands may induce fear-based behaviours. In the narrow confines of the handling situation, this increases the risk of aversion and injury to the handler.

Horses are great readers of body language, and an upright posture with a relaxed approach to the horse's shoulder should be practised. They are generally habituated to being approached in this way, and this takes account of their visual field. A direct approach to the front of the horse is acceptable only when it and the handler are familiar, with the latter allowing the hand to be sniffed for identification.

As much as horses usually appreciate being scratched on the neck or withers (Fig. 14.4), they generally do not like to be handled in the poll region. They are often sensitive to being touched under the belly, over the lower flank and between the hindlimbs. When it is necessary to touch the belly or lower flank, a hand is placed on the neck or withers and run firmly but gently along the back to the hindquarters, on the way down to the limbs. The legs and feet should be touched last in handling and grooming. This approach trains the horse to accept handling and grooming procedures. To lift a hind leg the handler stands beside the limb, facing the rear, grasps the fetlock and draws it forward and upwards. The hoof is taken in the other cupped hand. While bent over and holding the hoof, a step is taken to the horse's rear so that the cannon rests on the handler's thigh. The arm towards the horse is then put over the animal's hock so that the elbow helps to control the horse's leg. The upturned hind hoof can then be held, cleaned and inspected. Any signs of threat in a horse should be known and heeded as a warning of the probable reaction of the animal. Failure to heed the warning risks injury. The handler should clearly signal to the horse any intended handling procedure (Fraser, 2010).

Any location where the horse is restrained for examination, or a special procedure, should have non-slip flooring. Examination places may become slippery with manure and urine of a horse being

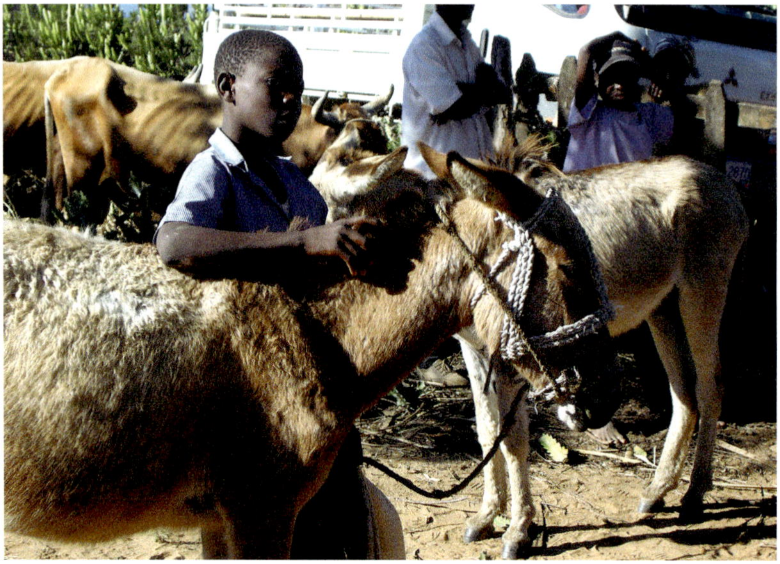

Fig. 14.4. A scratch on the neck is preferred to a pat. Photo: author.

examined and should be kept clean. In the general handling of horses, appropriate use and choice of the bit and bridle, if necessary, are of critical importance. Horses should be accustomed to this means of head control by appropriate training. This conditions them for the circumstances of handling. For example, to control the head and hold the mouth open for a dental examination, the horse's tongue can be grasped and held outside the corner of the mouth.

In handling and controlling horses, it is necessary to apply knowledge of their natural mechanics of movement. The horse can use its head and strong neck to resist handling. Therefore, it is essential for the head to be secured as a first step in the control of the animal. In some circumstances raising the head can be used to control attempts by the horse to move forward. A common method of head control is to back the horse into a stall and crosstie its halter to the stall posts. The unhabituated horse should not be left alone in this position. In addition, control over the muzzle restrains the horse very effectively. Fig. 14.5 illustrates one method of control using the Chifney bit, frequently used with stallions.

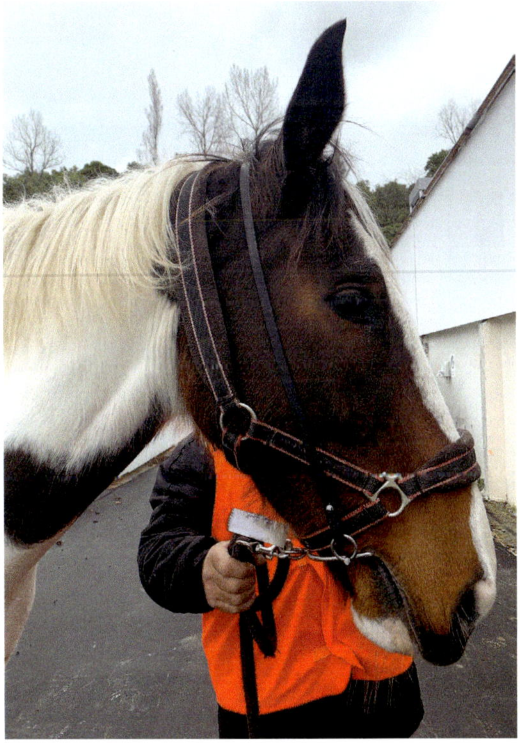

Fig. 14.5. Stallion led with a Chifney bit to assist with control. This ring bit applies direct force and is not weakened by joints, as on the snaffle bit. Photo: author.

Leg restraint

The limb movements of a horse require control in a variety of circumstances. In its simplest form, the forefoot is held with the knee flexed while the toe of the hoof is grasped by one hand with the bridle-rein held with the other or steadied by catching hold of the mane. This is a precaution against being struck. A physically effective means of controlling kicking with the hindlimbs uses a sideline or hobbles (see Figs 14.6a and 14.6b). Here, a leather hobble or noose on a rope is placed around the fetlock region of each hind leg and the rope, secured to a collar, placed around the base of the neck. Training horses to this and other mechanical limb constraints rely upon flooding, as the horse cannot escape. Sidelines are commonly used on studs and are popular in regions where horses cannot be tied or confined, such as open rangelands. However, there has not been a critical review of their use and effect on equine welfare. A recent workshop on applying the five domains to equine welfare did not consider this form of restraint (McGreevy *et al.*, 2018a). Strapping a forelimb in the flexed position by means of a leather strap applied around the pastern and forearm and tying them in this fashion with a piece of rope falls within the same category (Fig.14.6c). The forelimb may be held briefly, avoiding compromising blood circulation, in the flexed position by means of a rope tied around the pastern and passed over the horse's withers but risks a rope burn or worse for an uncooperative horse.

The upper lip twitch

The judicious application of an upper lip twitch to provide a brief period of restraint should only be performed by a skilled person. The standard twitch is a loop on the end of a wooden shaft or hollow plastic tube. The loop is put around the horse's upper lip, and the handle/shaft is twisted to snare the lip firmly (Fig. 14.7). The twitch should enclose an adequate portion of the upper lip. It is then quickly tightened until the horse shows the first sign of rigidity in the way the head is held. The person applying the twitch must judge the exact amount of time and pressure based on the horse's behaviour. If the horse continues to resist the twitch once it has

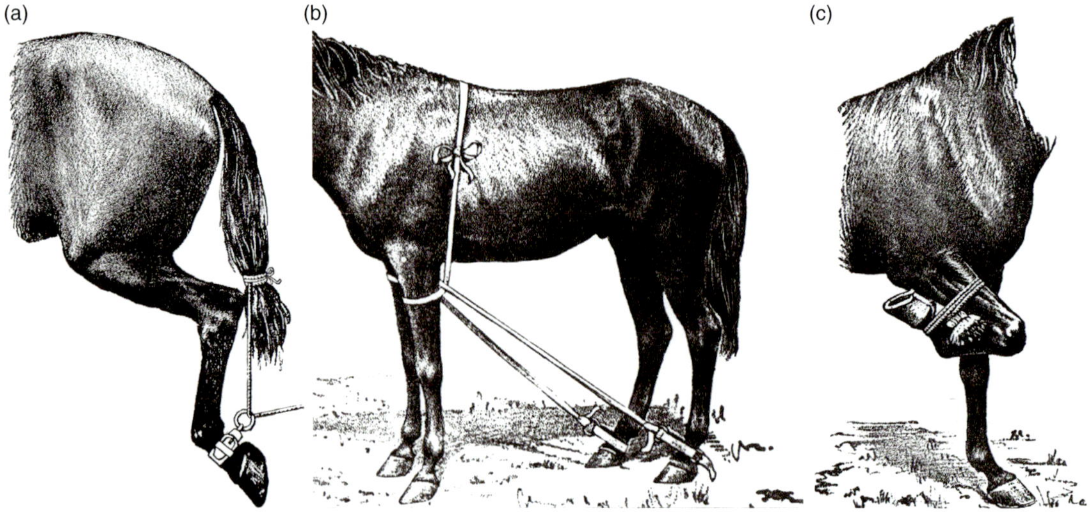

Fig. 14.6. (a) Control of hind leg with rope tie. (b) Sidelines. (c) Control of foreleg with rope tie. Drawings: D. Cody.

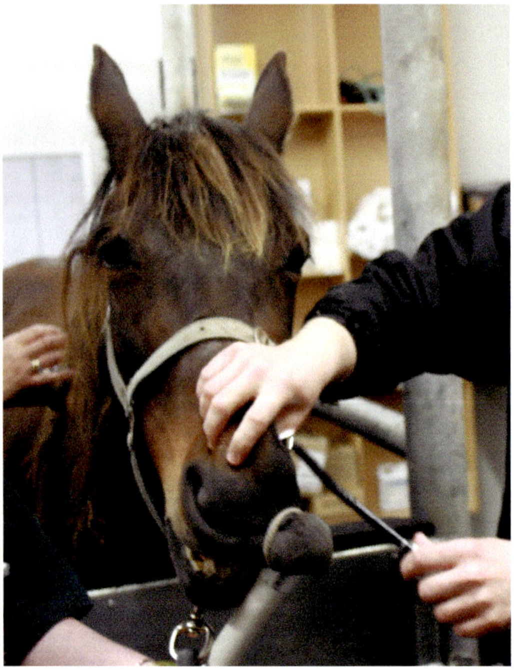

Fig. 14.7. An upper lip twitch has been applied to facilitate the safe passage of an endoscope through the nares to examine the airways. Photo: author.

been appropriately tightened, it should be removed, and the horse restrained by some other means. The twitch should only be used for short procedures of 5 minutes or less because, after this time, restraint causes pain rather than the initial beta-endorphin release associated with its use (Flaköll *et al.*, 2017). Experienced horses show no aversion to repeated twitching, but horses with a history of aversion should not be twitched. Recent research confirms that the restraint effects of an ear twitch are mediated by fear or pain, and this should not be used as a method of restraint (Flaköl *et al.*, 2017).

Stocks

Stocks (crushes) are sometimes used in the control of horses for veterinary examination and procedures. If constructed of solid posts and side pieces such stocks are useful in protecting the horse and people working with it. Procedures such as rectal examination and attention to the feet can be performed more effectively on a horse restrained within stocks. They should be appropriate in size for the horse being examined to ensure close restraint, ensuring the least amount of movement. The stocks should also be structurally secure yet have removable sides should the horse fall. The sidebars should not be at a height that would permit the horse to kick over the top of them and entrap a leg. Some horses may tend to panic when firmly restrained in stocks and must be gradually trained or conditioned to their use. It should never be assumed that the stocks fully protect the handler; many human injuries occur from distressed horses in stocks.

Chemical restraint

Chemical restraint uses drugs to influence or modify a horse's behaviour, reduce fear and increase the threshold to noxious stimuli. Modern chemical agents of varied pharmacological activities make it possible to alter a horse's behaviour by tranquillization or sedation. These drugs are commonly used when a horse is subjected, for a period, to forms of total restraint or handling to which they are unaccustomed and could induce a state of panic detrimental to their health. Tranquillizers induce calm in anxious horses without physiological depression or clouding of consciousness. They are more effective if given before the horse is stimulated.

The most commonly used drugs are acepromazine and the alpha-adrenergic agonists xylazine, detomidine and romifidine. Acepromazine provides a longer tranquillization period but rarely results in complications affecting the penis of stallions and geldings. Xylazine provides predictable short-term sedation as well as short-term pain relief for some gastrointestinal conditions. However, it is not recommended for noxious procedures of the hindlimbs. Some horses under the influence of xylazine may be hypersensitive to touch in this region. Detomidine provides more profound and prolonged sedation and is commonly used for more noxious or fear-inducing procedures. However, some horses struggle to maintain an upright posture at higher doses. Both acepromazine and detomidine come in oral formulations that may be dispensed by a veterinarian and given by the owner or trainer. Like all medications, a thorough knowledge of their use and associated complications is critical, and thus they should only be administered with veterinary guidance. They do not replace the need for appropriate expertise in the handling of horses and do not eliminate the risk of injury associated with painful or fear-inducing procedures.

Recumbent restraint

Drugs administered by a veterinarian are more frequently used today to assist in getting the horse to lie down. Resultant recumbency can be hazardous and requires supervision by an experienced veterinarian. This method of control is usually used out of necessity for major surgical operations when total restraint is essential for success and safety (Fig. 14.8). This ensures the safety of both the veterinarian and the animal. The obsolete process of casting the conscious horse with ropes and hobbles is a source of stress and alarm to the animal and exposes it to injury while struggling. The use of muscle paralysing drugs alone to cast the conscious horse is both inhumane and dangerous for the animal. The availability of modern drugs that induce very transient periods of unconsciousness enables necessary noxious procedures to be performed in a way that should be safe and humane.

Preventative Health and Welfare Programmes

A modern and advisable system of horse care involves a health programme for a single horse or several under the same management. A health and welfare programme provides assurance and guidance on matters of preventative medicine for the horse caregiver. This operates by having veterinary input into horse husbandry and routine practices to maintain health through preventive medicine. Related visits can be for a prescribed appointment, during which time routine matters such as pregnancy testing, nutrition, teeth checking and floating, health checks, special examination, blood and faecal sampling, deworming, and vaccination advice is obtained on a preventive basis. Preventive health programmes vary widely depending on the number of horses, their ages, how they are housed and used, and their geographic location (Sandoval and True, 2012; Thompson *et al.*, 2018).

An important part of infectious disease control is a vaccination programme based on known risks and regional circumstances (Waller, 2014). Effective vaccines are available to protect against many serious, transmissible diseases of horses. Sometimes the immunity obtained by vaccination is of short duration, and annual or semi-annual re-vaccination is necessary. Proper vaccination enables horses to resist or recover more rapidly from common infections. Vaccination against equine influenza, equine herpes and rhinopneumonitis viruses, tetanus, and strangles are most recommended. A veterinarian working in your geographic region is best able to assist in weighing the risks of infection by these organisms with the need for vaccination. Biosecurity protocols and the risk of contact with other horses (e.g. on breeding properties or at competitive horse events) are other considerations.

Routine faecal testing and deworming timetables are other necessary components of an equine health programme. Parasite control involves regular deworming of all the horses at the same time in

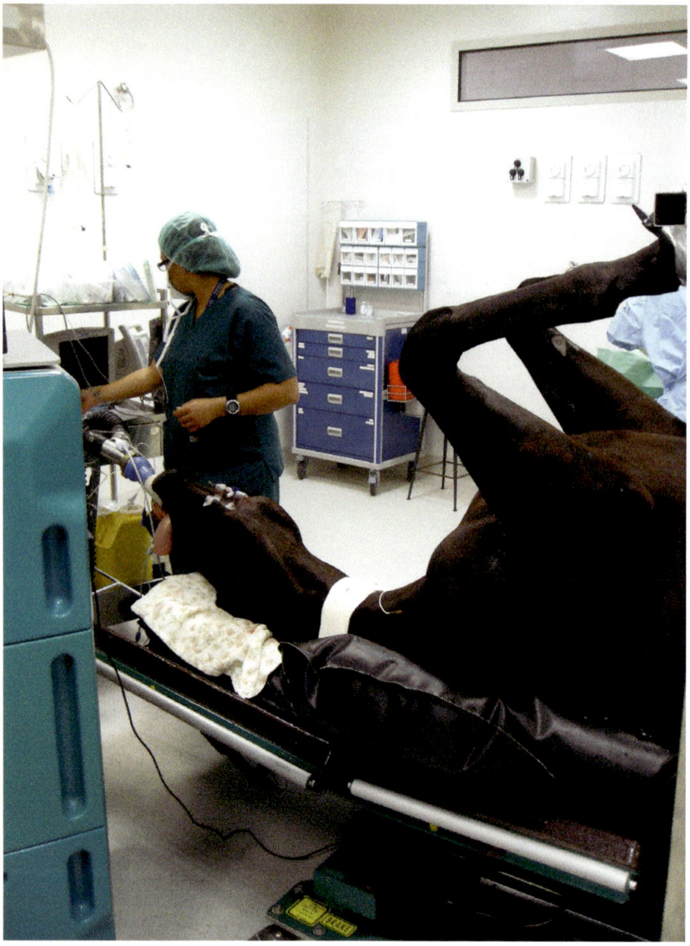

Fig. 14.8. A horse anaesthetized and placed in dorsal recumbency for a surgical procedure. Photo: author.

response to the results of faecal monitoring of a given facility. Faecal examination of any new horse, and periodic faecal examinations of each resident horse, determine the type and amount of parasite infestation. Large strongyles (bloodworms) and roundworms are the most dangerous. Other internal parasites that can depress or endanger a horse's health include small strongyles, pinworms, tapeworms, stomach worms and bots. Modern broad-spectrum anthelmintics are available to kill such internal parasites, but they must be properly selected and accurately dosed. The programme's veterinarian determines a schedule of deworming with recommendations of the anthelmintic used according to factors such as horse condition, the types of parasites found on periodical faecal examinations and the response to deworming.

Horse managers can play a major part in parasite control via pasture management and suitable segregation of animals. Newly weaned horses are very susceptible and should be kept separate from other older horses. Yearlings should be confined to the cleanest possible grazing and have a carefully executed deworming strategy. Newcomers should be quarantined as recommended above for infection control.

End-of-life Welfare

The decision to end the life of an equine companion is perhaps the most difficult one faced by horse carers (Clough *et al.*, 2021). Euthanasia, or 'a good death', describes ending the life of a horse in such a way that pain and stress are minimized or eliminated (Leary *et al.*, 2020). Humane euthanasia means that death is induced in a manner in the animal's interest and/or because of welfare concerns, in a rapid, painless and as distress-free manner as possible. It is the horse owner's responsibility to make this decision, aided in the case of a severe, sudden, or chronic ailment by a veterinarian. In the case of the unwanted horse or one that cannot be rehomed, abandonment is not a humane option and may lead to a prolonged and painful death. Perhaps because of the difficulty in making these decisions, delayed euthanasia (and therefore continued suffering) is considered one of the most pressing modern equine welfare issues (Horseman *et al.*, 2016). Owners have cited costs associated with the termination of life and carcass disposal (i.e. financial reason) as reasons for the delay; these do not justify prolonged suffering for the horse.

Owens (2019) has suggested that sending a horse to slaughter is an approach to euthanasia of unwanted horses that allows owners to get a small financial return to cover transport costs. However, this option must be critically weighed against the considerable welfare costs (i.e. injury and psychosocial distress) associated with transporting the horse, especially if it is ill, debilitated or unaccustomed to transport.

Carcass disposal is a major concern for many owners. In many cases, owners do not have a property on which the horse can be buried, or local waste management statutes prohibit burial. Furthermore, for horses euthanized with chemical agents, these residues may pose a hazard to wildlife and domestic animals. Cremation is available in some jurisdictions, but it's often expensive, requires transport of the horse carcass to the facility and is performed at a substantial environmental cost. Animal composting is also available in some locations.

The slaughter of horses for meat employs euthanasia within a different context than that when considering end-of-life decisions for a horse suffering from an acute or chronic painful condition. These are usually otherwise healthy horses, euthanized to produce an agricultural product. Here, the focus should be on reducing any pain and suffering before the horse's final moments and using handling techniques that minimize stress. Humane slaughter is defined as the animal being killed instantly or rendered insensible until death ensues (Browning and Veit, 2020). Welfare codes of practice require that stunning methods are used to render the horse insensible prior to the final act of killing. The most common stunning methods used to render the horse unconscious are either the penetrating captive bolt (PCB) or a gunshot directly into the brain. In the case of the PCB, an explosive charge drives a bolt into the skull and renders the animal unconscious. Whereas some PCBs stun the horse, it is preferred to use those that drive through the skull and cause brain death. Once the horse is stunned or killed, it is hoisted, and the vessels within the neck severed to allow the animal to bleed out. It is critical that this procedure is monitored and audited regularly to ensure that it is consistently performed, and that the termination of life is humane.

There are several methods for humane euthanasia. During the procedure, the horse may fall unpredictably or start flailing and thrashing during its final moments. This poses a risk of injury to people facilitating euthanasia of the horse. Although these responses frequently occur, they do not reflect pain or distress in the animal. Nevertheless, they can be distressing to an already upset owner and the person euthanizing the horse. The area for performing euthanasia should be quiet and sheltered and provide an escape route for people should the horse become excited or fall. A soft halter and lead rope are recommended, with the person holding the horse (in the case of intravenous injection) wearing leather gloves to prevent rope burn.

Lethal injection with pentobarbital or a pentobarbital combination is the preferred choice in veterinary performed euthanasia (Christensen, 2013). To ensure the entire volume of the drug is injected quickly, an intravenous catheter can be placed. The horse can then be sedated with acepromazine, xylazine or detomidine. These assist with the horse that is frightened or uncooperative but also has effects on the circulation that may prolong the time to loss of consciousness (Leary *et al.*, 2020). Some veterinarians administer an intravenous anaesthetic protocol before administration of the pentobarbital (Gehlen *et al.*, 2020). This reduces flailing and thrashing but adds to the expense of euthanasia. The entire volume of the lethal agent is injected quickly, and the handler steps away from the horse to a safe distance. When administered at the correct dose, pentobarbital results in loss of cortical electric activity within one minute and brainstem reflexes in 1.5 minutes (Aleman *et al.*, 2015). Heart sounds stop within a minute and electrical activity shortly thereafter. Visible and audible breath sounds stop immediately after injection, although sometimes there are one or two agonal gasps. Death is confirmed by auscultation of the chest to confirm the absence of a heartbeat and the elimination of other bodily reflexes. There are other chemical means for euthanasia available to veterinarians where pentobarbital cannot be used, but these should only be given after induction of general anaesthesia by a veterinarian. Methods that rely on paralysing drugs in a conscious animal are unacceptable (Gehlen *et al.*, 2020).

As indicated above, euthanasia by a PCB or gunshot are considered acceptable methods. However, they should only be performed by well-trained and licensed personnel. Accuracy and safety are paramount. They may be used in circumstances where the disposal of carcasses with barbiturate is prohibited, the meat is to be used for pet food, when appropriate amounts of drugs for euthanasia are unavailable, or multiple animals are to be euthanized. The use of the PCB requires appropriate restraint. Human safety is critical when using a firearm, and the horse should not be manually restrained by a person during its use. If restraint is necessary, the horse should be tied to a wooden structure. Alternatively, food can be placed on the ground to lower the horse's head. In cases where there is stress or distress for the horse and/or the owner, sedation with acepromazine may be performed first. The horse is euthanized with a single bullet placed in the centre of the forehead, just above the eyes. The horse will drop suddenly to the ground. The sound of the gunshot and the sight of the blood may be distressing to owners. There may be twitches, muscle spasms and limited paddling for a short time after the shot.

Irrespective of the method of euthanasia, the process should be carefully discussed and planned with the owner. The owner should be informed as to the steps to be taken, what to expect, and where they are best located to remain safe. After death, the owner may wish to spend some time with the horse. Grief, misgivings and self-doubt are common responses by owners and may require the support of a veterinarian, family, social contacts or a counsellor (Endenburg *et al.*, 1999). There is increasing evidence that the mental well-being of veterinarians that provide these services to horse owners is also affected.

References

Aleman, M., Williams, D.C, Guedes, A. and Madigan, J.E. (2015) Cerebral and brainstem electrophysiologic activity during euthanasia with pentobarbital sodium in horses. *Journal of Veterinary Internal Medicine* 29, 663–672.

Baragli, P., Padalino, B. and Telatin, A. (2015) The role of associative and non-associative learning in the training of horses and implications for the [sic] welfare (a review). *Annali Dell'Istituto Superiore di Sanità* 51, 40–51.

Beaver, B.V. (2019) *Equine Behavioral Medicine.* Academic Press, London.

Browning, H. and Veit, W. (2020) Is humane slaughter possible? *Animals* 10, 799.

Christensen, J.W. (2013) Object habituation in horses: The effect of voluntary versus negatively reinforced approach to frightening stimuli. *Equine Veterinary Journal* 45, 298301.

Christensen, J.W. (2016) Early-life object exposure with a habituated mother reduces fear reactions in foals. *Animal Cognition* 19, 171–179.

Clough, H., Roshier, M., England, G., Burford, J. and Freeman, S. (2021) Qualitative study of the influence of horse-owner relationship during some key events within a horse's lifetime. *Veterinary Record* e79.

Endenburg, N., Kirpensteijn, J. and Sanders, N. (1999) Equine euthanasia: the veterinarian's role in providing owners support. *Anthrozoös* 12, 138–141.

Flaköll, B., Ali, A.B. and Saab, C.Y. (2017) Twitching in veterinary procedures: How does this technique subdue horses? *Journal of Veterinary Behavior* 18, 23–28.

Fraser, A.F. (2010) *The Behaviour and Welfare of the Horse,* 2nd edition. CAB International, Wallingford, UK.

Gehlen, H., Loschelder, J., Merle, R. and Walther, M. (2020) Evaluation of stress response and a standard euthanasia protocol in horses using analysis of heart rate variability. *Animals* 10, 485.

Hall, C., Randle, H., Pearson, G., Preshaw, L. and Waran, N. (2018) Assessing equine emotional state. *Applied Animal Behaviour Science* 205, 183–193.

Hancock, E., Redgate, S. and Hall, C. (2014) The effects of patting and withers scratching on behaviour and heart rate of domestic horses. In: *Proceedings 10th International Equitation Science Conference*, Denmark, p. 38.

Hayes, M.H. (1889) *Illustrated Horse Breaking.* Hurst and Blackett, London.

Henshall, C. and McGreevy, P.D. (2014) The role of ethology in round pen horse training – A review. *Applied Animal Behaviour Science* 155, 1–11.

Horseman, S., Whay, B., Mullan, S., Knowles, T., Barr, A. *et al.* (2016) *Horses in our Hands*. University of Bristol. Available at: www.worldhorsewelfare.org/what-we-do/research/horses-in-our-hands (accessed 5 June 2020).

Houpt, K.A. and Wickens, C.L. (2019) Handling and transport of horses. In: Grandin, T. (ed.) *Livestock Handling and Transport,* 5th edn. CAB International, Wallingford, UK.

Innes, L. and McBride, S. (2008) Negative versus positive reinforcement: An evaluation of training strategies for rehabilitated horses. *Applied Animal Behavior Science* 112, 357–368.

ISES (2018) *ISES 10 Training Principles.* Available at: https://equitationscience.com/learningtheory/ (accessed 4 July 2020).
King, S., Wills, L. and Randle, H. (2018) Early training of foals using the ISES training principles. *Journal of Veterinary Behavior* 29, 140–146.
Kydd, E., Padalino, B., Henshall, C. and McGreevy, P. (2017) An analysis of equine round pen training videos posted online: Differences between amateur and professional trainers. *PloS ONE* 12 (9), e 0184851.
Lansade L., Bouissou, M-F. and Erhard, H.W. (2008) Fearfulness in horses: A temperament trait stable across time and situations. *Applied Animal Behavior Science* 115, 182–200.
Leary S., Underwood, W., Anthony, R., Cartner, S., Grandin. *et al.* (2020) AVMA Guidelines for the euthanasia of animals. Available at: www.avma.org/sites/default/files/2020-01/2020-Euthanasia-Final-1-17-20.pdf (accessed 5 July 2020).
Leiner, L. and Fendt, M. (2011) Behavioural fear and heart rate responses of horses after exposure to novel objects: Effects of habituation. *Applied Animal Behavior Science* 131, 104–109.
Marlborough, L.C. and Knottenbelt, D.C. (2001) Basic management. In: Coumbe, K.M. (ed.) *The Equine Veterinary Nursing Manual.* Blackwell Science Ltd, Oxford, pp. 1–24.
McDonnell, S.M. (2017) Preventing and rehabilitating common healthcare procedure aversions. *Proceedings of the American Association of Equine Practitioners* 63, 262–268.
McGreevy, P.D. and McLean, A.N. (2009) Punishment in horse-training and the concept of ethical equitation. *Journal of Veterinary Behaviour* 4, 193–197.
McGreevy, P., Berger, J., de Brauwere, N., Doherty, O., Harrison, A. *et al.* (2018a) Using the five domains model to assess the adverse impacts of husbandry, veterinary, and equitation interventions on horse welfare. *Animals* 8, 41.
McGreevy, P., Christensen, J.W., König von Borstel, U. and McLean, A. (2018b) *Equitation Science*, 2nd edn. John Wiley & Sons Ltd, Oxford.
McLean, A.N. (2008) Overshadowing: A silver lining to a dark cloud in horse training. *Journal of Applied Animal Welfare Science* 11, 236–248.
McLean, A.N. and Christensen, J.W. (2017) The application of learning theory in horse training. *Applied Animal Behavior Science* 190, 18–27.
Owens, R. (2019) Should we slaughter horses at abattoirs? *Veterinary Record* 185, 577.
Pearson, G. (2015) Practical application of equine learning theory, part 2. *In Practice* 37, 286–292.
Preshaw, L., Kirton, R. and Randle, H. (2017) Application of learning theory in horse rescues in England and Wales. *Applied Animal Behavior Science* 190, 82– 89.
Randle, H. and Waran, N. (2019) Equitation science in practice: how collaboration, communication and change can improve equine welfare. *Journal of Veterinary Behavior* 29, viii–x.
Sandoval, C. and True, C. (2012) Equine wellness care in ambulatory practice. *Veterinary Clinics of North America: Equine Practice* 28, 189–205.
Schomber, J., McLean, A. and König von Borstel, U. (2018) Horses' learning performance when using different training schedules (daily vs. every three days training sessions) to train novel tasks via negative reinforcement. *Proceedings 14th International Conference International Society of Equitation Science*, p. 30.
Smith, A.V., Proops, L., Grounds, K., Wathan, J., Scott, S.K. and McComb, K. (2018) Domestic horses (*Equus caballus*) discriminate between negative and positive human nonverbal vocalisations. *Scientific Reports* 8, 13052.
Starling, M., McLean, A. and McGreevy, P. (2016) The contribution of equitation science to minimising horse-related risks to humans. *Animals* 6, 15.
Thompson, K.R. and Haigh, L. (2018) Perceptions of equitation science revealed in an online forum: Improving equine health and welfare by communicating science to equestrians and equestrians to scientists. *Journal of Veterinary Behavior* 25, 1–8.
Thompson, K.R., Clarkson, L., Riley, C.B. and van den Berg, M. (2018) Horse husbandry and preventive health practices in Australia: An online survey of horse guardians. *Journal of Applied Animal Welfare Science* 21, 347–361.
Thorbergson, Z.W., Nielsen, S.G., Beaulieu, R.J. and Doyle, R.E. (2015) Physiological and behavioural responses of horses to wither scratching and patting the neck when under saddle. *Journal of Applied Animal Welfare Science* 19, 245–259.
Visser, E.K., van Dierendonck, M., Ellis, A.D., Rijksen, C. and van Reenen, C. (2009) A comparison of sympathetic and conventional training methods on responses to initial horse training. *The Veterinary Journal* 181, 48–52.
Waller, A.S. (2014) New Perspectives for the diagnosis, control, treatment, and prevention of strangles in horses. *Veterinary Clinics of North America: Equine Practice* 30, 591–607.
Warren-Smith, A. and McGreevy, P.D. (2007) The use of blended positive and negative reinforcement in shaping the halt response of horses (*Equus caballus*). *Animal Welfare* 16, 481–488.
Warren-Smith, A.K. and McGreevy, P.D. (2008) Preliminary investigations into the ecological relevance of round-pen (round-yard) training of horses. *Journal of Applied Animal Welfare Science* 11, 285–298.

15 Evacuation and Rescue Welfare

Rebecca Husted, BS, PhD*

Technical Large Animal Rescue®, Inc., Macon, Georgia, USA

Introduction 211
Background 211
How Horses Get into Trouble 212
  Human responsibility 212
Risk Management 213
  Horses don't comprehend human intent 213
  Not magic – it's language 214
  Flight distance, critical distance as social reactive distance 214
  Positioning people for safety 215
  Anxiety and fear 216
Triage at the Scene 216
What to Do in an Emergency 216
  First, situational awareness 216
  Second, call a veterinarian 217
  Third, personal protective equipment 217
  Fourth, make a rescue plan 217
The Horse's Perspective 218
  Pain 218
  The opposition reflex 218
  Horses are always horses 218
  Senses 218
    Smell 218
    Taste 219
    Hearing 219
    Vision 220
    Touch 220
    Proprioception 221
    Thermoregulation 221
Practical Application of Equine Rescue Theory 221
  Help them help themselves 221
  Approach zone 221
  Catching loose horses 222
  Danger zones 222
  Entrapped recumbent horse behavior 223
  Learned helplessness in TLAER® 223
Tools and Physical Techniques 224
  Halters and control 224
  Twitches 224
  Blindfold 225

*Corresponding author e-mail: delphiacres@hotmail.com

 Fraser's the Behaviour and Welfare of the Horse (eds C.B. Riley, S.E. Cregier and A.F. Fraser)
DOI: 10.1079/9781789242133.0015

Legacy method – recumbent horse restraint 225
TLAER® method – recumbent horse restraint 225
Pressure on the chest and abdomen 225
Euthanasia 226
Myths of Animal Rescue 226
Fear of trailers after wrecks 226
Leading from boats 226
Training Horses for Large-animal Rescue 227
Climate Change 227
Welfare Concerns in Emergencies 227
References 228

Introduction

As a prey animal, the horse needs to be desensitized rapidly to things that aren't genuinely frightening or dangerous, or they'd never stop running, observes veterinarian Robert Miller (Gaumnitz, 2017). In other words, if the handler can convince the horse it is not being hurt, it may allow humans to do otherwise alarming manipulations such as riding, rescue extrication or lifts.

Fundamental behavioural concepts are common to many types of emergencies. Understanding equine ethology directly improves success, whether catching a loose horse on the highway, extricating it after a trailer, van, or float wreck, or calming one trapped in a septic tank or sinkhole. Identifying poor animal welfare helps in early decision making to aggressively treat or field euthanize the victim. The goal is to limit the exposure of rescuers to injury and improve the efficiency and successful outcomes for the team on scene, while optimizing the animal's welfare.

This chapter outlines horse behaviour characteristics applicable to safer Technical Large Animal Emergency Rescue (TLAER®), including evacuation and technical rescue. (See Fig. 15.1 for an example of a safe intervention.)

Background

On TLAER® scenes, there are few normal behaviour patterns, and injuries happen to both owners and veterinarians regardless of experience. Predicting what a horse might do is difficult. Most people know what an agitated horse looks like: head high, wide-eyed, staring with unblinking eyes, flickering ears, tight mouth, wide nostrils, tight neck and body muscles, tail tight, loose bowel movement, and legs animated with quick tense movements and irregular rhythms. Yet some or all these behaviours are impossible to evaluate or express when a horse is entrapped, entombed, recumbent or upside down, etc.

Agitation, frustration, fear or a combination thereof can elevate to aggression in the animal's panicked attempts to get free by struggling, attempting to raise the body to move its legs (rear), head slinging, stamping or pawing. Uninformed handlers or responders may assess these reactions as angry when the horse is actually agitated and panicked. The biological and chemical changes (e.g. hyper- or hypothermia, neurologic, enzymatic and hormonal) within an entrapped horse's body can affect its behaviour much like combative humans with head injuries.

Compounding the hazards of large animal rescue are the decades of film and media popularization of profoundly dangerous scenarios and responses. Owner expectations, procedures and animal welfare concerns are ill-served by urban lore unacquainted with rescue protocols developed for human and animal safety and good welfare outcomes for the horse (Fiedler and McGreevy, 2016). Live social media rescues are not subject to the scrutiny of animal welfare, equestrian or veterinary science, or someone with heavy rescue expertise. Uncritical viewers or untrained rescuers think it correct to rope an animal and use a truck to pull it out of the mud, across the pasture by the feet, tail, neck or head, risking separated joints, crushed tissue and asphyxiation. These approaches indicate no clear understanding of horse behaviour, medical concerns or fear responses. Although well-intentioned, these mechanical methods cause iatrogenic injury in equine victims, including traumatic amputations, lacerations, asphyxiation, corneal damage, myopathy, neurologic injury, etc. Trained responders understand that media's anthropomorphic interpretation of rescue events leads to popular beliefs that horses in peril comprehend our efforts to help, when science shows they do not.

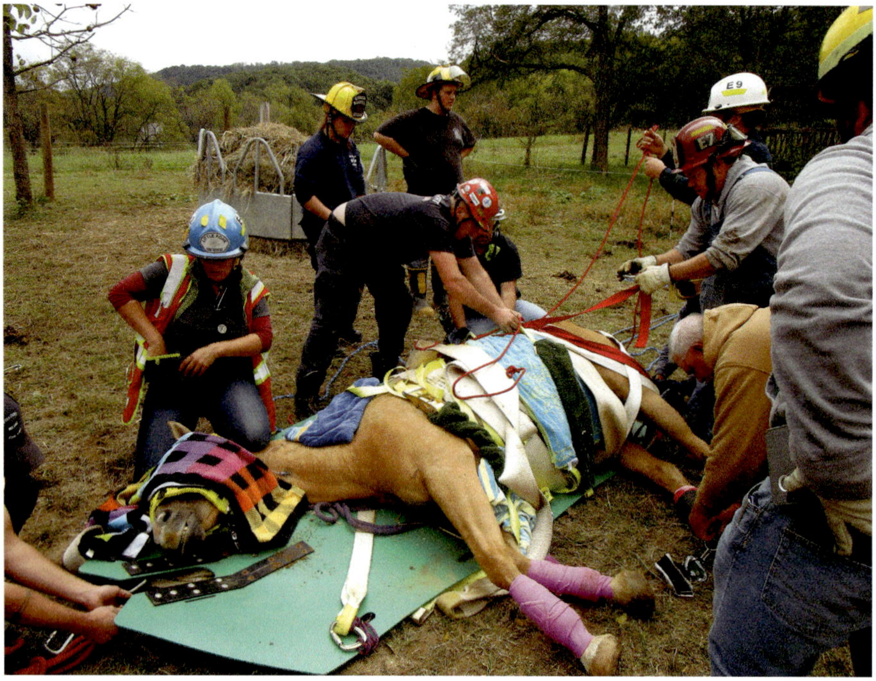

Fig. 15.1. Horse strapped onto a rescue glide for transport to veterinary care. Photo: Little Fork Fire Department, Virginia.

Well-intentioned rescuers also sustain injuries with debilitating long-term effects. Today, specialized methods and procedures, including physical and chemical control of the patient, are basic to TLAER®, a dedicated form of heavy rescue in fire and rescue services intimately tied to the veterinary practitioner's expertise.

How Horses Get into Trouble

Unlike the human brain, the horse has no well-defined frontal lobe function for executive functions. In people, these processes are responsible for planning, cognitive flexibility, abstract thinking, rule acquisition, initiating appropriate actions, inhibiting inappropriate actions and selecting relevant sensory information. Horses don't ask: 'What would happen if I walk across that pool cover?' or 'How do I get out of this pool without hurting myself?' Instead of rational puzzle-solving, their primal instinct is to react by crashing through fences, kicking the sides of a trailer or stall until injured or struggling to escape until they break a bone or choke.

Horses are curious, contributing to their ending up in situations that humans assume they would never enter. For example, attempting to climb the stairs to a hayloft or stepping into a muddy pond. Curious horses use their forefeet and senses to explore. They sniff and tap things for soundness before stepping in or on them. Anything not previously experienced causes some horses to startle, but curiosity is engendered by novelty. It is a part of the learning processes and positive behavioural patterns. Exploration is an aspect of horse behaviour used in training for equestrian disciplines, but it can contribute to entrapment in TLAER® situations.

Entrapments may be credited to poor facility maintenance or design, dominance by other horses, curiosity or novelty-seeking, or even attempting to self-medicate (Fig. 15.2). In the latter case, it is anecdotally speculated that some animals initially enter the unsafe environment on purpose. For example, older, infirm animals in pain may go into watercourses, muddy areas, or similar environments in attempts to get relief for laminitis of the hooves, generalized inflammation and fever, or relief from biting insects.

Human responsibility

Other TLAER® situations are fully the fault of the humans who put the horse into a dangerous situation,

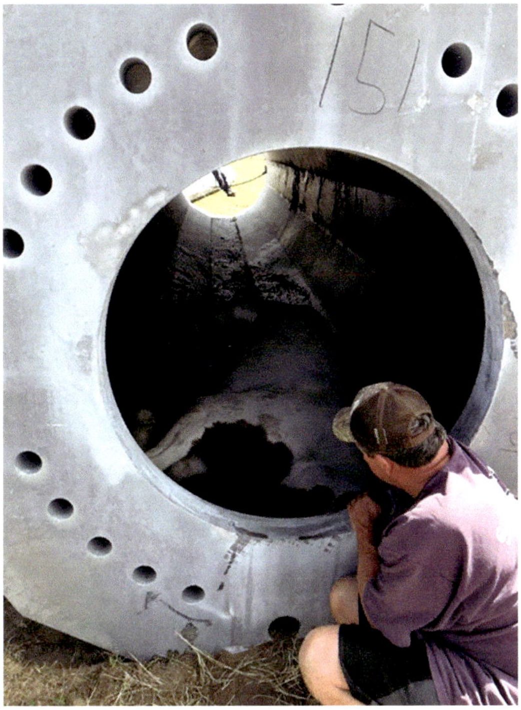

Fig. 15.2. A horse inside a utility pole dropped off into his pasture. He climbed in the other end (curiosity), slipped down, then panicked (fear and motion) and wiggled his way to this end. Exhausted, he could not get up to climb out. A rear drag or slide is the technical approach recommended for extrication. Photo: Charleston SC Rescue Squad.

such as riding over a poorly constructed bridge, off the correct trail, failing to hitch the trailer properly, or leaving the pond unfenced with surface ice forming. The prevention, mitigation and instruction of the horse industry participants in safer ways to cope with climate change, build facilities, fencing, veterinary clinics having fire prevention, evacuation and defence in place, disaster planning, safer transport to prevent injuries both in road incidents, and loading and unloading situations, are on-going educational effort well covered elsewhere (Gimenez *et al.*, 2008; Cregier and Gimenez, 2015).

Risk Management

Risk assessment and management, especially at the corporate level, are fundamental to emergency response agencies. Potential liabilities documented include frantic attempts by owners and bystanders to assist, responders intimidated by horses, lack of protective equipment (e.g. helmet, gloves, reflective jacket on roadways, etc.), civilians unfamiliar with incident command training and ignorance of best practices (Langley and Hunter, 2001).

Given that horses have the fastest reaction time of any domestic animal or human, hazards associated with horses are dynamic and rapidly changing. Consider, for example, the entrapped horse's tendency to struggle, appear to lay quietly, then struggle again with no warning. Fear for personal and scene safety, lack of training and liability concerns prevent some veterinarians and professional rescuers from responding. Risk-averse uninformed policies treat rescues as an expendable service. Getting responders involved in large animal rescue training and adoption of best practices increases understanding of emergency scene roles, safety protocols and acceptance of rescue responsibilities. Essentials of behaviour and handling for emergencies have been taught to urban firefighters, law enforcement, military personnel, civilians and animal control officers internationally with success. Fig. 15.3 is an example of a fully trained veterinarian-aided rescue.

Horses don't comprehend human intent

Humans usually have the intention to do helpful things. Horses have never stopped to help another entombed in mud, held down by a predator, or trapped upside down in a ditch; they do not conceive solutions to these problems. Horses do not and cannot rely on other horses to save them. They instinctively rely on themselves for survival. The actions based on human intent to help are perceived as a new pattern, and horses react in unpredictable ways. Like trying to catch a cat for a trip to the veterinary clinic, they know something is different.

Since fear drives horses' seemingly illogical reactions and behaviour, learning to identify and shape behaviour protects the emergency responder from horses' specialized weaponry: weight, teeth, hooves and lightning-fast reflexes. Fear is a primitive, fundamental emotion generated by neuroendocrine effects of the amygdala in all mammals and directs survival's primary response – a fight for life. In situations where the animal is trapped in mud, a deep hole, or an overturned trailer and cannot move away to feel safety and comfort, responders often have to work inside the critical distance (danger zone). This makes the positioning of animal handlers

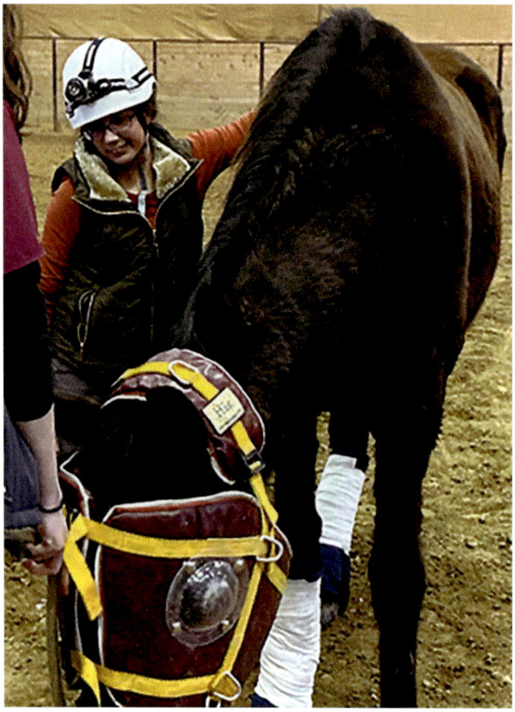

Fig. 15.3. An equine veterinarian with full personal protection equipment supervising a horse waking up from sedation after rescue from entrapment. Photo: author.

and operational personnel when rescuing horses even more contingent on safety.

Not magic – it's language

Although horses respond to the tone and timbre of the human voice, they do not understand spoken words. They use body language and limited vocalization to communicate. Showing the rear end to another horse could mean not paying attention, signalling distance increase (go away!), not giving respect, sickness or exhaustion or injury, inability to move, or it has fled as far as it can and is ready to fight. Understanding the horse's body language and behaviour is the most important skill to interact with horses safely. Even in the direst circumstances, such as drowning in ice holes, horses still act true to their evolved nature.

Knowing what is normal for horses raises awareness of abnormal medical, emotional or physical states. Postural changes express body language and are consistent but can be incorrectly interpreted by humans. Behaviours that we assume are similar to humans' (e.g. yawning) can actually mean the animal is trying to deal with stress.

Human facial expressions affect horse behaviour. A human's intense focus with direct eye contact may be interpreted as aggression since many humans have tunnel vision and closed body postures when focusing on a task. Use of a smiling, open-body posture is less intimidating, as is a soft focus and avoiding direct eye contact. The horse's ability to accurately perceive human facial expressions and body language is uncanny. Through associative learning, they often know what humans are going to do even before they act. Research shows that horses react to details humans are unaware of including the angle of the body, eyebrow positions, voice pitch and measured tread. They also know when humans are scared, happy, worried or angry.

Although safer and less damaging equipment and methods of vertical lifts, drags and extrication are available, human factors have a major effect on the success, or not, of technical rescue. Understanding human and horse behaviour on the scene, and appropriate use of the animals' anatomical features, contribute to greater success than using any power tool. This understanding continues to develop on applying learning theory, managing human behaviour and accommodating the horses' reactions on emergency scenes such as trailer accidents, cast, entombed in mud, barn fires, floods, wildfire evacuations, hurricane destruction, etc.

Flight distance, critical distance as social reactive distance

The flight distance is the distance to which a threatened animal runs until it feels safe and then turns to evaluate the situation. When stressed, its flight distance increases. Just as personal space varies in humans, horses have a personal flight distance. Even a few inches (cm) can make the difference between the horse perceiving safety or becoming stressed, trapped and fearful.

Attacking humans is not normal equine behaviour. Most incidents of horse–human conflict are defensive behaviours driven by fear, where the person is too close. Since the critical distance is inside the action zone, where animals perceive no escape route, their fear increases, and they are motivated to fight. When a human uses direct eye contact and quick, direct line approaches, normal for humans but predatory in nature, the horse's instinctive fears increase. Crouching or sneaking up while attempting to put on a halter or lifting sling is instantly recognized as predatory behaviour when inside the horse's perceptive distance.

Giving more distance reduces stress, especially in tight situations inside barns, trailers, stalls or corrals. The challenge on TLAER® scenes is crossing into the animal's action zone and critical distance to put webbing or equipment onto the horse safely, while concurrently attempting to get it to manage the stress of the situation. Understanding the horse's perceptions and how to accommodate them safely is vital for overall scene safety.

Positioning people for safety

Where people stand relative to the horse can contribute to success or failure during a rescue. Dangerous places for humans include directly in front of the legs, head and neck of standing or recumbent horses; between the legs of recumbent horses; above a recumbent horse; or within 3.5 m (12 ft) behind a horse to drive it forward. Note the positions of people in Fig. 15.4.

The safest place to stand when leading a horse is adjacent to the shoulder area or working it in a circle at least 3.5 m (12 ft) away. Safe manipulation requires knowledge of anatomy and physiology to prevent injury when emplacing webbing or slings, proper personnel positioning and consideration of horse dominance hierarchies. Responders should plan for the containment of loose horses and have an escape plan for humans inside the action zone.

When placing equipment, tools or appliances, no rescuers should be positioned between the animal and solid objects such as a trailer, wall, gate, fence, tree or vehicle in case the animal moves. Its bodyweight can crush a human. However, handler and operational personnel may strive for body contact during extrication because, at specific times, proximity increases rescuer safety. For example, a kick gets more leverage and is more lethal as distance increases. If possible, handlers should keep one hand on the animal to feel changes in musculature as an early warning before seeing body movement. In order of occurrence, the horse decides the intended action (often quickly), tenses its muscles, shifts its weight, and moves one foot, before moving the whole body.

With experience, handlers and veterinarians learn to assess horse body language to react in a timely manner and determine the required physical or chemical restraint.

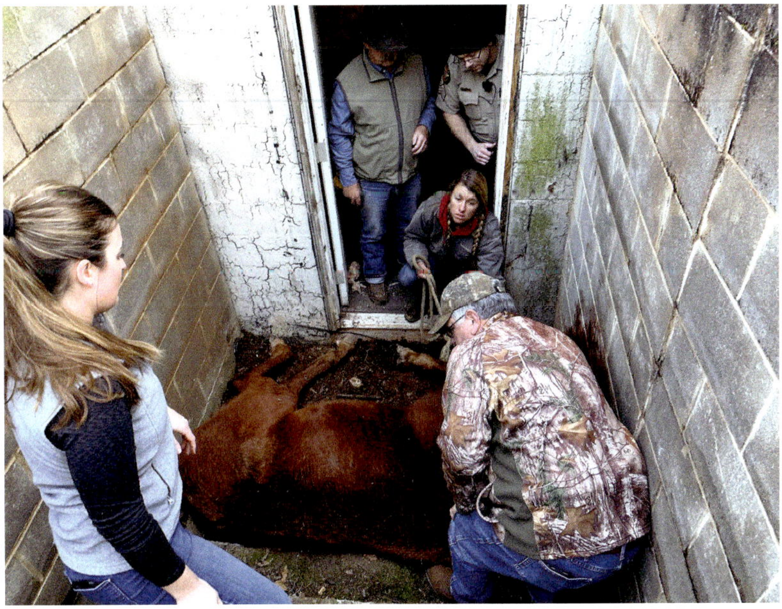

Fig. 15.4. A horse trapped at the bottom of the stairs is injured and exhausted from struggling. The responding team must determine a plan for safe extrication. Photo: Elbert County Fire Rescue, Georgia.

Anxiety and fear

Anticipating an unidentified threat raises a horse's fear, especially if escape routes are blocked or they are unable to see or return to a conspecific. Fear responses to sudden threats usually include avoiding an object, person, or a specific place, backing up and acute stress. Fear-inducing situations include confinement and tightly restricted movement (e.g. stall, horse trailer, veterinary stocks, etc.). Survival responses ingrained in the horse occur irrespective of human efforts to calm the animal and may injure handlers.

Once the horse exhibits a fearful response, it takes 20–30 minutes to calm it down. Responses can be documented using an objective numerical scale of indicators (e.g. restlessness, uncomfortable actions, aggression) that parallel measured fluctuations in physiological or haematological factors such as cortisol. Long-term stress, physiologic, psychologic, or both, is not a normal part of TLAER® situations but may be a predisposing factor for entrapment or injury.

There are two general types of stress responses noted at the rescue scene: (1) active flighty, reactive horses, and (2) passive coping behaviour and movement-inhibited horses (see learned helplessness below). Acute stress reactions such as startle, shying, or attempts to flee, are associated with an immediate rise in heart rate and reactivity. It is difficult to get past fear, but reactive horses can be desensitized and learn fast. Good handlers use treats to encourage positive behaviours, and horses can be successfully taught on the scene to accept even bizarre situations. If the horse can approach, sniff and investigate, it may decide all is safe and relax. Learning theory involving habituation, overshadowing, desensitization, positive and negative reinforcement is taught to veterinarians to reduce stress and reactivity in treatment situations and is fully applicable to large animal rescue (Dehorty *et al.*, 2017). However, the time and place to learn these scientifically validated techniques is not on the scene, but prior, with an instructor well versed in the timing and efficacy of these techniques.

If approached too quickly or directly or by an unfamiliar person or object, separated from companions, pressured to perform by the handler, harassed, chased or restricted in movement, horses can become panicked. Standard scene management involving responders, tool noises, tarps, sounds and lights can scare horses. Success is improved by using curiosity, treats or forage to help introduce new aspects of the rescue attempt, such as equipment, harnesses, slings and loud noises.

Triage at the Scene

Primary health and welfare triage is best done by a veterinarian conducting an initial inspection of all animals, who then assists the team in extrication of animals that are easiest to treat, have cooperative dispositions, and present the least threatening injuries. Secondary triage is conducted once out of the danger zone or at the clinic. Severely injured horses may not be transported to the definitive treatment location without appropriate methods for medical support. For example, an animal with a fracture must not be loaded on a trailer without a properly applied limb splint, pain treatment and medication to combat shock.

Injury types that are uncommon in other areas of equine veterinary practice are found in TLAER® scenarios. Horses entrapped in abnormal positions (dorsal, posterior, lateral recumbency) are subject to various consequences based on pre- and post-extrication examination and treatment efficiency. They are known to stand up and walk after extrication, even eat, yet the same horse may die a few hours later. Even when a trained large animal rescue team effects an efficient rescue and the on-scene veterinarian treats the animal immediately, the animal can still have a prolonged recovery or die. Untreated crush injuries, compartment syndrome, traumatic brain injury, hyperthermia, or accidental hypothermia, pneumonia and colic are common causes of death.

What to Do in an Emergency

First, situational awareness

The first action is to call emergency services. The responder must stay calm, breathe, and not panic. Clear thinking requires breathing, and panic interferes with rationality.

Situational awareness (SA) is a military term for the perception of the surrounding dynamic elements, how a person's actions can change that, making estimates of how influences may transform with changing variables such as time, responders or space. Whether difficult or seemingly easy, performing any task requires SA of changing conditions and planning for possible worst case outcomes. Under normal circumstances leading a horse requires a multitude of tasks and intense concentration. Leading an injured horse alone on a busy roadway in the dark requires command and control at another level of complication and skills.

As the on-scene eyes and ears, the first on the scene must prepare to give needed information to the telecommunicator or dispatcher when calling for assistance. For example, yelling 'There's a trailer wreck' is much less informative than 'I'm southbound on Interstate 85 at the 26-mile marker. There is an overturned two-horse trailer. The driver is out of the truck, and at least one horse is injured. One is also loose'. To a veterinarian, telling them, 'My horse is trapped' is quite different from 'My aged mare is down in the trailer after a 2-hour haul. Her rectal temperature is 102 °F (38.9 °C). She has minimal gut sounds and her leg is through the trailer wall'. Details allow responders of any type to assign resources more efficiently.

Second, call a veterinarian

Once emergency agencies have been alerted, it is vital that an equine veterinarian is called to the scene before efforts are made to extricate an animal. The horse must also be seen by a veterinarian after extrication because medical issues must be evaluated, treated, or euthanasia provided.

The veterinarian is an advisor to the Incident Commander (IC: the person in charge of directing the rescue team) as to making decisions about saveability, extrication options, and physical and chemical methods of restraint useful to the extrication effort. While their primary concern is the animal, he/she must work inside the constraints of the Incident Command System for everyone's safety. Similar operational systems govern such operations in the USA, Australia (AIMS), Canada (ICS), New Zealand (CIMS), the United Kingdom (FICCS) and many other countries. Veterinarians have the training to remain calm, make rational decisions, offer definitive treatment and to handle animals professionally. Close coordination with owners can ensure better outcomes based on diagnosis and early treatment options or selecting euthanasia at a rational point.

Third, personal protective equipment

Personnel safety on the scene is of utmost importance. At a minimum, responders should wear a helmet with chinstrap, safety boots and heavy gloves for TLAER® scenarios. A brightly coloured reflective vest is required near roadways or if personnel are on the road for any reason (e.g. chasing loose horses, changing a tyre, checking for trailering issues, etc.). Vests on people, reflective tape on vehicles and equipment, and use of cones and/or signage are especially vital at roadside incidents where impacts from other vehicles are far more dangerous than the task at hand. People in other vehicles can see the vest, and although that doesn't make it safe for someone to be in the road chasing a horse, it does make it possible for the other driver to see them and slow down. That may help prevent horrific tragedies to people helping horses. However, due to safety concerns on roadsides, responders should identify dangerous situations and contact qualified human resources (fire/rescue, law enforcement) for assistance.

Fourth, make a rescue plan

Responders with some equine first aid training can perform basic medical tasks and update the veterinarian even before he/she arrives on scene. Document and communicate the rectal temperature, pulse rate, respiration rate and the character of breathing, movement, attitude and the possible degree of pain. Photos and short videos can be captured and sent via a mobile phone.

While planning extrication, get all humans out of the animal's critical distance after offering forage and water when possible to do so safely. Keep bystanders and onlookers away (the police can assist with this). When trapped and unable to flee or fight, some animals appear to lay quietly, but they can move quickly and injure a person. This periodic struggle to escape, violent reactions to small stimuli or perceived escape opportunities will exhaust and injure the animal. Some horses realize they are out of options and wait for human assistance, often due to prior desensitization training.

There are a few forbidden methods of TLAER® extrication. These can cause severe injury or death and greatly compromise welfare. These are based on behavioural, anatomical and welfare concerns:

Ropes around the head or neck
Failing to protect the head or eyes during a rescue attempt
Ropes around the legs without padding
Pulling an entire animal by the tail or neck

Winches attached to any body part
Chasing horses (e.g. on foot, vehicles, etc.)
Dragging on abrasive surfaces without protection (e.g. gravel, asphalt, etc.)
Using incorrect landmarks on the skull for a field euthanasia
Tying an animal on scene and/or leaving an animal unattended

The Horse's Perspective

Pain

Our understanding of trauma-related pain in animals has improved over the last two decades. Pain sensitizes the horse to stress, so veterinary attendance and timely administration of analgesia should improve welfare, the experience of pain, and behaviour, maximizing the ease of handling. Inadequate pain management at the point of injury has deleterious effects on patient recovery. Horses rarely vocalize even when in extreme pain; no noise does not mean the absence of pain.

Pain is not a good training tool as it causes intense stress, and although horses may mask pain, they can explosively attempt escape or thrash without warning. Especially in acute pain, their brain releases pain-reducing endorphins, so when later exposed to physical pressure (e.g. twitch or sling or the pressure of mud), they may appear quiescent but are still reactive.

Physiological, pharmacological and haematological indicators of pain are difficult to assess on scene. It is better to use the equine pain grimace scale or equine pain scale (Gleerup and Lindegaard, 2016). However, if the horse is trapped, it cannot be easily assessed for most activities, positions or behaviours discussed on pain scales. Generally, changes from normal postures, such as holding up a leg, arching the back, transferring weight, can be assessed along with increased or no sweat, hyper- or hyposensitivity, stiffness of ears, the tension of the eyelid, the shape of the nostril, restlessness and tooth grinding. Lack of interest in food is a strong indicator of pain, stress and fear.

The opposition reflex

The opposition reflex is a self-defence strategy where prey animals push or lean against pressure placed anywhere on their bodies. The reflex is seen as horse handlers put pressure on the top of the head (often unintentionally), pulling on a halter. The horse fights this pressure by rearing or falling backwards in opposition to the expected result and preferred forward action. It is counterintuitive to humans but pulling on a rope around a leg or neck used as an anchor causes the animal to frantically fight the pressure or pull the rope out of the hands, causing injury to both human and horse. Another example is the common mistake of pulling on the head of a recumbent horse just as it organizes its body to stand up. Pulling on the head causes it to go off-balance and fall back down. Instead, get the animal to the sternal recovery position. Then let the animal stand when it feels comfortable and strong enough to do so (Fig. 15.5).

Horses are always horses

More dominant equines continue to exhibit aggressive behaviours towards less dominant animals within the range of teeth, hooves and express threatening behaviours, irrespective of how dire humans perceive the situation. Horses assert their dominance over conspecifics forcing or inhibiting their movement. For example, horse to horse injuries are common in trailers, where desperate attempts to get away from dominant animals cause injury and panic. They can also happen when one horse attempting to escape another horse runs over the handler.

Senses

Horses rely on their senses of vision, smell and hearing or combine them with other senses to assess the environment. The brain judges their significance, and the horse reacts, or not, to the stimuli. Their sensitivity to movement, sounds and strange objects makes large animal rescue scenes overwhelming, and can induce fear responses that may injure people and the horse. The senses have been covered in detail in Chapter 2. This section focuses on aspects of senses relevant to technical rescue scenarios.

Smell

As obligate nose breathers, horses are used as excellent tracking animals for mounted search and rescue and are exquisitely sensitive to smells (e.g. smoke, equipment, sweat, blood) unusual to horses. Allowing the horse to sniff and recognize you are a

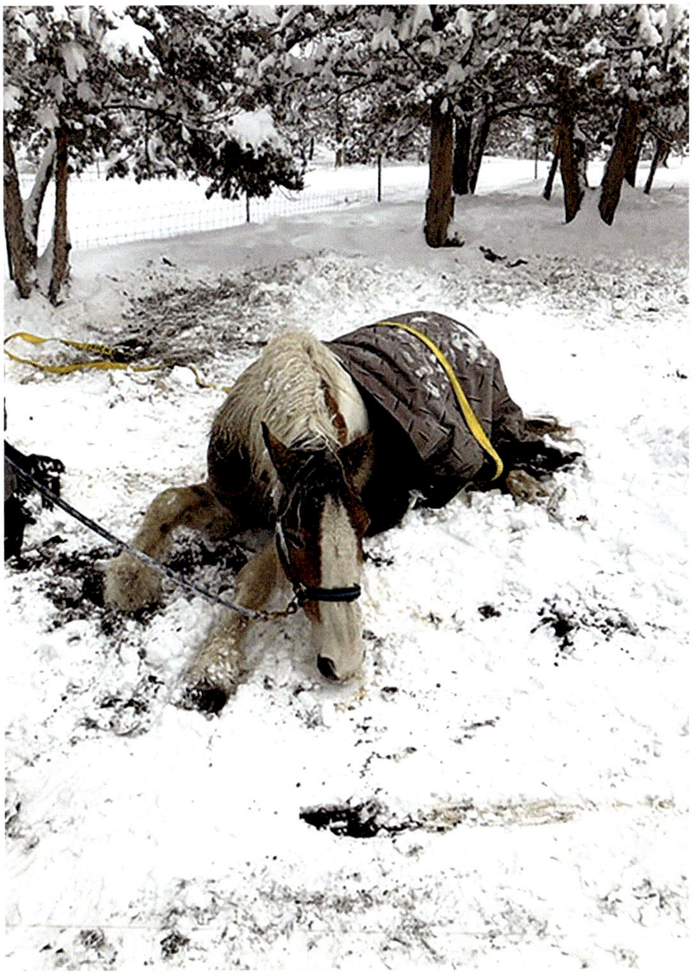

Fig. 15.5. A horse cast in the snow has been rolled to the recovery position (sternal recumbency) and can recover and stand when it is ready. Photo: Kate Beardsley.

human can calm it, especially if associated with a treat, although food is not a priority to fearful animals. Loose animals may be coaxed using smell to follow food or forage into safe areas or enclosures.

Taste

Taste is not commonly used to the advantage of rescuers, but to reduce stress responders can coax animals to graze or offer forage or feed, even while trapped. Many domesticated horses know the sound of plastic wrapped around a treat and may come to investigate. Loose horses have successfully been distracted inside overturned trailers, and those entrapped in mud and loose on busy highways attracted with flakes of good quality hay. When the head and neck are down in the grazing position, heart rate and blood pressure are reduced, cortisol levels decline over time, the animal calms down and may be easier to capture or handle.

Hearing

Vocalization is atypical, but when horses do so, it is low pitched wuffles, nickers, grunts or loud alarm snorts. Bellowing or whinnying or screaming indicate severe stress such as that expressed on separation from herd mates or attack by a predator. Grunts, groans and sighs by recumbent or downed horses are due to exhaustion, the limited function of the downside lung and prolonged discomfort. These sounds are recognizable by humans as similar to how we might sound in a similar situation.

Horses hear everything – voices, tool use, vehicles, footsteps, extrication equipment – even if they can't see it. Sirens induce fearful responses and raise acute stress levels. Thus, a silent approach with strobe or warning lights is encouraged. Animals acclimate quickly, and the lights increase scene safety. During a rescue, responders should limit loud sounds from cutting equipment or engines until necessary and make tool selection based on the needed results. Certain tools – air chisel, reciprocating saw and chain saw – are extremely loud but efficient. Others (e.g. hydraulic tools) are silent but cut jagged edges. Generally, the use of cutting tools is the responsibility and expertise of the fire department. All require different strategies to overcome.

Although horses are nonverbal, responders should continue attempting to make a connection using voice. Responders and bystanders should remain calm with limited loud voices, and handlers should use a low, rhythmic voice when handling the horse. Requirements to talk and direct a safe rescue means that responders need to converse on the scene. By simply being mindful of the overwhelming amount and intensity of sound, they can reduce stress to the animal.

Vision

The horse's ability to see in low light is due to its tapetum that gives a green/yellow eye glow reflection. Rods in the retina do not accommodate sudden changes in light intensity, making them suspicious of dark or light patches on the floor, white lines on a dark road, darkened horse trailers and building interiors. However, once adjusted to the dark, they can see better than humans. In any light condition, their horizontal pupil aligns with the horizon as they raise and lower their heads, giving them a stable view with minimal light scattering from the sun into their eyes, assisted by the corpora nigra of the pupil.

The equine eyes are widely placed and up high on a long skull, allowing eating while keeping eyes above the grass, with greater peripheral vision to survey their environment. Since horses cannot see between their eyes, touching them on the head may generate a fear response. They cannot see directly behind themselves without turning their heads and may become concerned if they detect something behind them that they cannot turn to see.

Horses turn their heads to use binocular vision (both eyes and depth perception) to look at novel stimuli. They have better depth perception in a small area directly in front of the skull and will raise or lower their heads to focus on an object. Stationary objects (e.g. parked fire trucks/heavy equipment) may be intimidating but less scary than flapping movements (plastic, flapping flags or arms). Colour vision is poor and dichromatic. They see shades of grey or pastel blue/yellow, but they do not react to clothing colour or firetrucks on scenes. Because they are rhythmical and predictable, horses quickly desensitize or habituate to strobe or flashing rescue lights; flash photography and flashlights may startle them. On emergency scenes, the choice of bright reflective colours is recommended for human safety, not to assist the horse visually.

Fladry and knowledge of the horse's aversion to contrast can be used to control their movements. For example, a series of cut lengths of fire hose or planks arranged in parallel across an egress point may deter prey animals from attempting to cross, or string with short streamers of surveyors' or caution tape at about a meter high provide a funnel or makeshift fence.

Touch

The head, face and ears are extremely sensitive but tend to be where laypeople want to touch. While in physical contact with horses, find areas to calmly stroke the neck and shoulder or scratch or groom the withers or under the chin in circular motions to help the horse perceive you as friendly. Flat-handed slaps or patting is aggressive and makes the horse more nervous. Grooming, scratching and stroking are preferred.

Horses detect sensations through their hooves and react to vibrations in the ground (e.g. vibrations from rescue tools for extrication). Rescuers must balance the need for equipment with the reactions of the animal. For example, percussion tools vibrate by design. As hydraulic tools, they are slow, cumbersome, quiet and leave a jagged edge. As air chisels, they are fast, very loud and leave a smooth edge. Is it better to finish the job fast without a jagged edge? The operational personnel on the scene makes these decisions.

Proprioception

Proprioception is the ability to detect body position and movement with respect to gravity. Prey animals do not like to lie down except when necessary to sleep and when they feel safe. Staying upright and balanced with respect to gravity is an instinctual priority. If they find themselves upside down, lying down or trapped, they will incessantly fight to stand, even if severely injured. If trapped in recumbency positions for an extended time, proprioception is disturbed. Even when righted, they may fall while attempting to stand. It is always best to allow the animal to remain in the rescue sternal relaxed position until they are comfortable trying to stand.

Thermoregulation

The large body size of a horse makes it capable of withstanding a wide range of temperatures. Still, it is quickly compromised under the stress of entrapment, unusual body positioning or posture, or environmental conditions beyond its control. Horses can lose their ability to thermoregulate under conditions complicated by water, stress, wind, mud, exposure and recumbency. Under all such conditions, they become hypo- or hyperthermic very quickly (e.g. on their sides in an overturned trailer in a muddy flowing creek).

Practical Application of Equine Rescue Theory

Help them help themselves

Animals under stress rely on instinct, overriding rational reaction. Humans cannot reason a horse out of a hazardous position. On scene, the handler has just one opportunity to show the horse that he/she knows something about behaviour and increase chances of success. Inconsistent cues reward incorrect behaviour. Patiently convincing the horse it is its idea to do what you want leads to success.

The best solution is to use their behaviour patterns and instincts to help them save themselves. Fighting a horse's instinct results in injury to the animal and possibly to rescuers. Because of the animal's reactivity, best practice strives to get it into a better position for self-rescue, then determines an approach that allows the animal to help itself.

Approach zone

Awareness of the human's location relevant to the compromised animal is described by three zones extending around every animal as it is approached. These dynamic zones can expand or contract based on interactions and reactions. By manipulating these zones, handlers can control a herd of horses and particularly single horses. The handler can increase his or her ability to catch the animal using approach and retreat concepts and keep it calmer. The work of Lamm (2020) demonstrates that large animal containment and handling techniques are fully applicable to mustangs, wild, free-roaming or feral horses. Due to its excellent senses, horses become alarmed if you sneak (stalk); do not try this! Instead, speak in soft tones, make sure it is aware of your presence and use relaxed body language in the approach.

On first approach, the rescuer steps into the **awareness zone** (the safest zone for human and horse), where the animal smells, hears or sees the rescuer. Usually, the animal's reaction is to flick an ear toward the person, raising the head and using the senses to gain information about you. Slowing your approach and spending more time, even just a few seconds, in this zone allows the animal to observe you. You are using eye pressure on the animal at this point.

Next, the rescuer steps closer into the **alertness zone**. Here the horse turns to face the human and, by direct observation, gains information by focusing the ears, eyes and nose. It uses these sensory inputs to make an instant judgment as to its safety or endangerment. Perceptions of danger, even subtle body language cues, cause prey animals to flee. Anything perceived as non-threatening is evaluated continuously to confirm it is still safe. At the slightest hint of danger, a fear response is stimulated. In this zone, an animal may not be able to turn and face the responder physically so that it will become stressed and take action; scrambling or struggling is an attempt to do so. Help the horse relax with a calm, soothing voice by backing away a few steps to relieve pressure while synthesizing a plan. The need for social contact can be used to advantage here because isolation is a stressor. A buddy horse standing quietly within sight of the trapped horse may help to calm it and stop its struggling.

Once approached within its **action zone**, the animal responds (i.e. takes action). This may be standing still, running away (forward, backward, sideways), rearing, or attacking with the front or hind end. A horse walking away from you is technically fleeing, just slowly. It flees to the end of its flight distance, then turns to verify what it was that caused it to flee. Flight responses can be extreme such as crashing through fences, jumping over obstacles or hurtling over rocks. Uninformed rescuers get into trouble with trapped horses. The horse can appear to be sedate, the nervous system under stress having released neuroendocrine products that quell pain and calm the animal. However, they quickly react when stimulated; they still seek to flee but cannot (Fig. 15.6).

Catching loose horses

A common response scenario is horses loose on the road. Well camouflaged and erratic in behaviour, many horses are hit by vehicles each year. Chasing is not an option, but humans can out plan and outsmart horses for containment.

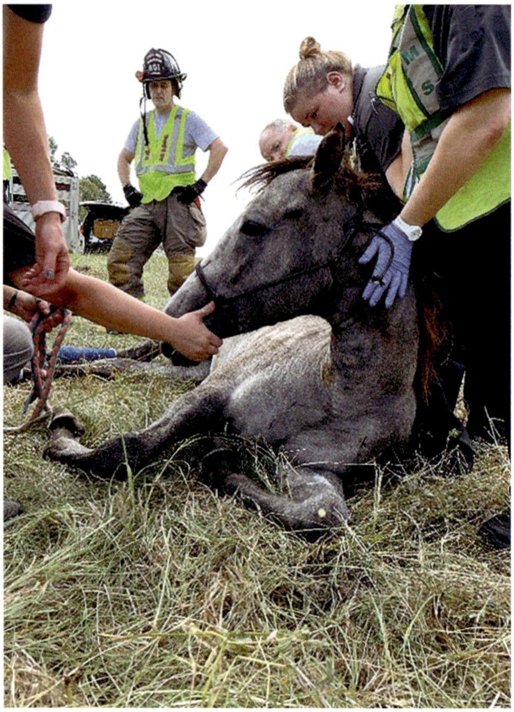

Fig. 15.6. A horse trapped in an overturned trailer on an interstate highway. There are too many people close to this young, injured horse (inside the action zone) while waking up from sedation. Photo: Rebecca Galeazzo.

The best animal handler available should attempt to catch the horse with a soft approach. Prey animals are sensitive to direct line thought processes and approaches. They know when humans are trying to catch them and are perfectly aware of how close a human has to be to do so. A good handler is non-aggressive, calm and confident, alert to the animal's emotional state by understanding the mental pressure experienced by the animal. They can use reactions to this pressure to move the animal in the direction wanted or slightly retreat to help it relax.

Food, treats or a conspecific (i.e. Judas horse) can attract the horse close enough to be contained. If possible, catch and lead one animal of the group, halter it and then walk away toward containment. Horses want to be part of a herd. Bringing a buddy horse to the scene may attract other loose horses, often following the led horse into containment. Mares and foals have a strong natural desire to be together. If you catch one, the other will follow closely.

Danger zones

Several studies have shown that one of the most dangerous jobs for occupational injuries is that of an equine veterinarian. When trapped, the response of the horse is fear, panic or fight motivated. The dangerous nature of large animal rescues has been the subject of governmental efforts to educate responders. As a result, planning at national levels for animals in disasters has improved since the late 1980s (Farm Animal Welfare Committee, 2012; Husted and McConnico, 2019).

Similar to hazardous materials incidents, a TLAER® scene has designated or imaginary zones. The hot zone is the high-risk area within the horse's kicking, biting, or lunging distance. The animal handler, essential operational personnel, and the veterinarian are usually required to be located here. The warm zone is where the Incident Commander, owner, logistics personnel and equipment should be located. The cold zone is the lowest risk area where spectators, transportation, vehicles and media are located (Fig. 15.7). Note, these zones are for humans to understand the safety limits and are NOT the same as the equine awareness, alertness and action zones of flight as described above.

A human cannot physically dominate a horse; the strength and weight ratios favour the equine. In the hot zone, responders should stay in a safe

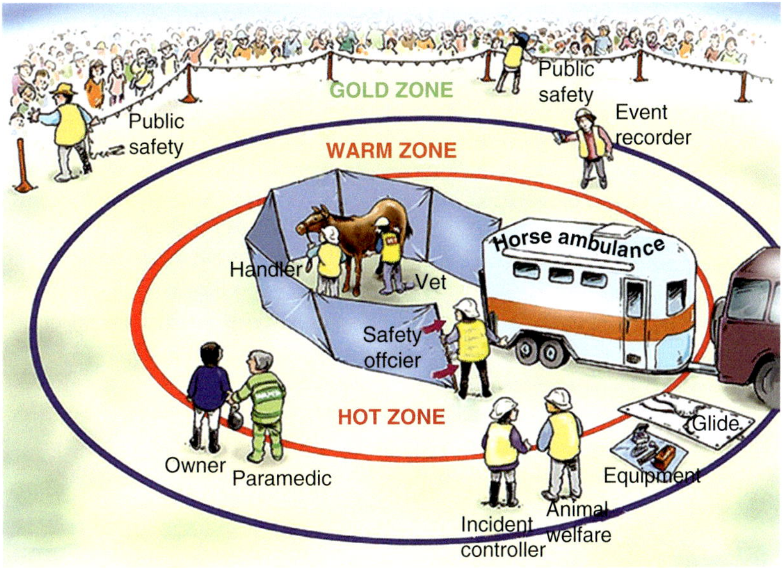

Fig. 15.7. Hot, cold and warm zones. Figure: modified from Horse SA, Australia.

position and have a planned escape route away from the struggling equine. Under duress, horses will try to go through spaces that are too tight or too small for their bodies, whether attempting to jump out of horse trailer, horsebox or stall windows, or squeezing past a human in a horse trailer or stall. The confined spaces where horses are trapped, inside stalls, trailers or ravines, require appropriate personal protective equipment such as helmets, and may entail the use of reaching, prying and cutting tools.

Entrapped recumbent horse behaviour

Entrapped recumbent horses have already tried to get up. If able to get up, they do so immediately. If still recumbent upon arrival, there is a reason. Slapping or stimulating a downed horse that is entrapped and not able to move is not helpful and engages fear responses. For example, short trailer ties that do not break will guarantee that the horse cannot get up. Slick floors, obstacles, lack of leverage or space may contribute to a horse's failure to rise as much as injuries and must be evaluated. Horses tend to fight to stand if physically possible. When a horse is recumbent, it is fractious, difficult and dangerous to handle with a tendency to thrash in an attempt to stand, leading to further injury. When manipulated out of the entrapment or enabled to roll to sternal position, many animals will rise and stand on their own. Thus, facilitating self-rescue is the best use of manipulation methods.

Horses commonly get cast in various positions against a stall wall, in pasture depressions or ditches, or trapped with legs into fences or other obstacles where they cannot right themselves. They may not be injured or sick and are fully enabled and capable of easily injuring a person.

Learned helplessness in TLAER®

A poorly understood psychological state occurs in horses when they cannot control their situation, and even valiant efforts can make no difference (e.g. struggling, calling, etc.). Learned helplessness is defined as 'When individuals learn that they have no control over unpleasant or harmful conditions, that their actions are futile, and that they are helpless' (Hall *et al.*, 2008). As a result, horses shut down and often show no interaction with their environment or other attendees to the incident but are not predictable as to explosive reactions (Fig. 15.8). Scientists believe this tonic immobility, a state of paralysis of the horse's flight response, is a last-ditch defence response of prey species (usually to a predator).

Forced tonic immobility in mud or other inescapable entrapment (e.g. under a collapsed structure, entanglement in fencing, down in a trailer or stall)

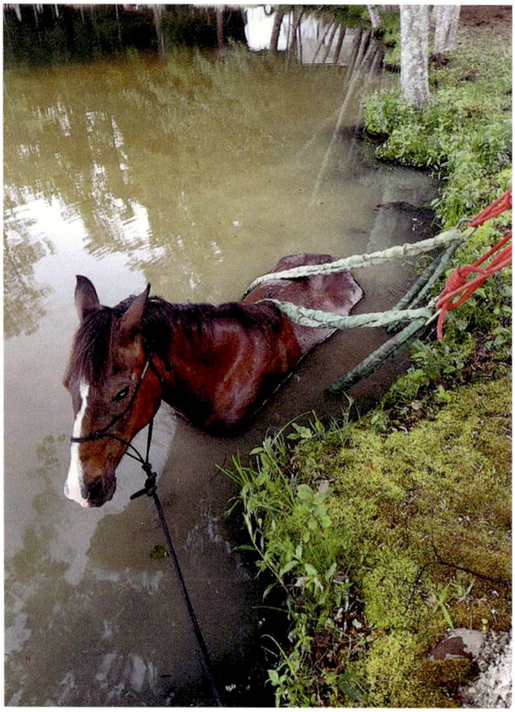

Fig. 15.8. A trapped horse is overwhelmed by the stress of the entrapment and humans responding. These animals may require significant veterinary treatment to prevent shock. Photo: author.

is commonly encountered in large animal rescue. Here the animal's movement is severely limited, and their initial anxiety motivates their attempts to move or change the conditions. When self-resolution is frustrated, regardless of the level of effort, this causes a serious compromise of their welfare, similar to learned helplessness. When their behavioural responses fail to result in escape, and in the case of mud, may make their entrapment even tighter, a state of learned helplessness akin to despair in humans occurs.

These situations have physiological effects. It is common for a trapped horse to be described as passive, listless, unmotivated, dull and even non-reactive to stimuli, or by veterinarians as displaying signs of anhedonia and depression. Since TLAER® situations are often accompanied by hypothermia, poor perfusion in the downside lung, exertional rhabdomyolysis (muscle damage) due to the extreme weight of a horse on the downside muscle (compartment syndrome), extreme stress or accompanying pain, the overall picture is of an animal totally giving up.

Tools and Physical Techniques

Humane control with simple tools is detailed elsewhere (Gimenez *et al.*, 2008). This section summarizes advice on their use. Despite the variety of 'quick fixes' that people attempt to apply to keep horses calm (including twitches, training devices, bridles and blindfolds), fear cannot be reduced by punishment, force or pain. The devices do not stop their explosive attempts at escape. The author asserts that a simple rope halter and good long lead rope 3.5–6.5 m (12–22 ft) is best for handling horses and reducing injuries to people at rescue scenes.

Halters and control

During urgent situations such as a barn fire, responders do not have time or may lack the dexterity to halter a horse intent on avoiding them. Most trained horses will follow the direction given by a loose lead rope looped around the neck (Fig. 15.9). Do not make a lasso or other locking loop. Emergency halter configurations are described in other publications (Gimenez *et al.*, 2008).

A simple rope halter and a long lead rope are best for guidance and control. It is not an anchor point for pulling or holding. If the horse is dangerously fractious, aggressive or difficult, a veterinarian should provide chemical restraint via sedation or anaesthesia during the use of rescue equipment and procedures, or euthanize the animal.

Horses establish dominance within seconds. Aggressive greeting and squealing are normal behaviours but can be terrifying and dangerous to inexperienced handlers. Aggressive animals, mares protecting foals, feral horses or stallions, should be handled for containment or by qualified individuals. When dealing with multiple animals, separate them by at least 4.5 m (15 ft) when holding or leading.

Twitches

Twitches may be used by qualified personnel who are familiar with the device and its use. Incorrectly used, the handle can become a dangerous flailing baton. Removed incorrectly, it teaches the horse never to let someone apply it again. Gathering the skin into a temporary shoulder twitch can easily be used to distract a horse for a short procedure. Picking up one front leg for simple restraint may

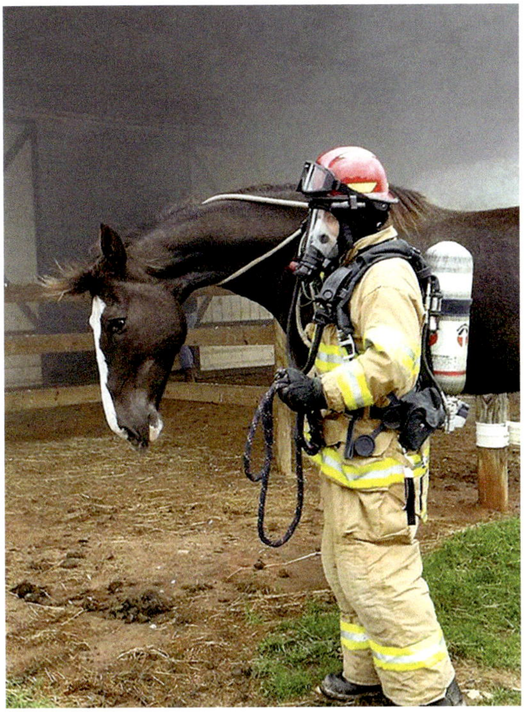

Fig. 15.9. A horse in a practice smoke situation is led from the stall by a firefighter in full gear. She caught the horse by looping a rope around the neck and leads it by walking forward. Photo: Tori McLeod.

prevent an injured or stressed horse from moving around and further injuring itself until chemical restraint is administered.

Blindfold

Contrary to what horse enthusiasts project as common knowledge about the use of blindfolds, their use is restricted to recumbent horses in TLAER® scenarios for two reasons: to protect the downside eye from injury, and to keep the animal calm by limiting visual stimuli by covering the upside eye. Any soft, nonabrasive material can be used as a blindfold.

Blindfolds are not recommended for standing horses. They are extremely dangerous if the horse gets away from the handler. If frightened, it may run in a straight line until it slams into an obstacle or falls into a ditch. It is ill-advised to consider leading blindfolded horses from barn fires. It usually takes longer to get the blindfold on than it would be to simply catch and lead the horse.

Legacy method – recumbent horse restraint

The legacy method of attempting to hold a recumbent horse down was to place the handler on his or her knees on the neck of the horse. Obviously, the larger and stronger the person the greater the odds of success, but it places the handler in a questionable position of safety with minimal leverage to tip the nose skyward. It limits the handler's ability to get out of the way quickly if the horse lunges to get up. Handlers have been kicked by the rear leg striking forward and have been pulled down by the struggling horse into the area between the forelegs. Proponents say that it is easier for the animal handler to cover the eye, get pulse, respirations and capillary refill times on the oral mucosa. However, in rescue, the handler's job is to focus on the animal handling to keep the other people safe, not to attempt other tasks.

TLAER® method – recumbent horse restraint

Large animal rescuers use a safer, more ergonomic method that allows the handler to use the lead rope for better leverage to tip the nose skyward by placing the bottom of the foot on the horse's neck right behind the horse atlantooccipital joint. By using the weight and pressure of a person to physically restrain the horse from a position that provides better leverage, the handler can move if the horse flails. Tipping the nose slightly up makes it more difficult for the horse to get up, keeping the animal handler away from the neck so that the veterinarian has better access to the jugular vein for catheter insertion and drug administration, and the facial area to assess capillary refill times, facial artery pulse, orbital and oral mucous membranes. It is still possible for a trained animal handler to assess respiration rate by watching chest rise or nostril movements, assess ear and eye reactions, and cover the eye with a blindfold while holding in this manner (Fig. 15.10).

Pressure on the chest and abdomen

When pressure is applied on a horse's chest and abdomen, for example, with a simple vertical lift webbing sling such as the Becker, U.C. Davis Large Animal Lift, or Anderson sling, an immediate physiological response minimizes struggling. However, the effect is short term and not every horse responds the same way. This apparent physical sedative effect

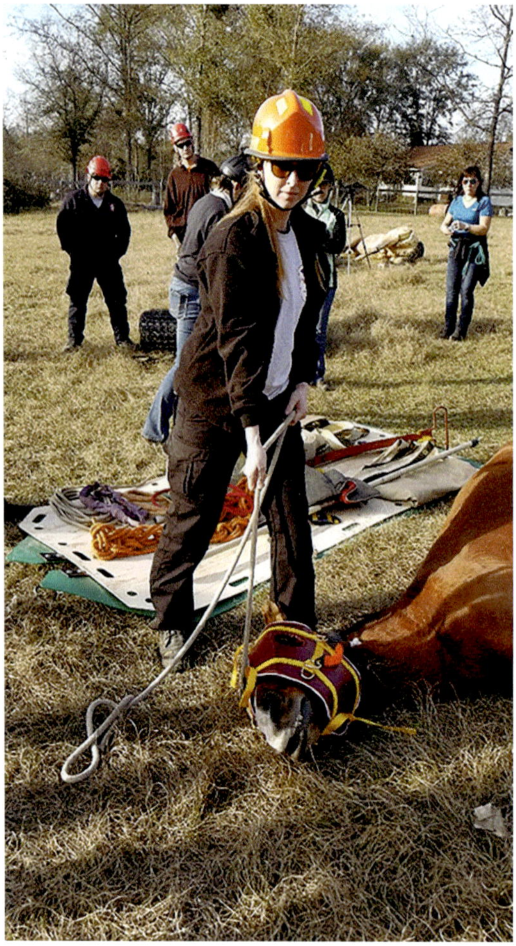

Fig. 15.10. Using the standing method, even a smaller person can hold down the head and neck of a horse safely with better leverage. Here the horse has on a Becker Head Protector for facial protection. Photo: author.

has been used by farriers, veterinarians and horsemen throughout history to cause horses to become quiescent for various procedures using tilt-turn tables and stocks, slings or side-line hobbles.

Euthanasia

Before providing euthanasia, the veterinarian consults with the owner or agent about possible treatments, cost, long-term welfare and prognosis. Euthanasia should be considered for horses with a poor to grave prognosis after triage and veterinary examination. Indications include severe, extensive injuries, multiple organ or system involvement, severe shock or blood loss, amputation, organ evisceration, nonresponsiveness to pain management, dangerously combative or aggressive, or neurologically impaired.

Euthanasia should be performed in a logical manner to achieve insentience, minimize pain and suffering in the animal, and reduce the chance of injury to personnel. In the field, humane euthanasia with a firearm or penetrating captive bolt can be performed safely by emergency personnel, owners or veterinarians who are trained to identify correct skull landmarks, proper placement and angle of introduction. Alternatively, euthanasia is induced by intrathecal lidocaine injection into the atlanto-occipital space or barbiturate overdose in sedated animals by a veterinarian.

Myths of Animal Rescue

Fear of trailers after wrecks

It is a common misconception that horses that will not load into trailers must have been in past trailer accidents (wrecks). However, numerous anecdotal and documented cases show horses in serious collisions immediately reloading into trailers (floats) after extrication. Therefore, the author and others speculate that horses do not associate acute collisions with fear of trailers. Instead, it is persistently poor driving, panic associated with being injured, bitten or kicked by others, inability to spread the legs base wide or raise and lower the head and neck to balance, that may be associated with long-term trailering phobias. This is an important field for further research.

Leading from boats

Under the threat of drowning, horses can swim. However, for untrained horses, swimming is a difficult, tiring and dangerous activity. Swimming for hours is impossible for a horse due to the energy expenditures required. Their hooves, like tiny paddles at the end of very long toothpicks, are not made for swimming. The horse is forced to hold its nostrils above the water while swimming, requiring the extension of the neck, then extension of the head, while the pressure of the water acts like a corset on its chest. Dragging a haltered horse through the water by a boat is hazardous because when the halter pulls on its head, the opposition reflex causes it to pull back into the water or resist and refuse to swim.

Training Horses for Large-animal Rescue

The amount of work in preparing animals to deal with an emergency is rewarded with less stress, better handleability and less reactivity. Prevention strategies involve habituation or desensitization of horses to get them used to webbing around their bodies and legs, teaching them to accept having their bodies handled, and exposure to novel situations. Teaching a horse to lower the head, relax and turn off the flight reaction is the basis of good horsemanship.

Most horses are naïve to TLAER® situations (i.e. they haven't been in a trailer accident before, been stuck in the mud before, or trapped in a barn fire before), so any opportunity to simulate visual, auditory, tactile or kinesthetic learning modalities BEFORE an incident is useful. For example, train horses to:

Load into a trailer readily in all conditions (snow, rain, dark, windy). Take them places (show grounds or a friend's barn) to get used to new surroundings, the trailhead for a hack, give them treats or allow them to graze and praise their efforts to investigate and adapt. The MOST common evacuation that horse owners make is to take their sick or injured horse to the veterinarian. That is not the time to be teaching them to get onto a trailer.

Accept ropes and hobbles around their legs and bodies. Use webbing on their bodies to get them used to the feel and asking them to 'give' to a slight pull (e.g. forward assist, etc.). This is preparation for manipulations that might be performed in an extrication.

Be relaxed around loud sounds and excitement. Carriage and police horses in city centres are desensitized to crowds of people, loud and unexpected sounds, unusual smells and sights. Take horses to events, parades, or even board them for a month in a pasture right next to a busy roadway or train track.

Come to you and be easy to catch on command at liberty (loose). Practise these skills regularly. Have other people practise catching and haltering your horse, then giving a treat so that they associate people with good things.

Accept handling of their legs, tail, face, ears, lips, tongue. Teach them to lower their heads and turn off the flight reactions. This pays off when veterinary and farrier procedures must be accomplished and ensures that horses don't get as stressed or excited by the handling of these parts of their body in TLAER® situations.

Climate Change

Scientific evidence suggests that with climate change, droughts, windstorms, floods, heat, cold and wildfires are increasing in frequency, reach and intensity, meaning that TLAER® situations are more common. An evacuation plan, or, sadly, triage plan, for every contingency, should be in place for every animal (Riley, 2012) even when the necessity is not immediately apparent. For example, drifting toxic smoke from wildfires can affect the health and welfare of horses hundreds or more miles (kilometers) from the fire. Airborne particulates may inflame the cornea and affect vision. Horses suffering smoke inhalation become lethargic, unresponsive, ignore feed and are susceptible to bronchitis and pneumonia.

Competitive events have been cancelled because of heat waves and smoke. However, if the event is cancelled mid-day, horses transported from the event suffer even hotter conditions in the trailers and vans. High ambient temperatures and humidity, conditions within the transport environment and performance activities conducted under adverse environmental conditions all impact horse welfare. As do marathon runners, horses with even mild dehydration and hyperthermia will have compromised cognitive function (Rebbeck, 2011).

Where transport or evacuation is necessary, it must be conducted outside the hottest times of day and well before the highways become clogged with traffic or cut off by flood or fire. Planning for these contingencies saves time and horses should the worst happen.

Welfare Concerns in Emergencies

Horses in emergency scenarios have special medical concerns: severe injuries, stress, hyper- or hypothermia, dehydration, shock and exhaustion. Coordination between the veterinarian and response team is important to increase treatment efficiency on the scene, facilitate extrication and allow transport to definitive care. In general, if the animal has been trapped for more than 4 hours, its medical situation becomes very fragile. After 24 hours, very few animals survive entrapment even with heroic veterinary efforts.

Euthanasia should be considered early in the rescue effort, not later (American Veterinary Medical Association, 2020). If welfare is related to how a horse is coping (physically and emotionally) with its environment, then the ability of an entrapped animal to survive the extrication should be closely evaluated to ensure that the animal does not suffer any more than necessary. If the medical prognosis is poor, the horse dangerously combative, or pain cannot be limited, these are excellent reasons to consider euthanasia before an extrication attempt. Additionally, use of the Five Freedoms Guidelines (freedom from hunger and thirst; freedom from pain, injury or disease; freedom from discomfort, freedom from fear and distress, and freedom to express normal behaviour) or the Five Domains model (optimum nutrition, environment, health, behaviour and mental states) for evaluating an animal's welfare more objectively assists with making good decisions for the horse in these situations. Some animals will need to be euthanized based on the extent of their injuries. The advice of the attending veterinarian is mandatory. Leaving an animal to suffer and die without treatment or euthanasia is inhumane and, in most jurisdictions, illegal. Subjecting an animal to the stress of an extrication simply to euthanize it soon afterwards is not humane.

The use of sedation should be carefully evaluated when horses are recumbent in wet or muddy environments because the sedated horse could drown or suffer thermal maintenance issues. An increased chance of shock occurs when combining sedation with rescues, and the veterinarian cannot be present to treat the animal until several hours after the incident.

Some rescue situations arise with older, arthritic horses that cannot rise. These horses instinctively know they may not be able to get up. They are often sleep deprived and stressed. Eventually, their reticular system forces them into lateral recumbency. Owners may unintentionally leave them down for hours. This is a welfare issue that sometimes can be solved by allowing a larger stall with in/out privileges to a paddock. They get to choose where to lie down so that they can get up. Modern use of slings to lift horses is a valuable tool in the rescue box, but some owners have taken the concept of saving their debilitated horse too far. Quality of life must always be evaluated before making successive lifts.

References

American Veterinary Medical Association (2020) *AVMA Guidelines for the Euthanasia of Animals*. American Veterinary Medical Association, Schaumburg, IL. Available at: www.avma.org/sites/default/files/2020-01/2020-Euthanasia-Final-1-17-20.pdf (accessed 5 September 2020).

Cregier, S. and Gimenez, R. (2015) *Noncommercial Horse Transport: The Need for Standards Cheiron's Court*. Montague, Prince Edward Island. Available at: www.academia.edu/18507742/Non_Commercial_Horse_Transport_The_need_for_standards (accessed 5 September 2020).

Dehorty, O., McGreevy, P.D. and Pearson, G. (2017) The importance of learning theory and equitation science to the veterinarian. *Applied Animal Behavior Science* 190, 111–112.

Farm Animal Welfare Committee (2012) *Opinion on Contingency Planning for Farm Animal Welfare in Disasters and Emergencies*. Department for Environment, Food and Rural Affairs, London.

Fiedler, J.M. and McGreevy, P.D. (2016) Reconciling horse welfare, worker safety and public expectations: Horse event incident management systems in Australia. *Animals* 6, 16.

Gaumnitz, J. (2017) *Understanding the Mind of the Horse*. Available at: www.dvm360.com/view/understanding-mind-horse (accessed 5 September 2020).

Gimenez, R., Gimenez, T. and May, K.A. (2008) *Technical Large Animal Emergency Rescue*. Wiley-Blackwell, Ames, Iowa.

Gleerup, K.B and Lindegaard, C. (2016) Recognition and quantification of pain in horses: A tutorial review. *Equine Veterinary Education* 1, 47–57.

Hall, C., Goodwin, D., Heleski, C., Randle, H. and Waran, N. (2008) Is there evidence of learned helplessness in horses? *Journal of Applied Animal Welfare Science* 11, 249–266.

Husted, R. and McConnico, R. (2019). How to develop an equine veterinary facility all-hazards sheltering and evacuation plan. In: Ross, C. (ed.) *Proceedings of the 64th American Association of Equine Practitioners* 64, 74–86.

Lamm, W. (2020) *Nevada Animal Emergency Network*. Available at: www.facebook.com/groups/2910005 11045603/ (accessed 6 September 2020).

Langley, R.L. and Hunter, J.L. (2001) Occupational fatalities due to animal related events. *Wilderness and Environmental Medicine* 12, 168–174.

Rebbeck, M.A. (2011) *Impact of Climate Change on Horses and the Horse Industries*. South Australian Research and Development Institute, Adelaide, South Australia. Available at: www.horsefx.com.au/wp-content/uploads/2013/01/Impact-of-Climate-Change-on-horses-SARDI.pdf (accessed 5 September 2020).

Riley, C.B. (2012) Emergency management of horses and food animals involved in disasters. In: *Proceedings of the Australian Veterinary Association Northern Territory Conference*, Darwin, Northern Territory, pp. 4–7.

Index

Note: The page references in italics and bold represents figures and tables respectively.

abdominal pain 10
abnormal ingestion
 bolting food 184–185
 bruxism 183
 chewing 183–184
 eating faeces 184
 exhibited annoyance *188*
 horses **187**
 litter eating 184
 quidding 183
 stabled horses **187**
accelerometers 58
active behaviour
 exercise 55–56
 explorative 54
 feeding 54
 grooming 55
 locomotion 55–56
 play 55
 social 54–55
adaptive mechanisms 4
adrenocorticotropic hormone (ACTH) 45
allogrooming *74*
animal intelligence 18
applied ethology 2
Arab horse *12*
archetypal behaviour 3
autonomic nervous system 44–45, 51

bacterial bronchopneumonia 155
behavioural appraisals 7–8
 clinical conditions 10–11
 early experience 13–14
 mechanical conditions 11
 methods 8
 neurological conditions 11
 open-field test 8–9
 technology *see* technological advances
behavioural templates 6
behavioural welfare problems
 loading 117
 phases of transport 116
 physical injuries and fatalities 116
 pre-loading 116–117
 in transit 117
 unloading 117
behaviour tests 9–10
biogenic amine system 47
birth (parturition)
 bladder or urachus 151
 definition 151
 human error 151
 meconium 152
 meconium impaction 152, 153
 miniature foal strains 151, 152
 rib fractures/costochondral dislocation 151
blindfold 225
bruxism 183

canter 84–85
capillary refill time (CRT) 114, 115
catecholamines 47
cellular homeostatic phenomena 50
central nervous system (CNS) 36
 anatomy
  cerebral cortex 40–42
  3D model *40*
  neuroglia 39–40
  neurons *37*, 37–39, *38*
 functions **41, 42**
classical learning 14–15
cognitive bias 18–19
cold-blooded horse 3, 5
comfort
 grooming
  behaviour 72–73
  welfare 73–74, *74*
 pandiculation 74–75, **75**
 thermoregulatory
  behaviour 75–77, *76, 77*
  welfare 77
corticoids 45
corticotropin-releasing hormone (CRH) 45
crib-biting 181–182
cursorial browser concept 81

deep-water rushes 5
desensitization 16
deslorelin 132

diagonal limb 84
domestication 4–6
dominant individuals 174–175
dopamine 46–47
drinking
  behaviour 70
  welfare 70
dystocia 141–142

early locomotory behaviour 166–167
ecological niche 81
electrocardiogram (ECG) 56
electroencephalography (EEG) 57
elimination
  behaviour 70–71
  defecation 71
  urination 71–72, *72*
  welfare 72
embryo transfer (ET) 134
emotionality 18, 33–34
endocrine systems 45–46, 51
endocrinological studies 47
entrapped recumbent horses 223
epidemiology studies 90
equine forelimb 82, *83*
equine intelligence 33, **33**
equine species
  classification of **2**
  reproductive success *4*
  varietal extremes *3*
equine transport
  after the journey 113
  air 117, 118
  confinement and isolation 109
  dehydration and weight loss 114, 115
  direction of travel 110–111, 112, 113
  duration of travel 111, 112, 114
  environment 109–110
  gastrointestinal and respiratory systems 115–116
  horse 104
  laminitis, heatstroke and muscular problems 115
  land 104
  loading 108–109
  noise 110
  non-commercial 106, 107
  oar-/sail-powered ships 104
  physical welfare 113
  pre-loading 107, 108
  for racing 105, 106
  road 104
  slaughter 104–105
  space 109
  traumatic injuries 113, 114
  vehicle movement stressors 109
  water 118–119
  watering and feeding 110
equine welfare 19
  colt and mare showing full attention *20*
  fear-provoking events 20
  foal watching and learning, moving *21*
EquiWatch System® (EWS) 58
ethogram 47
euthanasia 226, 227
evacuation/rescue welfare
  agitation/frustration/fear 211
  animal rescue 226
  anxiety/fear 216
  approach zone 221, 222
  catching loose horses 222
  comprehend human intent 213
  danger zones 222, 223
  emergency
    call veterinarian 217
    personal protective equipment 217
    rescue plan 217, 218
    SA 216, 217
  flight distance 214
  fundamental behavioural 211
  gtrapped horse *224*
  halters/control 224
  horse's perspective
    hearing 219, 220
    pain 218
    senses 218
    smell 218
    taste 219
    touch 220, 221
    vision 220
  horse strapped onto rescue glide *212*
  horse, trouble 212
  human responsibility 212, 213
  language and limited vocalization 214
  large-animal rescue 211, 227
  learned helplessness 223, 224
  personal protection equipment *214*
  positioning people, safety 215
  primary welfare/health triage 216
  risk management 213
  safe extrication *215*
  standing method 225
  utility pole dropped *213*
  welfare concerns 227, 228
evolutionary adaptations 82

Federation Equestre Internationale (FEI) 109
fixed action patterns 3
fixed behaviour patterns 2
flexor tendons 82
foal
  activity/behavioural norms and maintenance behaviours
    elimination behaviours 159

feeding/drinking 158, 159
grooming 161
laterality 160, 161
pandiculation 160
play behaviour 161
stretching foal behaviour **158,** *160*
behaviour/early training 162, 163
biological dam 151
birth trauma (*see* birth (parturition)
common non-infectious conditions (*see* non-infectious conditions)
definition 148
foals at play *163*
health 148
herpes virus or strangles 148
human intervention 148
lick and nuzzle *149*
locomotor activity 150
neonatal functions, breeds **150**
neonatal immunity/health conditions *see* neonatal immunity
newboen foal, progression **148**
pories, neonatal functions **150**
reflexive allogrooming *161*
social and behavioural development 149
young horse behaviours **162**
follicle-stimulating hormone (FSH) 45
food ingestion
behaviour and motivation *62,* 62–63
concentrates **68,** 68–69
grazing *63,* 63–67, *64, 65,* **66,** *67*
welfare **69,** 69–70

gaits of locomotion
asymmetrical 83
classification 88
canter *86,* 87
gallop 87–88, *88*
genetic regulation 83
jumping 88–89
Milton Hildebrand's diagram 83, *84*
phases 83, *84*
stride cycle 83
symmetrical 83
trot 86–87
walk 85
gallop 85
genetic code 6
global positioning satellite (GPS) tracking units 96
glycogenolysis 45
gonadotropin 45
grazing *63,* 63–67, *64, 65,* **66,** *67*
grooming 55

habituation 15–16
heartbeat-to-beat (RR) 57
heart rate (HR) 56
heart rate variability (HRV) 56
homeostasis 6–7, 51
homozygous form 2
horse
basic structure 82
daily exercise
circumstances 93
distal limb 92
environments 92
locomotor activity 92
lungeing 93
riding 93–94
welfare codes 93
distal limb 82
equine limb 82
harmonic frequency 83
muscular effort 82
observations 85
racing behaviour and welfare
galloping 89, 90
hobbles 91
opponents 90
organizations 90
recovery pattern 90
whip 91
Standardbred 91
swimming 91–92
training 89–90
velocity 81
horse- human dyad 176–178
horse play
definition 167
features 172
function 168–172
interactive 169
leaping upward *171*
playful partnership 168–169
racing *171*
'serious' adult activities 169
social 169–170
survival functions 170–171
vascularization 172
welfare *168–170*
hot-blooded horse 3
human chorionic gonadotrophin (hCG) 132
human control training/husbandary
associative learning 199, 200
carcass disposal 207
chemical restraint 205
domesticated horse 196
effective restraint 195
euthanasia/gun shot 208
handling/restraint 201, 202, 203

human control training/husbandary (*continued*)
harsh restraint 195
horse anaesthetized *206*
horse tied *196*
husbandary procedures 198
learning principles 196
leg restraint 202
lethal injection 207
non-associative learning 196, 198, 199
prevention health/welfare programmes 205, 206
recumbent restraint 205
round pen (ring) breaking 201
scratch on neck *202*
stallion led *202*
stocks 204
training principles 200, 201
upper lip twitch 202, 203, *204*
hyperthyroid 46
hypothalamus 144
hypothyroid 46

imprinting 13
inactive behaviour 53
innate behaviour 5, 12–13
innate releasing mechanism (IRM) 13
instinctive behaviours 11–12
instrumental learning 15
International Society for Equestrian Science (ISES) 196, **197, 198**
Intracytoplasmic sperm injection (ICSI) 134

lameness 93
learning
classical 14–15
desensitization 16
habituation 15–16
motivation 16
operant 15
punishment 18
reinforcement 16–17
learning theory *177*
limbic system 42–43
basal ganglia 43
brainstem 43
cerebellum 43
hypothalamus 43
spinal cord 43–44
locomotor behaviour 11
luteinizing hormone (LH) 45
lying 51

maintenance behaviour 7
mare/foal dynamics
after birth 146
aggression 142
ambivalence 143
dystocia 141–142
fear of the foal 143
foster mares 143
free-ranging situations 142
geldings and stallions 142
gestation 139–140
gestation length 138–139
normal functions 144
noxious/aversive stimuli 143
nursing avoidance 143
parturition 140
pregnancy 139
savaging 143
stages of parturition 140, 141
stealing foals 143
strong maternal protectiveness 142–143
suckling behaviour 144, 145
welfare implications 138
meconium aspiration syndrome 152
Milton Hildebrand's diagram 83, *84*
motivation 16, 46–48
muscular contraction 82

negative reinforcement 16–17, *17*
neonatal immunity
abnormal transfer, passive immunity 153
bacterial bronchopneumonia 155
infections 154
isoerythrolysis 154, *154*
passive immunity 153
septic arthritis and osteomyeliti 155, 156
umbilical infection 155, *155*
neonate foal 3
neuroendocrine system
behavioural responses 191
chronic stress 191
neuroethology 47
neurologic faculties
emotionality 33–34
intelligence 33, **33**
memory 32
welfare 34
neurophysiological research 47
newborn foal *4*
non-associative learning 15, 196, 197
non-infectious conditions
angular limb deformity 157
congenital flexural contracture deformities 156
congenital tendon laxity 156
cuboidal bone hypoplasia 156, *157*
osteochondrosis 157, 158
normal eye expression 19, *19*
nuclear transfusion techniques 134

oestrous behaviour 9
open-field test 8–9
operant learning 15
overshadowing 101, 199
oxytocin 45, 144

pandiculation 8, 160
parasympathetic innervation 44
pedometers 58
perinatal asphyxia syndrome 151, 152
physiological studies 47
pineal gland 46
positive reinforcement 16–17
posterior pituitary 144
postural signs *10*
precision livestock farming (PLF) 56, 57
proprioception 222
psychogenic polydipsia 185

quidding 183

rapid eye movement (REM) 53, 186
recurrent airway obstruction (RAO) 110
Red blood cells (RBCs) 154
reinforcement 16–17
reproduction and breeding
  aggression 135
  artificial insemination (AI) 133–134
  castration 135–136
  clitoral winking 127, 128
  cloning 134
  colt foals 136
  embryo transfer (ET) 134
  feral horses 125
  horse 125
  human control 124
  in-hand breeding 129–131
  intracytoplasmic sperm injection (ICSI) 134
  lights 131
  local anaesthetic 132
  low libido 135
  masturbation 135
  non-oestrus mares 134
  older horses 131
  oocyte retrieval 134
  paddock breeding 128
  palpation and scanning 131
  prolonged oestrus behaviour 134–135
  self-mutilation 135
  social isolation 125
  stallion-like behaviour 135
  stallions 125, 126
  stallion semen collection 133–134
  teasing mares 131
  Thoroughbred industry 131, 132
  ultrasound 132
  unruly stallions 135
resting/sleeping 53
resting time 51
roll on/roll off' (RORO) transport. 119

seasonal oestrus *46*
sea transport 118–119
self-stimulation behaviour 47
sensory faculties
  hearing and balance 27–29, *28, 29*
  olfaction and taste 29–31, *30, 31*
  pain 31–32
  somatic sensation 31–32
  touch 31–32
  vision 24–27, *25, 26, 27*
septicaemia 154
situational awareness (SA) 216
slow-wave sleep (SWS) 53
social behaviour
  avoidance behaviour 174–175
  avoidance order 175
  colts and fillies 173
  general 172–173
  grazing associates 175
  group effect 172
  groups and housing 175–176
  horse-human dyad 176–178
  isolation *177*
  learning theory *177*
  mutual exploration *176*
  play *see* (Horse play)
  early locomotory behaviour 166–167
  foal play 169
  social facilitation 172, 173
  structure and communication 173–174
  under-hoof pads 166
spatial factors
  agonistic behaviours 100
  core home range 96–97
  domestic horses at pasture 97–98, 99
  feral horses 96, 99
  herds 96
  home range 96–97
  home range estimates 97
  management and sport 101–102
  minimal standards/optimal environment 101
  noxious 101
  social and spatial behaviour patterns 96
  stabling and stall environment 98, 99
  stocking density 100
stereotypical behaviours 180, 181
stimulus blending 199
stocks 204
stress 10

stress (*continued*)
  autonomic nervous system 190
  behavioural and physiological responses 189
  clinical behavioural expressions 191, 192
  depression/learned helpness 193
  minimizing stress response 191
  pain/suffering 192
  standard stress model 189
  welfare 192
stride frequency 83
stride length 84
suck reflex 2
superficial digital flexor tendon (SDFT) 82
survival 6–7
sympathetic innervation 44
systematic desensitization 199

teaser stallion 129
technological advances 56
  accelerometers 58
  EWS 58
  pedometers 58
  slow and automatic feeders 56
  wearable EEG 57
  wearable GPS 58
  wearable heart rate monitors 56–57
  welfare implications 58
The Humane Society International (2012) 105
thermoregulation 222
  horse cast *219*
  opposition reflex 218
thigmotaxic stimuli 3
thyroxine 46
time budget 51–53, *52*
TLAER® method 225
tongue-dragging 183
transport-related behavioural problems (TRBPs) 116
twitches 224, 225

undesirable behaviour
  abnormal behaviours 180
  abnormal ingestion (*see* abnormal ingestion)
  abnormal oral activities, horses **181**
  bolting 188
  chronic standing 185, 186
  cognitive underperformance 180
  conflict behaviour 180, 187, **191**
  crib-biting *181*
  crib-whetting 183
  crowding, barging and crushing 188, **191**
  head-tossing or nodding 182, 183
  jibbing/baulking/napping 188, 189
  kicking **191**
  pawing 182
  self mutilation 186, 187
  shying 188
  stall-walking/box-walking 182
  tail rubbing 186
  tongue-dragging **181**, 183
  weaving 182

waxing up 2

Zeitgeber 51